Atlas of Orthodontic Case Reviews

Atlas of Orthodontic Case Reviews

Marjan Askari, DMD, MS
Assistant Clinical Professor
Tufts University School of Dental Medicine
Boston MA, USA, and
The Smile Institute
Brookline, MA, USA

Stanley A. Alexander, DMD
Distinguished Teaching Professor
Emeritus, Stony Brook University School of Dental Medicine
Stony Brook, NY, USA, and
The Smile Institute
Brookline, MA, USA

WILEY Blackwell

This edition first published 2017
© 2017 John Wiley & Sons, Inc.

The right of Marjan Askari and Stanley A. Alexander to be identified as the authors of this work has been asserted in accordance with law.

Registered Office
John Wiley & Sons, Inc., 111 River Street, Hoboken, NJ 07030, USA

Editorial Office
111 River Street, Hoboken, NJ 07030, USA

For details of our global editorial offices, customer services, and more information about Wiley products visit us at www.wiley.com.

Wiley also publishes its books in a variety of electronic formats and by print-on-demand. Some content that appears in standard print versions of this book may not be available in other formats.

Limit of Liability/Disclaimer of Warranty
The contents of this work are intended to further general scientific research, understanding, and discussion only and are not intended and should not be relied upon as recommending or promoting scientific method, diagnosis, or treatment by physicians for any particular patient. In view of ongoing research, equipment modifications, changes in governmental regulations, and the constant flow of information relating to the use of medicines, equipment, and devices, the reader is urged to review and evaluate the information provided in the package insert or instructions for each medicine, equipment, or device for, among other things, any changes in the instructions or indication of usage and for added warnings and precautions. While the publisher and authors have used their best efforts in preparing this work, they make no representations or warranties with respect to the accuracy or completeness of the contents of this work and specifically disclaim all warranties, including without limitation any implied warranties of merchantability or fitness for a particular purpose. No warranty may be created or extended by sales representatives, written sales materials or promotional statements for this work. The fact that an organization, website, or product is referred to in this work as a citation and/or potential source of further information does not mean that the publisher and authors endorse the information or services the organization, website, or product may provide or recommendations it may make. This work is sold with the understanding that the publisher is not engaged in rendering professional services. The advice and strategies contained herein may not be suitable for your situation. You should consult with a specialist where appropriate. Further, readers should be aware that websites listed in this work may have changed or disappeared between when this work was written and when it is read. Neither the publisher nor authors shall be liable for any loss of profit or any other commercial damages, including but not limited to special, incidental, consequential, or other damages.

Library of Congress Cataloging-in-Publication Data
Names: Askari, Marjan, author. | Alexander, Stanley A., author.
Title: Atlas of orthodontic case reviews / by Marjan Askari, Stanley A. Alexander.
Description: Hoboken, NJ : Wiley, 2017. | Includes bibliographical references and index. |
Identifiers: LCCN 2017015699 (print) | LCCN 2017016072 (ebook) | ISBN 9781119303763 (pdf) |
    ISBN 9781119303770 (epub) | ISBN 9781119303756 (pbk.)
Subjects: | MESH: Orthodontics–methods | Malocclusion | Case Reports | Atlases
Classification: LCC RK521 (ebook) | LCC RK521 (print) | NLM WU 417 |
    DDC 617.6/43–dc23
LC record available at https://lccn.loc.gov/2017015699

Cover Design: Wiley
Cover Image: © Marjan Askari and Stanley A. Alexander

Set in 10/12pt Warnock by SPi Global, Pondicherry, India
Printed and bound in Singapore by Markono Print Media Pte Ltd

10 9 8 7 6 5 4 3 2 1

Contents

Preface   *xiii*
Acknowledgments   *xv*

1   Interceptive (Mixed Dentition): Case 1   *1*
Interview Data   *1*
Clinical Examination   *1*
    Dentition   *2*
        Right Buccal View   *2*
        Left Buccal View   *2*
        Maxillary Arch   *2*
        Mandibular Arch   *2*
Function   *3*
Diagnosis and Treatment Plan   *3*
Treatment Objectives   *5*
Treatment Options   *5*
First Active Appointment with Quad-Helix in Place   *6*
Second to Fourth Active Appointments   *7*
Six Months after Initial Placement of the Appliance   *8*
Commentary   *9*
Review Questions   *10*
Suggested References   *10*

2   Interceptive (Mixed Dentition): Case 2   *11*
Interview Data   *11*
Clinical Examination   *11*
    Dentition   *12*
        Right Buccal View   *12*
        Left Buccal View   *12*
        Maxillary Arch   *13*
        Mandibular Arch   *13*
Function   *13*
Diagnosis and Treatment Plan   *14*
Treatment Objectives   *15*
Treatment Options   *15*
First Active Appointment   *16*
Second Active Appointment   *17*
Third Active Appointment   *17*
Fourth Active Appointment   *18*
Fifth Active Appointment   *18*
Phase I Completed   *19*
Commentary   *21*
Review Questions   *21*
Suggested References   *21*

3 Phase I Treatment: Class III Skeletal and Class I Dental with Posterior and Anterior Crossbites *23*
Interview Data *23*
Clinical Examination *23*
Dentition *24*
Right Buccal View *24*
Left Buccal View *24*
Maxillary Arch *25*
Mandibular Arch *25*
Function *25*
Diagnosis and Treatment Plan *26*
Treatment Objectives *27*
Treatment Options *27*
First Active Appointment *28*
Second Active Appointment *29*
Third Active Appointment *30*
Fourth Active Appointment *31*
Fifth Active Appointment *32*
Sixth Active Appointment *32*
Seventh and Eighth Active Appointments *33*
Ninth and 10th Active Appointments *34*
Eleventh Active Appointment *35*
Twelfth Active Appointment *36*
Thirteenth Appointment *36*
Commentary *39*
Review Questions *40*
Suggested References *40*

4 Class I Skeletal and Class I Dental with Blocked-Out Maxillary Canine: Non-Extraction *41*
Interview Data *41*
Clinical Examination *41*
Dentition *42*
Right Buccal View *42*
Left Buccal View *42*
Maxillary Arch *43*
Mandibular Arch *43*
Function *43*
Diagnosis and Treatment Plan *44*
Treatment Objectives *45*
Treatment Options *45*
First Active Appointment *46*
Second Active Appointment *47*
Third to Fifth Active Appointments *48*
Sixth Appointment *49*
Commentary *53*
Review Questions *53*
Suggested References *53*

5 Class I Skeletal and Class I Dental with a Deep Bite *55*
Interview Data *55*
Clinical Examination *55*
Dentition *56*
Right Buccal View *56*
Left Buccal View *56*
Maxillary Arch *57*
Mandibular Arch *57*

Function   *57*
Treatment Objectives   *59*
Treatment Options   *59*
First and Second Active Appointments   *60*
Third Active Appointment   *61*
Fourth Active appointment   *62*
Fifth Active Appointment   *63*
Sixth Active Appointment   *64*
Seventh Active Appointment   *66*
Eighth and Ninth Active Appointments   *67*
Tenth Active Appointment   *68*
Eleventh and 12th Active Appointments   *69*
Thirteenth Active Appointment   *69*
Fourteenth Active Appointment   *70*
Fifteenth Appointment   *71*
Commentary   *74*
Review Questions   *74*
Suggested References   *74*

6   **Class I Skeletal and Class I Dental with Asymmetry: Non-Extraction**   *75*
Interview Data   *75*
Clinical Examination   *75*
   Dentition   *76*
      Right Buccal View   *76*
      Left Buccal View   *76*
      Maxillary Arch   *77*
      Mandibular Arch   *77*
Function   *77*
Diagnosis and Treatment Plan   *78*
Treatment Objectives   *79*
Treatment Options   *79*
First Active Appointment   *80*
Second Active Appointment   *81*
Third Active Appointment   *82*
Fourth Active Appointment   *83*
Fifth Active Appointment   *84*
Sixth and Seventh Active Appointments   *85*
Eighth Active Appointment   *85*
Ninth Appointment   *86*
Commentary   *90*
Review Questions   *90*
Suggested References   *90*

7   **Class II Skeletal and Class II Dental: Extraction of Maxillary First Premolars**   *91*
Interview Data   *91*
Clinical Examination   *91*
   Dentition   *92*
      Right Buccal View   *92*
      Left Buccal View   *92*
      Maxillary Arch   *93*
      Mandibular Arch   *93*
Function   *93*
Diagnosis and Treatment Plan   *94*
Treatment Objectives   *95*
Treatment Options   *96*

First Active Appointment *96*
Second Active Appointment *98*
Third Active Appointment *99*
Fourth Active Appointment *100*
Fifth Active Appointment *101*
Sixth and Seventh Active Appointments *102*
Eighth Active Appointment *103*
Ninth and 10th Active Appointments *104*
Eleventh and 12th Active Appointments *105*
Thirteenth Appointment (Debond and Retainer Delivery) *105*
Commentary *108*
Review Questions *108*
Suggested References *108*

8   Class II Skeletal and Class II Dental: Non-Compliant *109*
Interview Data *109*
Clinical Examination *109*
  Dentition *110*
    Right Buccal View *110*
    Left Buccal View *110*
    Maxillary Arch *111*
    Mandibular Arch *111*
Function *111*
Diagnosis and Treatment Plan *112*
Treatment Objectives *113*
Treatment Options *113*
First Active Appointment *114*
Second and Third Active Appointments *115*
Fourth and Fifth Active Appointments *116*
Sixth Active Appointment *117*
Seventh and Eighth Active Appointments *118*
Ninth to 12th Active Appointments *119*
Thirteenth Appointment *120*
Fourteenth Active Appointment *122*
Fifteenth Appointment *122*
Commentary *125*
Review Questions *126*
Suggested References *126*

9   Skeletal Class II and Dental Class II Division 1 Subdivision: Four Premolar Extractions *127*
Interview Data *127*
Clinical Examination *127*
  Dentition *128*
    Right Buccal View *128*
    Left Buccal View *128*
    Maxillary Arch *129*
    Mandibular Arch *129*
Function *129*
Diagnosis and Treatment Plan *130*
Treatment Objectives *131*
Treatment Options *131*
First Active Appointment *131*
Second Active Appointment *133*
Third Active Appointment *134*

Fourth and Fifth Active Appointments   *135*
Sixth Active Appointment   *136*
Seventh Active Appointment   *137*
Eighth Active Appointment   *137*
Ninth Active Appointment   *138*
Tenth Active Appointment   *139*
Eleventh Active Appointment   *140*
Twelfth Active Appointment   *141*
Thirteenth Active Appointment   *142*
Fourteenth Active Appointment   *142*
Fifteenth to 17th Active Appointments   *143*
Eighteenth Appointment   *143*
Commentary   *145*
Review Questions   *147*
Suggested References   *147*

10   Class III Skeletal Tendency and Class I Dental: Four Premolar Extractions   *149*
Interview Data   *149*
Clinical Examination   *149*
   Dentition   *150*
      Right Buccal View   *150*
      Left Buccal View   *150*
      Maxillary Arch   *151*
      Mandibular Arch   *151*
Function   *151*
Diagnosis and Treatment Plan   *152*
Treatment Objectives   *153*
Treatment Options   *153*
Passive Appointments   *153*
First Active Appointment   *154*
Second Active Appointment   *155*
Third Active Appointment   *156*
Fourth Active Appointment   *157*
Fifth Active Appointment   *158*
Sixth to Eighth Active Appointments   *159*
Ninth Active Appointment   *160*
Tenth to 11th Active Appointments   *161*
Twelfth to 13th Active Appointments   *162*
Fourteenth Active Appointment   *163*
Fifteenth Active Appointment   *163*
Commentary   *167*
Review Questions   *167*
Suggested References   *167*

11   Class III Skeletal and Class III Dental: Non-Extraction and Non-Surgical   *169*
Interview Data   *169*
Clinical Examination   *169*
   Dentition   *170*
      Right Buccal View   *170*
      Left Buccal View   *170*
      Maxillary Arch   *171*
      Mandibular Arch   *171*
Function   *171*
Diagnosis and Treatment Plan   *172*

Treatment Objectives *173*
Treatment Options *173*
First Active Appointment with Full Appliances Placed *174*
Second Active Appointment *175*
Third Active Appointment *176*
Fourth Active Appointment *177*
Fifth Active Appointment *178*
Sixth Active Appointment *179*
Seventh Active Appointment *179*
Eighth and Ninth Active Appointments *180*
Commentary *183*
Review Questions *183*
Suggested References *183*

12 Class III Skeletal and Class III Dental: Non-Extraction *185*
Interview Data *185*
Clinical Examination *185*
  Dentition *186*
    Right Buccal View *186*
    Left Buccal View *186*
    Maxillary Arch *187*
    Mandibular Arch *187*
Function *187*
Diagnosis and Treatment Plan *188*
Treatment Objectives *189*
Treatment Options *189*
First Active Appointment *190*
Second Active Appointment *191*
Third Active Appointment *192*
Fourth Active Appointment *193*
Fifth Active Appointment *194*
Sixth Active Appointment *195*
Seventh to Eighth Active Appointments *196*
Ninth Active Appointment *196*
Tenth Active Appointment *197*
Tenth Appointment *198*
Commentary *201*
Review Questions *201*
Suggested Reference *201*

13 Class III Skeletal Pattern and Class II Dental: Non-Extraction *203*
Interview Data *203*
Clinical Examination *203*
  Dentition *204*
    Right Buccal View *204*
    Left Buccal View *204*
    Maxillary Arch *205*
    Mandibular Arch *205*
Function *205*
Diagnosis and Treatment Plan *206*
Treatment Objectives *207*
Treatment Options *207*
First Active Appointment *207*
Second Active Appointment *208*

Third to Fourth Active Appointment   *209*
Fifth Active Appointment   *210*
Sixth Active Appointment   *211*
Seventh Active Appointment   *212*
Eighth Active Appointment   *213*
Ninth Appointment   *213*
Commentary   *216*
Review Questions   *217*
Suggested References   *217*

14   Class III Skeletal and Class I Dental: Four Premolar Extractions   *219*
Interview Data   *219*
Clinical Examination   *219*
  Dentition   *220*
    Right Buccal View   *220*
    Left Buccal View   *220*
    Maxillary Arch   *221*
    Mandibular Arch   *221*
Function   *221*
Diagnosis and Treatment Plan   *222*
Treatment Objectives   *223*
Treatment Options   *223*
First Active Appointment   *223*
Second Active Appointment   *224*
Third Active Appointment   *225*
Fourth Active Appointment   *226*
Fifth Active Appointment   *227*
Sixth Active Appointment   *228*
Seventh Active Appointment   *229*
Eighth Active Appointment   *230*
Ninth Active Appointment   *231*
Tenth Active Appointment   *232*
Eleventh to 12th Active Appointments   *233*
Thirteenth Active Appointment   *234*
Fourteenth Active Appointment   *235*
Fifteenth Appointment   *236*
Commentary   *239*
Review Questions   *239*
Suggested References   *239*

15   Class III Surgical   *241*
Interview Data   *241*
Clinical Examination   *241*
  Dentition   *242*
    Right Buccal View   *242*
    Left Buccal View   *242*
    Maxillary Arch   *243*
    Mandibular Arch   *243*
Function   *243*
Diagnosis and Treatment Plan   *244*
Treatment Objectives   *244*
Treatment Options   *245*
First Active Appointment   *247*
Second and Third Active Appointments   *248*

Fourth Active Appointment   *248*
Fifth and Sixth Active Appointments   *248*
Seventh Active Appointment   *250*
Eighth Active Appointment   *250*
First Post-Surgical Appointment   *251*
Second Post-Surgical Appointment   *253*
Third Post-Surgical Appointment   *253*
Commentary   *256*
Review Questions   *256*
Suggested References   *256*

Index   *257*

Preface

The interest in orthodontic care amongst dental students, general dental practitioners and young, newly trained orthodontists has increased dramatically over the past 50 years and continues to rise as dental schools have trained an increasing number of new practitioners on an annual basis. It becomes imperative when the decision is made to treat a patient requiring orthodontics that clinicians base their judgment on an accurate diagnosis and treatment plan, which includes the treatment objectives and options for care. Such information should be easily accessible to students and useful for new graduates and seasoned practitioners.

This book is organized into 15 chapters, with the first three devoted to interceptive or mixed dentition treatment. The remaining chapters are arranged in order from Class I to Class III malocclusions; however, each chapter incorporates both the skeletal and dental components of the specific malocclusion. Each chapter is devoted to a specific case report supported by sequential photographic documentation visit by visit until the treated case is completed.

What is unique in regard to this atlas of case reports is that every chapter or case was treated by the same individual, Dr. Marjan Askari. The mechanics remain straightforward and classical, without incorporating or relying upon invasive techniques such as temporary anchorage devices to achieve their goals. Each sequence can be easily followed and applied to cases of a similar nature with regard to the skeletal and dental components of the patient's problem list.

Unlike most treatment plan schemes, which incorporate stainless steel or β-titanium wires as a predominant component of the mechanical design of the appliance, the use of round and rectangular nickel-titanium wires provides the majority implementation described in each case. Only when a rigid wire is necessary, as in a surgical case, was stainless steel routinely used.

Dental students, private practitioners, and first-year orthodontic residents will find useful information in each case report description and the important aspects of each case. Simply applied, the mechanical feature of the case reports can achieve predictable results with patient cooperation.

Marjan Askari
Stanley A. Alexander
Brookline, MA, 2017

Acknowledgments

Our gratitude is directed to all of our patients who made this work possible, not only the individuals who appeared in the chapters of this text, but every patient treated under our direction during our professional careers. A special emphasis is directed to our teachers and classmates who gave us greater insight into our own thoughts and treatment plans, and to our former residents, whose questions often contributed to patient care in a way that a young mind assimilates information and illuminates a new perspective that is often overlooked by senior clinicians.

With the support of our individual families, this work was made possible with the generosity of their time and caring, which allowed us the freedom to complete this task.

1

Interceptive (Mixed Dentition): Case 1

LEARNING OBJECTIVES

- The records required for treatment of a mixed dentition
- The problem list for interceptive orthodontics: posterior crossbite
- The development of treatment objectives and formation of a treatment plan for a quad-helix appliance

---

Interview Data

This 8-year-old Caucasian male presented with maxillary constriction that manifested as a unilateral posterior crossbite of the mixed dentition.

- Development: pre-pubescent
- Motivation: good
- Medical history: non-contributory
- Dental history: seen regularly for dental visits
- Family history: no history of malocclusion
- Habits: none
- Limitations: none
- Facial form: mesoprosopic and ovoid
- Facial proportions: normal lower facial height

Clinical Examination

- Incisor-stomion (Figures 1.1 and 1.2):
  - At rest: 0 mm
  - Smiling: 6 mm
- Smile line: 0 mm gingival display
- Breathing: nasal
- Lips: together at rest
- Soft tissue profile: convex (Figure 1.3)
- Nasolabial angle: slightly obtuse
- Slightly high mandibular plane angle

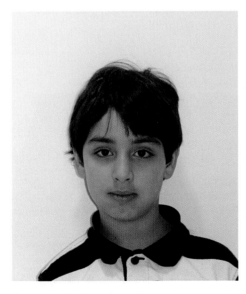

Figure 1.1 Full face at rest displaying a symmetric, ovoid face.

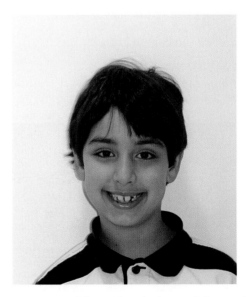

Figure 1.2 Full face with smile showing full enamel appearance of the incisors and no gingival display.

Atlas of Orthodontic Case Reviews, First Edition. Marjan Askari and Stanley A. Alexander.
© 2017 John Wiley & Sons, Inc. Published 2017 by John Wiley & Sons, Inc.

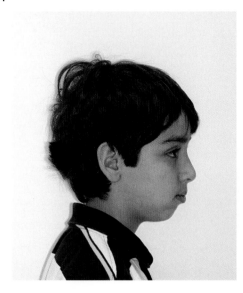

Figure 1.3 Right lateral view of profile indicating a convex appearance and obtuse nasolabial angle.

Dentition (Figure 1.4)

- Teeth present clinically:

6edc21	12cde6
6edc21	12cde6

- Overjet: 4 mm
- Overbite: 0 mm with open bite tendency
- Diastema: 3 mm
- Midlines: maxillary midline coincident with face; mandibular midline 2 mm to left

Right Buccal View

The right buccal view can be seen in Figure 1.5.

- Molar, right: end-on, mixed dentition
- Canine: Class I
- Curve of Spee: flat

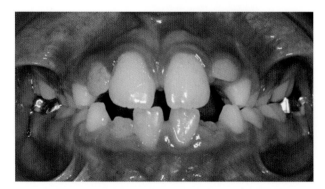

Figure 1.4 Anterior view of the dentition demonstrating midline diastema and mandibular shift to the left.

- Crossbite: none
- Caries: none

Left Buccal View

The left buccal view can be seen in Figure 1.6.

- Molar, left: Class II, mixed dentition
- Canine: cusp to cusp
- Curve of Spee: flat
- Crossbite: posterior crossbite
- Caries: none

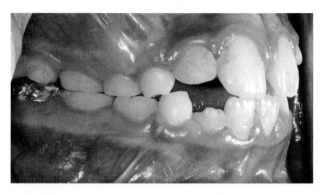

Figure 1.5 Right buccal view of dentition indicating an end-on mixed dentition molar relationship.

Maxillary Arch (Figure 1.7)

- Symmetric, catenary curve form with no crowding: elastic separator (arrow) still in place in the left quadrant from previous orthodontic consult
- No caries

Mandibular Arch (Figure 1.8)

- Ovoid arch form with lingual holding arch in place
- Slight rotation of erupting incisors
- No caries

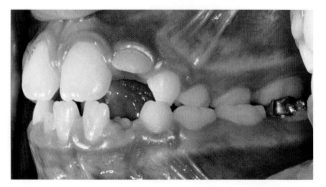

Figure 1.6 Left buccal view of dentition indicating a Class II mixed dentition molar relationship and posterior crossbite due to the functional shift of the mandible.

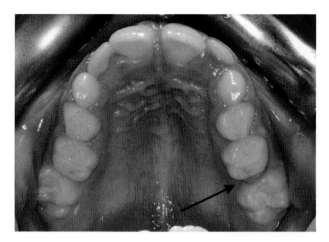

Figure 1.7 Occlusal view of the maxilla displaying a catenary arch form and rotated first permanent molars with separating elastic in place.

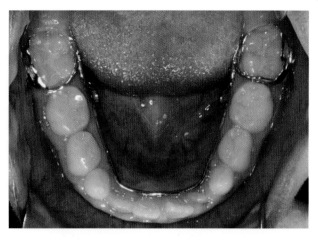

Figure 1.8 Occlusal view of the mandible displaying an ovoid arch form with a lingual holding arch in place.

Function

- Maximum opening = 40 mm
- Centric relation-centric occlusion (CR-CO): coincident
- Maximum excursive movements: right = 6 mm; left = 7 mm; protrusive = 5 mm
- Temporomandibular joint palpation: normal
- Right and left masseter: negative to palpation
- Habits: none
- Speech: normal
- Late mixed dentition with all 32 permanent teeth present or developing
- Root length and periodontium appear normal
- Condyles appear normal (Figure 1.9)

Diagnosis and Treatment Plan

As the patient is in the mixed dentition and displays a Class I skeletal and dental pattern (Figure 1.10; Tables 1.1 and 1.2), correction of the posterior crossbite is considered interceptive.

Maxilla – the maxillary first molars will be banded and a quad-helix appliance will be fabricated to rotate the molars and expand the palate. A lingual holding arch is presently on the mandibular arch to conserve leeway space and to maintain a non-extraction approach to further care in the future.

Once the posterior crossbite is over-corrected, the patient will be placed on a recall schedule and examined every 6 months for changes in the occlusion and eruption of the remaining permanent dentition.

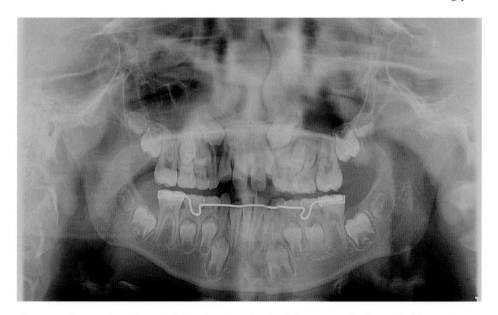

Figure 1.9 Panoramic radiograph indicating an early mixed dentition with a lingual holding arch present.

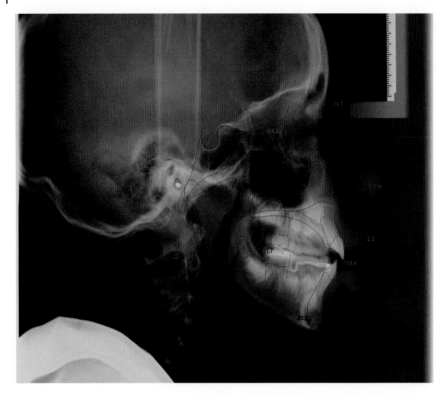

Figure 1.10 Digitized cephalogram of a Class I skeletal relationship and a high mandibular plane angle indicative of a vertical growing patient.

Table 1.1 Significant cephalometric values

	Norm	Patient pre-treatment
SNA	80°	83.2°
SNB	78°	76.7°
ANB	2°	+6.5°
WITS appraisal	−1 to +1 mm	+0.5 mm
FMA	21°	32.6°
SN-GoGn	32°	38.9°
Maxillary incisor to SN	105°	108.5°
Mandibular incisor to GoGn	95°	93.2°
Soft tissue		
Lower lip to E-plane	−2 mm	9.3 mm
Upper lip to E-plane	−1.6 mm	2.3 mm

SNA, sella-nasion-A point; SNB: sella-nasion-B point; ANB: A point-nasion-B point; WITS appraisal, Witwatersrand appraisal; FMA, Frankfort horizontal-mandibular plane (angle); SN-GoGn: sella nasion-gonion gnathion.

Table 1.2 The patient's problem list in three dimensions

	Transverse	Sagittal	Vertical
Soft tissue	Normal	Convex profile; full lower lip; obtuse nasolabial angle	Hyperdivergent
Dental	Bilateral posterior crossbite presenting as a unilateral crossbite due to the functional shift	Normal mixed dentition regarding molar and canine relationships	0 mm overbite
Skeletal	Maxillary constriction	Class I	Hyperdivergent

An argument may be made for an additional radiograph to be taken to aid in the diagnosis and treatment plan in patients with posterior crossbites who will require palatal expansion. The radiograph of choice is a posterior-anterior cephalogram, or PA radiograph as it is more commonly termed. In young, growing children where the clinical examination demonstrates no gross asymmetries and only functional shifts due to the crossbite, it is unnecessary to further expose the child to additional radiation that would have negligible clinical benefit.

Treatment Objectives

The patient's clinical problem in the mixed dentition will be addressed by correction of the posterior crossbite. Once corrected and maintained, the child will be evaluated annually for further orthodontic treatment if required. As the patient appears to be growing in a Class I direction both skeletally and dentally, it is anticipated that any further treatment would require only dental alignment.

Treatment Options

The options presented to the parent and patient were two-fold:

1) No treatment.
2) Interceptive treatment to correct the posterior crossbite through palatal expansion followed by comprehensive orthodontic care if it became necessary.

Both the patient and parent wanted option 2. Based upon the patient's skeletal and dental development, crossbite correction and palatal expansion would be undertaken with a quad-helix appliance, although other fixed appliances such as a rapid palatal expander could have been utilized as well. The quad-helix would also allow for the rotation of the maxillary molars in addition to the palatal expansion (Figures 1.11 and 1.12). The hyperdivergent tendency would also be evaluated during treatment, and further modifications to the appliance would be implemented if the overbite appeared to open excessively.

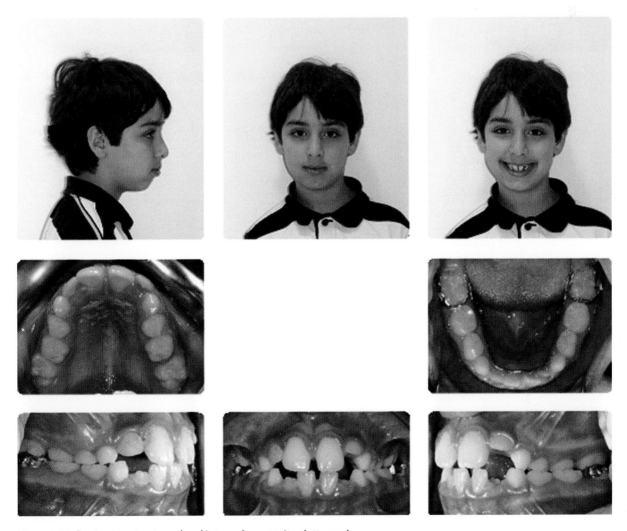

Figure 1.11 Pre-treatment extraoral and intraoral composite photograph.

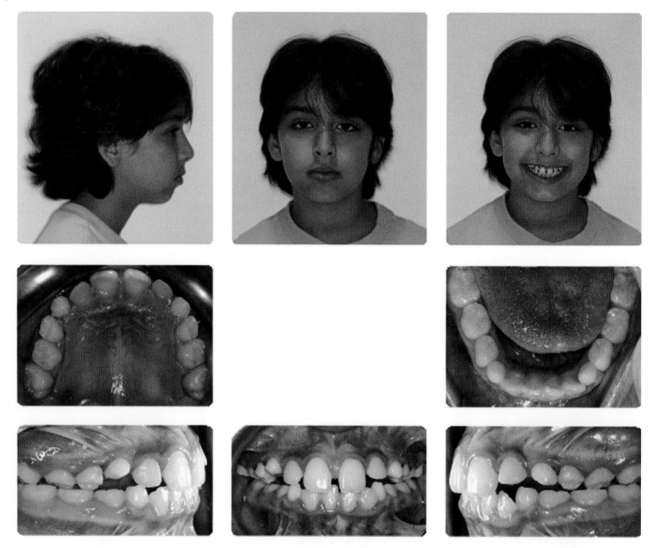

Figure 1.12 Post-treatment extraoral and intraoral composite photograph.

First Active Appointment with Quad-Helix in Place

The maxillary first molars were banded after 1 week prior to elastic separation and an iTero scan (Align Technology, Inc, San Jose, CA, USA) was done to fabricate a fixed quad-helix (Figure 1.13). The quad-helix was initially activated (arrows) 8 mm (to half the buccal-lingual width of each molar) and cemented into place with glass ionomer. The mandibular holding arch was kept in place (Figure 1.14).

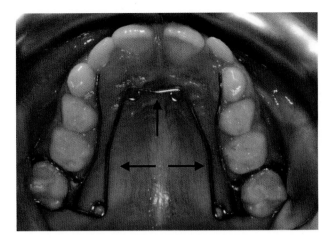

Figure 1.13 Occlusal view of the palate with initial insertion of the quad-helix. Note the anterior midline and lateral activations (arrows).

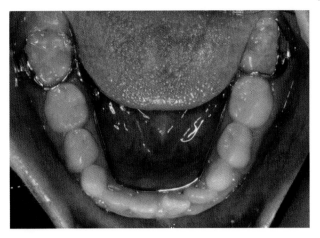

Figure 1.14 Occlusal view of the mandibular arch on the day the quad-helix was cemented to the maxillary arch.

Second to Fourth Active Appointments

The patient returned for two consecutive months after the initial activation and the appliance was expanded in the midline and along the lateral arms with three-pronged pliers; 3 months after the initial activation, the palatal form has changed to a broad ovoid configuration and the molars have rotated (Figure 1.15). Activation of only the arm between the two anterior helices would result in posterior expansion and further rotation of the maxillary molars; therefore the lateral arms were activated as well, to counteract this mesial-lingual rotation effect and to further rotate the molars to a correct position. The lingual holding arch had broken and it was decided not to continue lower maintenance due to minimal apparent crowding and differential mesial-distal size relationships between the primary and succedaneous teeth (Figure 1.16).

The crossbite has been over-corrected by expansion of the dental arch and tipping of the maxillary posterior dentition buccally (Figures 1.17–1.19). This will allow for relapse to a normal transverse relationship. During the procedure the overbite relationship did not open and therefore there was no need for correction of an open bite.

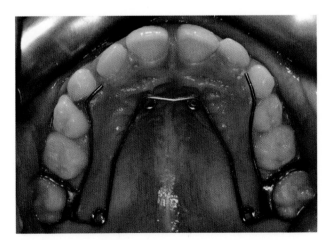

Figure 1.15 Occlusal view of the palate 2 months after the original activation. The arch form has changed to an ovoid form and the molars are being rotated to a correct position.

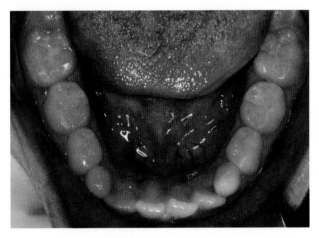

Figure 1.16 Two months after activation of the quad-helix, the lingual arch was broken and removed.

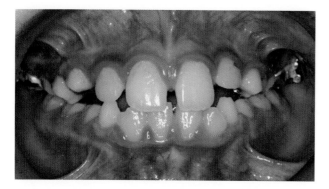

Figure 1.17 Anterior view of the dentition 2 months after the original activation. The crossbite has been over-corrected.

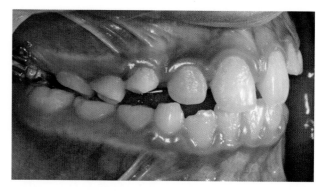

Figure 1.18 Right buccal view of the dentition indicating over-correction of the posterior crossbite.

Six Months after Initial Placement of the Appliance

The quad-helix has been removed and the crossbite has been corrected (Figures 1.20–1.24). The expansion has been over-corrected which will relapse through function to a normal transverse relationship. The width increased as measured from the gingival embrasures of the mesial-lingual cusps from 35 to 43 mm during the period of correction. No retention was necessary. The entire interceptive treatment occurred over a 6-month period.

Prior to the debanding procedure, a progress panoramic radiograph was taken. It was recommended that extraction of the maxillary primary canines and first primary molars be performed due to the eruption angulation of the permanent maxillary canines (Figure 1.25). Three months after appliance removal, the occlusion appeared stable in a normal mixed dentition position with a normal transverse relationship.

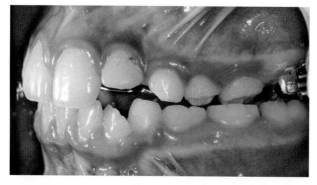

Figure 1.19 Left buccal view of the dentition indicating over-correction of the posterior crossbite.

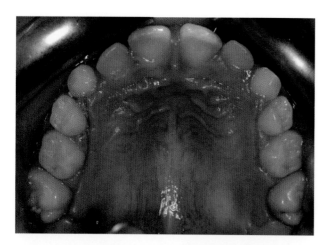

Figure 1.20 Occlusal view of the maxillary arch 6 months after the initial activation. The appliance has been removed and the over-correction is allowed to relapse to a normal relationship.

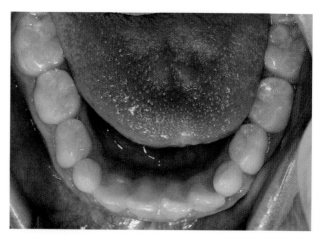

Figure 1.21 Occlusal view of the mandibular arch 6 months after the initial activation.

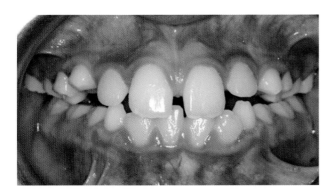

Figure 1.22 Anterior view of the dentition 6 months after the initial activation, displaying the over-corrected relationship of the posterior crossbite.

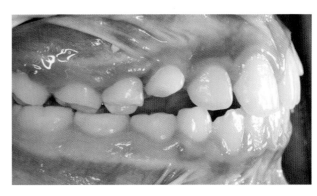

Figure 1.23 Right buccal view of the dentition 6 months after the initial activation, displaying the over-corrected posterior crossbite.

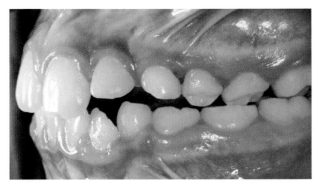

Figure 1.24 Left buccal view of the dentition 6 months after the initial activation, displaying the over-corrected posterior crossbite.

Commentary

The correction of posterior crossbites may be undertaken with fixed or removable appliances; the mechanics may be of rapid or slow design. The age of the patient very often will dictate the appliance of choice. The mixed dentition patient may be treated with a slow-expansion device, such as the quad-helix that was used in this case, and one that is capable of delivering forces in ounce increments, as opposed to the rapid palatal expander which is used more often in the late mixed or full permanent dentition when the maxillary sutures require greater force for separation (pounds). Both the rapid- and slow-expansion devices are capable of suture expansion; however, the appearance of a diastema is more commonly seen in rapid palatal

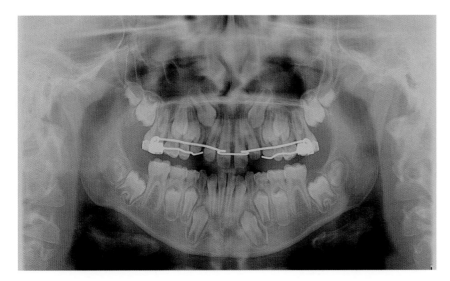

Figure 1.25 Progress panoramic radiograph taken prior to debanding. The angulation of the maxillary permanent canines indicated that extraction of the primary canines and first primary molars should be performed to aid in proper eruption.

expansion when forces are greater and the duration of treatment occurs over a much shorter time period, 2–3 weeks, rather than months as was seen with the quad-helix. It is also common for dental tipping to occur with slow expanders, but this is self-correcting because of over-expansion during treatment and as a result of uprighting of the dentition through function once the appliance is removed. Once growth is complete and the sutures are fully fused, posterior crossbites are usually corrected with a surgical assist, often called SARPE, which is the acronym for a surgically assisted rapid palatal expansion.

Review Questions

1 What material is used to create space for band placement?

2 How may a quad-helix be activated?

3 What type of force values does the quad-helix deliver during activation?

4 What form of palatal expander is the quad-helix considered to be – slow or rapid; fixed or removable?

Suggested References

Bell RA, LeCompte EJ. The effects of maxillary expansion using a quad-helix appliance during the deciduous and mixed dentitions. Am J Orthod 79: 152–157, 1981.

Dean, JA, Jones, JE, Vinson, LAW. Managing the developing dentition. In: McDonald and Avery's Dentistry for the Child and Adolescent, 10th edn. Elsevier, St. Louis, MO: Elsevier, 2016; pp. 449–452.

Fields HW, Proffit WR. Treatment of skeletal problems in children and preadolescents. In: Proffit WR, Fields HW, Sarver DM, eds. Contemporary Orthodontics, 5th edn. CV Mosby Co., 2013; pp. 476–480.

Kutin G, Hawes RR. Posterior crossbites in the deciduous and mixed dentitions. Am J Orthod 56: 491–504, 1969.

2

Interceptive (Mixed Dentition): Case 2

Interview Data

The parent's chief complaint was that, "Our daughter has a crossbite and spaces between the front teeth and we wanted it corrected before any other issues arose."

- Development: pre-pubescent
- Motivation: good
- Medical history: non-contributory
- Dental history: regularly seen for dental care
- Family history: no history of malocclusion
- Habits: none

Clinical Examination

- Incisor-stomion (Figures 2.1 and 2.2):
  – At rest: 4 mm
  – Smiling: 7 mm
- Smile line: 0 mm gingival show on smile
- Breathing: nasal
- Lips: together at rest
- Soft tissue profile: straight (Figure 2.3)
- Nasolabial angle: obtuse
- Normal mandibular plane angle

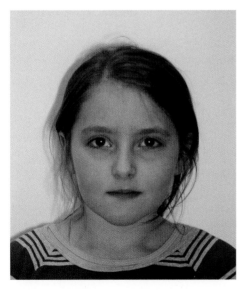

Figure 2.1 Full face at rest displaying an asymmetric, ovoid face due to a mandibular shift.

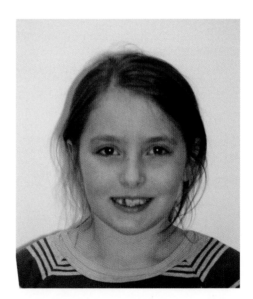

Figure 2.2 Full face with smile showing full enamel appearance of the incisors and no gingival display.

Atlas of Orthodontic Case Reviews, First Edition. Marjan Askari and Stanley A. Alexander.
© 2017 John Wiley & Sons, Inc. Published 2017 by John Wiley & Sons, Inc.

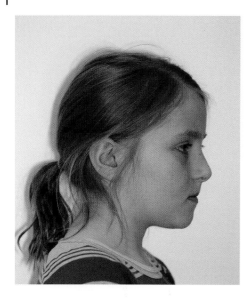

Figure 2.3 Right lateral view of the profile indicating a straight form with obtuse nasolabial angle.

Dentition (Figure 2.4)

- Teeth clinically present

6edc1	12cde6
6edc21	1bcde6

- Overjet: 2 mm
- Overbite: 3 mm
- Diastema: 1 mm maxillary midline
- Midlines: maxillary midline coincident with facial midline; mandibular midline 2 mm to right due to functional shift
- Anterior crossbite: none
- Posterior crossbite: right side due to maxillary constriction and functional shift
- Molar right: end-on mixed dentition with second primary molars present

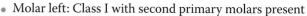

- Molar left: Class I with second primary molars present
- Canine right: Class II
- Canine left: Class I
- Caries: none

Right Buccal View

The right buccal view can be seen in Figure 2.5.

- Molar, right: end-on mixed dentition with second primary molar present
- Canine: Class II
- Curve of Spee: flat
- Crossbite: posterior crossbite
- Caries: none

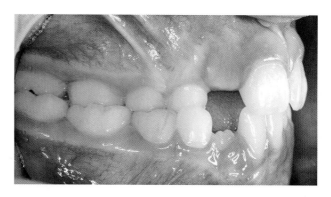

Figure 2.5 Right buccal view of the dentition displaying a posterior crossbite.

Left Buccal View (Figure 2.6)

- Molar, left: Class I with second primary molars present
- Canine: Class I
- Curve of Spee: flat
- Crossbite: none due to functional shift to right
- Caries: none

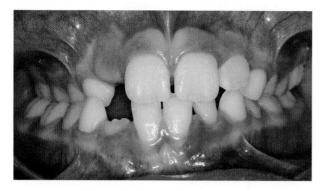

Figure 2.4 Anterior view of the mixed dentition with mandibular midline to the right due to a functional shift.

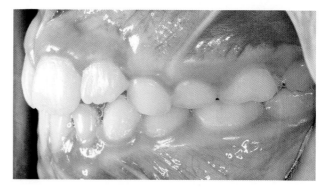

Figure 2.6 Left buccal view of the dentition displaying a normal transverse appearance due to the functional shift to the right.

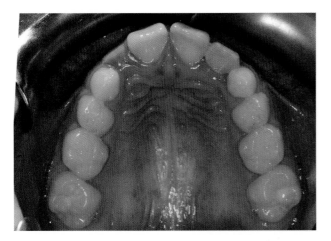

Figure 2.7 Occlusal view of the maxillary arch displaying a tapered, ovoid arch form of the maxilla with rotated molars.

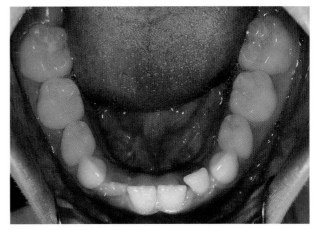

Figure 2.8 Occlusal view of the mandibular arch displaying a U-shaped arch form of the mandible with slight rotation of the incisors.

Maxillary Arch (Figure 2.7)
- Tapered, ovoid arch form with no crowding; rotated first permanent molars
- No caries

Mandibular Arch (Figure 2.8)
- U-shaped arch form
- Slight rotation of incisors
- No caries

Function

- Normal range of motion vertically, laterally, and protrusively; no pain upon excursions
- Centric relation-centric occlusion: coincident
- Early mixed dentition with second permanent molars developing (Figure 2.9)
- Root lengths and periodontium appear normal for age
- Condyles appear normal

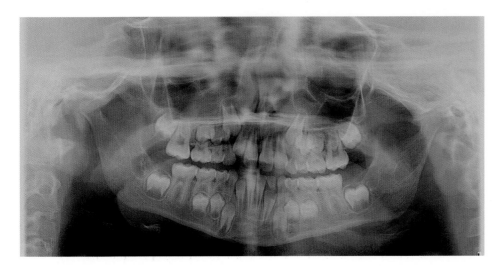

Figure 2.9 Panoramic radiograph indicating an early mixed dentition with development of the second permanent molars.

Diagnosis and Treatment Plan

The patient displays a Class I skeletal and dental pattern (Figure 2.10; Tables 2.1 and 2.2) and is in the early mixed dentition. The correction of the posterior crossbite and anterior spacing is considered interceptive. Treatment will be limited to the maxillary arch.

Maxilla – the maxillary first permanent molars will be banded and a quad-helix appliance will be soldered to the bands. The molars will be rotated and the bilateral crossbite corrected. Brackets will be bonded to the maxillary incisors once the posterior crossbite is corrected, and anterior space closure will be performed with arch wires and elastic chains. Based upon the length of time for correction, a retainer appliance may or may not be indicated at this age.

As described in Chapter 1, no posterior-anterior (PA) radiograph was taken to aid in the overall diagnosis owing to the clinical examination and the patient's age.

Table 2.1 Significant cephalometric values

	Norm	Patient pre-treatment
SNA	80°	82.2°
SNB	78°	80.1°
ANB	2°	+2.1°
WITS appraisal	−1 to +1 mm	−0.9 mm
FMA	21°	21.4°
SN-GoGn	32°	29.3°
Maxillary incisor to SN	105°	107.8°
Mandibular incisor to GoGn	95°	87.4°
Soft tissue		
Lower lip to E-plane	−2 mm	−2.8 mm
Upper lip to E-plane	−1.6 mm	−4.3 mm

SNA, sella-nasion-A point; SNB: sella-nasion-B point; ANB: A point-nasion-B point; WITS appraisal, Witwatersrand appraisal; FMA, Frankfort horizontal-mandibular plane; SN-GoGn: sella nasion-gonion gnathion.

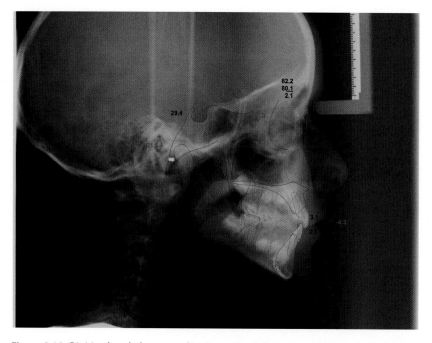

Figure 2.10 Digitized cephalogram indicating a Class I skeletal and dental relationship with normal vertical relationships.

Table 2.2 The patient's problem list in three dimensions

	Transverse	Sagittal	Vertical
Soft tissue	Normal	Straight profile; obtuse nasolabial angle	Normodivergent
Dental	Bilateral posterior crossbite represented as unilateral crossbite due to functional shift; maxillary midline spacing	Normal mixed dentition relationship of molars; Class I canine left and Class II canine right	3 mm overbite
Skeletal	Maxillary constriction	Class I	Normodivergent

Treatment Objectives

The patient's chief complaint for the mixed dentition will be addressed by the correction of the posterior crossbite and closure of the anterior maxillary spaces. Once corrected and maintained, the child will be evaluated annually for further orthodontic treatment. Growth appears in a Class I pattern both dentally and skeletally. Further orthodontic care would probably be limited to dental alignment.

Treatment Options

1) No treatment at this time – treatment to be provided during the late or permanent dentition period.

2) Interceptive treatment to correct the posterior cross-bite and anterior spacing (Figures 2.11 and 2.12).

Both the patient and parent chose option 2. Based upon the patient's age and development, the crossbite correction would be accomplished with a quad-helix appliance. The incorporation of the four helices allows the wire a greater range of activation over time and increases its springiness, thereby making it a more gentle form of movement, but also decreases its strength, which may cause it to break more easily during function. The quad-helix would also permit rotation of the maxillary first molars (Figure 2.7). Maxillary midline spaces will be corrected with a fixed 2×4 appliance (banded maxillary molars and bonded brackets to the four incisors).

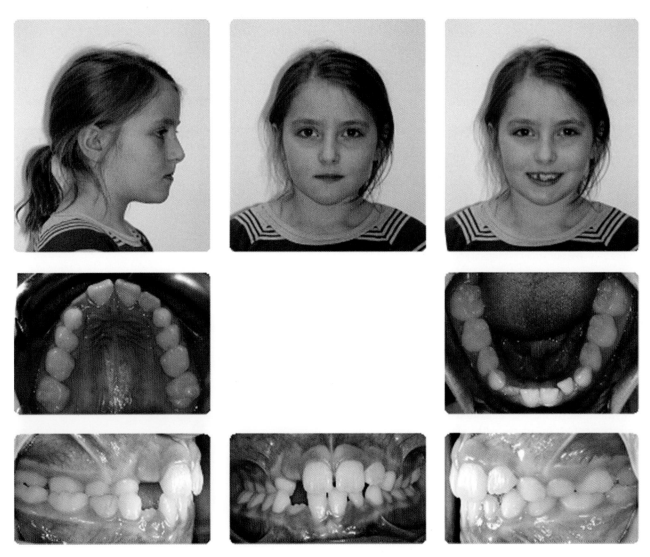

Figure 2.11 Pre-treatment extraoral and intraoral composite photograph.

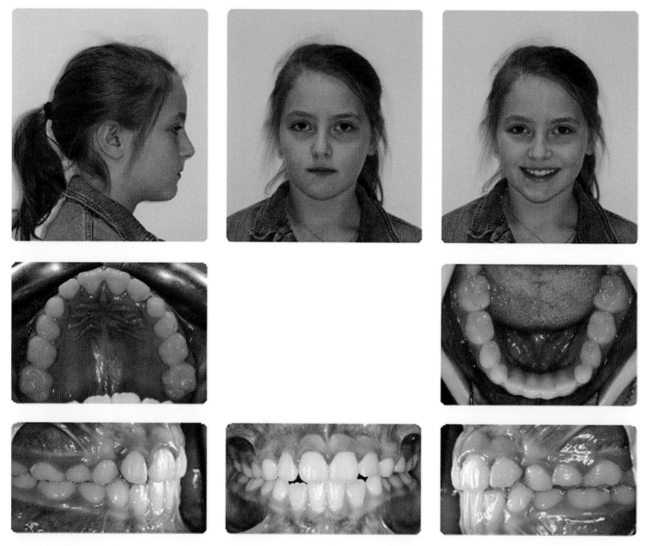

Figure 2.12 Post-treatment extraoral and intraoral composite photograph.

First Active Appointment

One week prior to this appointment, elastic separators were placed mesial to the maxillary first molars and an iTero scan (Align Technology, Inc, San Jose, CA, USA) was taken for the fabrication of a quad-helix. When fitted, the quad-helix was activated 8 mm for expansion and cemented in place with glass ionomer cement (Figure 2.13).

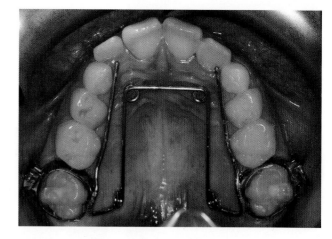

Figure 2.13 Occlusal view of the maxillary arch with initial placement of the quad-helix and activated 8 mm.

Second Active Appointment

The patient returned 8 weeks later after the initial activation with the crossbite corrected to a normal transverse relationship (Figures 2.14 and 2.15). The arch form has changed from an ovoid shape to a broad, U-shaped configuration as a result of the expansion. The lateral arms were beginning to become embedded in the palatal mucosa. The arms were shortened and the appliance was reactivated to over-expand the correction by approximately 20% and to rotate the maxillary molars in a disto-buccal direction.

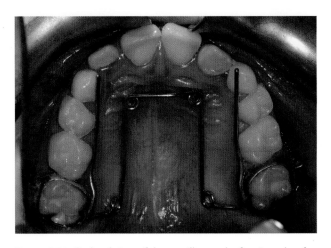

Figure 2.14 Occlusal view of the maxillary arch after 8 weeks of activation. The arch form has changed to a broad, U-shaped configuration.

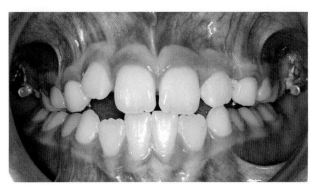

Figure 2.15 Anterior view of the dentition after 8 weeks. An improvement in the transverse relationship is apparent and the functional shift has been eliminated.

Third Active Appointment

The crossbite has been over-corrected within a 12-week period since appliance cementation and activation and the molars have been rotated (Figures 2.16–2.19). The lateral arms were now removed because they were constantly embedding into the mucosa.

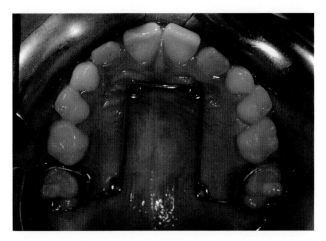

Figure 2.16 Occlusal view of the maxillary arch after 12 weeks of activation. The crossbite has been over-corrected, the molars have been rotated, and the lateral arms of the appliance were removed due to embedding into the palatal mucosa.

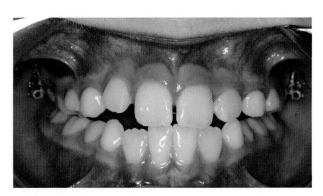

Figure 2.17 Anterior view of the dentition after the 12th week. The crossbite has been over-corrected and the functional shift was eliminated.

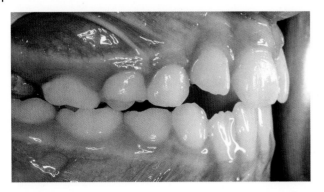

Figure 2.18 Right buccal view of the dentition indicating over-correction of the crossbite.

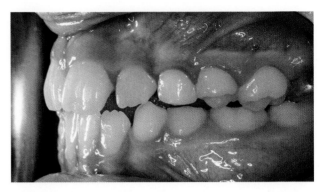

Figure 2.19 Left buccal view of the dentition indicating over-correction of the crossbite.

Fourth Active Appointment

Expansion remains over-corrected. The maxillary incisors have been bonded with brackets, and a .016 nickel-titanium wire was inserted to level the arch and to initiate anterior space closure (Figures 2.20 and 2.21).

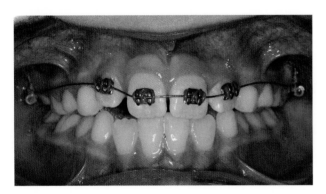

Figure 2.20 Anterior view of the dentition with brackets bonded to the maxillary incisors to initiate leveling of the arch and anterior space closure.

Fifth Active Appointment

Twenty weeks after the initial insertion of the quad-helix, the appliance was removed, with the over-correction of the crossbite maintained. A sectional .018 × .025 nickel-

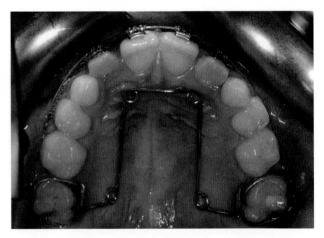

Figure 2.21 Occlusal view of the maxillary arch with appliance at the time of initiation of leveling and anterior space closure,

titanium archwire was inserted into the incisor brackets and the remaining space closure was attained with elastic modules to allow the teeth to approximate one another through sliding mechanics (Figures 2.22 and 2.23).

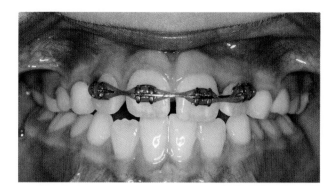

Figure 2.22 Anterior view of the dentition with a sectional .018×.025 nickel-titanium archwire and elastomeric chain stretching from the right lateral incisor to the left lateral incisor being used to close space.

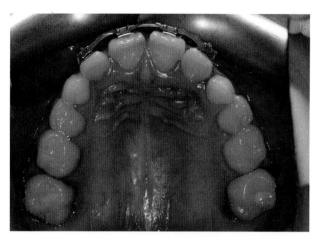

Figure 2.23 Occlusal view of the maxillary arch with a sectional nickel-titanium wire and elastomeric chain used to close space. Note that the quad-helix has been removed after the 20th week following placement.

Phase I Completed

Twenty-four weeks after the initiation of treatment, the patient was debanded and clinical photographs and a panoramic radiograph were taken (Figures 2.24–2.31). The posterior crossbite was corrected and anterior space closure was accomplished. Facial characteristics remained the same. The panoramic radiograph (Figure 2.32) indicated further normal development and no iatrogenic side-effects from the expansion or limited fixed appliance therapy. No retention appliance was fabricated. The patient was put on an annual recall for evaluation of further treatment in the future.

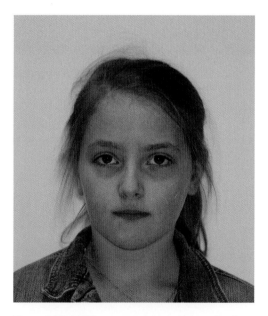

Figure 2.24 Full face post-treatment 24 weeks after appliance placement. Note the symmetry of the face compared with the pre-treatment situation.

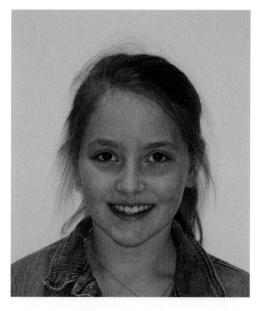

Figure 2.25 Full face smiling at post-treatment. Note the symmetry and balance without a functional shift of the mandible.

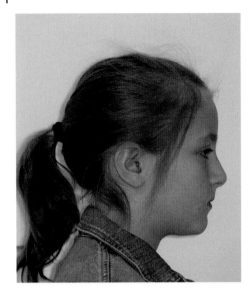

Figure 2.26 Right lateral view of the profile at post-treatment. It remains straight and balanced.

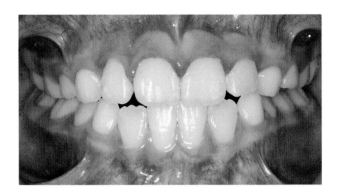

Figure 2.27 Anterior view of the dentition at post-treatment, indicating anterior space closure and the correction of the posterior crossbite without the presence of a functional shift.

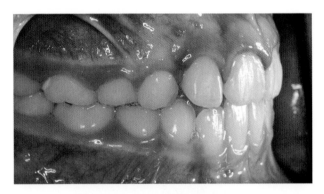

Figure 2.28 Right buccal view of the dentition at post-treatment, displaying a normal transverse relationship.

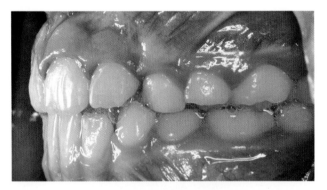

Figure 2.29 Left buccal view of the dentition at post-treatment, displaying a normal transverse relationship.

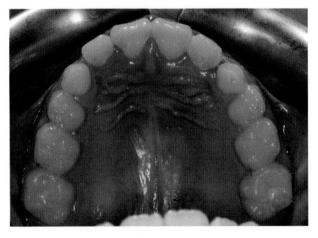

Figure 2.30 Occlusal view of the maxillary arch at post-treatment, displaying a broad, U-shaped configuration.

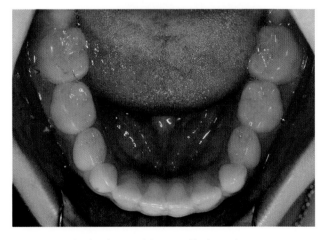

Figure 2.31 Occlusal view of the mandibular arch at post-treatment, displaying a U-shaped arch form.

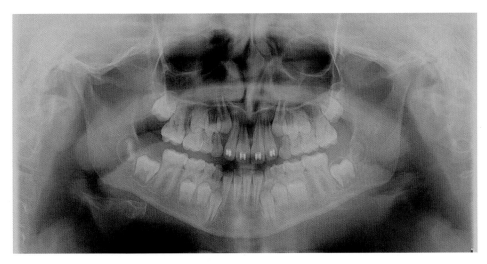

Figure 2.32 Post-treatment panoramic radiograph, indicating further normal development and no iatrogenic side-effects of the treatment.

Commentary

The terminology of phase I or interceptive treatment can often be misleading. In this case, the posterior crossbite was corrected, as well as the implementation of anterior space closure. In most circumstances, space closure is not considered interceptive treatment, but is adjunctive in nature, and this was performed at the request of the parent.

Review Questions

1   The quad-helix in this case demonstrated two types of orthodontic corrective capabilities. What are these capabilities observed here?

2   What characteristics do the four helices in the quad-helix appliance provide to the wire in terms of its mechanical properties?

3   How is space closure accomplished in this case?

Suggested References

Bell RA, LeCompte EJ. The effects of maxillary expansion using a quad-helix appliance during the deciduous and mixed dentitions. Am J Orthod 79: 152–157, 1981.

Bishara SE, Staley RN. Maxillary expansion: clinical implications. Am J Orthod Dentofac Orthop 91(1): 3–14, 1987.

Dean, JA, Jones, JE, Vinson, LAW. Managing the developing dentition. In: McDonald and Avery's Dentistry for the Child and Adolescent, 10th edn. Elsevier, St. Louis, MO: Elsevier, 2016; pp. 449–452.

Germa A, Clement C, Weissenbach M et al. Early risk factors for posterior crossbite and anterior open bite in the primary dentition. Angle Orthod 86 (5): 832–838, 2016.

Proffit WR. Contemporary Orthodontics, 5th edn. CV Mosby Co., 2013; pp. 476–480.

3

Phase I Treatment: Class III Skeletal and Class I Dental with Posterior and Anterior Crossbites

---

LEARNING OBJECTIVES

- The use of a rapid palatal expander (RPE) for crossbite correction
- The use of a protraction face mask in early Class III therapy

---

Interview Data

The parent's chief complaint for their 8-year-old son was the crossbite of the front teeth.

- Development: pre-pubescent
- Motivation: average
- Medical history: cardiac arrhythmia; no need for premedication
- Dental history: seen by a general dentist for routine care
- Family history: parents were treated for malocclusion with extractions; mother appears to have a Class III tendency
- Habits: none
- Facial form: ovoid, mesoprosopic asymmetric face
- Facial proportions: normal, but high mandibular plane angle

Clinical Examination

- Incisor-stomion (Figures 3.1 and 3.2):
  - At rest: 3 mm, with competent lips
  - Smiling: 10 mm, with 1 mm of gingival display
- Breathing: nasal
- Lips: apart at rest, but competent
- Soft tissue profile: straight (Figure 3.3)
- Nasolabial angle: obtuse
- High mandibular plane angle

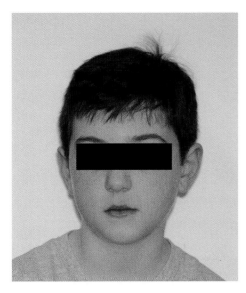

Figure 3.1 Full face at rest displaying an ovoid, asymmetric form.

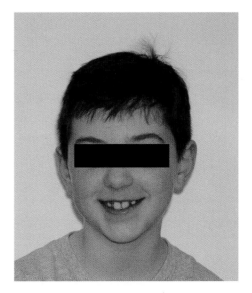

Figure 3.2 Full face with smile displaying 1 mm of gingiva.

Atlas of Orthodontic Case Reviews, First Edition. Marjan Askari and Stanley A. Alexander.
© 2017 John Wiley & Sons, Inc. Published 2017 by John Wiley & Sons, Inc.

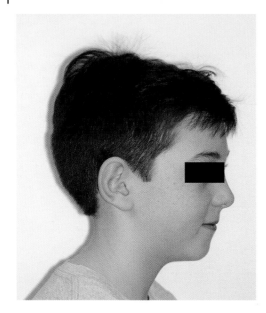

Figure 3.3 Right lateral view of profile indicating a straight form with an obtuse nasolabial angle and a steep mandibular plane.

Dentition (Figure 3.4)

- Teeth clinically present:

6edc21	12cde6
6edc21	12cde6

- Overjet: 1 mm
- Overbite: 1 mm
- Diastema: 2 mm
- Midlines: maxillary midline is coincident with the face; the mandibular midline is 2 mm to the patient's right

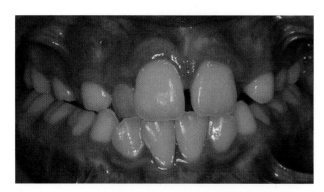

Figure 3.4 Anterior view of the dentition displaying a midline coincident with the face and a mandibuar midline shifted 2 mm to the right due to a functional shift.

Right Buccal View (Figure 3.5)

- Molar: 1/4 cusp Class II
- Canine: Class I
- Curve of Spee: flat
- Crossbite: posterior crossbite and anterior crossbite of lateral incisor
- Caries: none

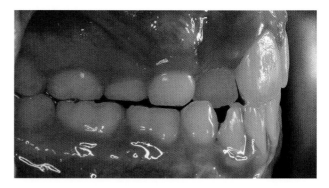

Figure 3.5 Right buccal view of the dentition indicating a molar end-on mixed dentition relationship, posterior crossbite, and anterior crossbite of the lateral incisor.

Left Buccal View (Figure 3.6)

- Molar: Class I
- Canine: Class III
- Curve of Spee: flat
- Crossbite: anterior crossbite of lateral incisor
- Caries: none

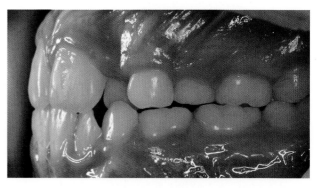

Figure 3.6 Left buccal view of the dentition indicating a Class I molar relationship and anterior crossbite of the lateral incisor.

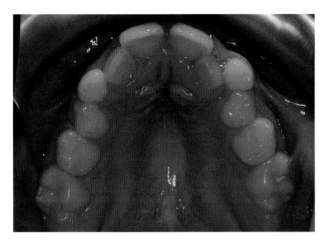 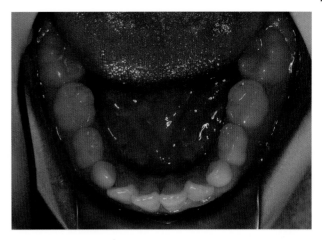

Figure 3.7 Occlusal view of the maxillary arch indicating a narrow, tapering, U-shaped arch form with lingually placed lateral incisors.

Figure 3.8 Occlusal view of the mandibular arch indicating a broad, U-shaped arch form.

Maxillary Arch (Figure 3.7)
- Narrow, tapered, U-shaped symmetric arch form with crowding
- No caries

Mandibular Arch (Figure 3.8)
- Broad, U-shaped symmetric arch form with anterior crowding
- No caries

Function

- Maximum opening = 35 mm
- Centric relation-centric occlusion: 2 mm discrepancy
- Maximum excursive movements: right = 6 mm; left = 5 mm; protrusive = 5 mm
- Temporomandibular joint palpation: normal without any signs of pain, popping or crepitus
- Early mixed dentition with developing second and third molars (Figure 3.9)
- Root length and periodontium appear normal
- Condyles appear normal

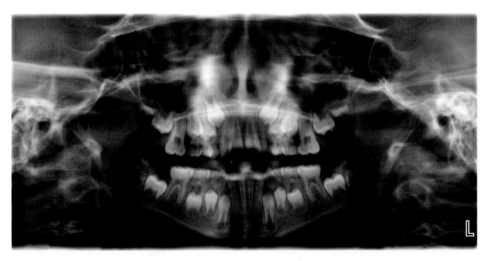

Figure 3.9 Panoramic radiograph indicating an early mixed dentition with the development of the second and third molars.

Diagnosis and Treatment Plan

The patient is in the early mixed dentition and displays a Class I dental malocclusion with both posterior and anterior crossbites and a skeletal Class III tendency (Figure 3.10; Tables 3.1 and 3.2). At this stage, any orthodontic correction would be considered interceptive.

The plan of treatment will include rapid palatal expansion, alignment of the anterior dentition, and correction of the crossbites with fixed appliances and a reverse pull face mask. Once the corrections are attained, the patient will be placed on an annual recall schedule to monitor the growth and future development.

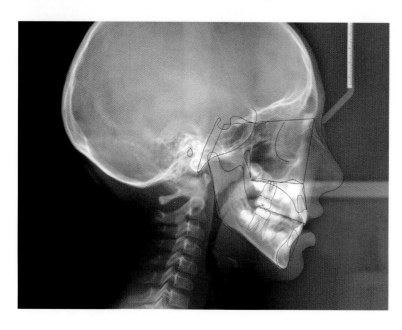

Figure 3.10 Digitized cephalogram indicating a Class III skeletal pattern, high mandibular plane angle, and upright incisors.

Table 3.1 Significant cephalometric values

	Norm	Patient pre-treatment
SNA	80°	78.6°
SNB	78°	75.9°
ANB	2°	+2.7°
WITS appraisal	−1 to +1 mm	−6.4 mm
FMA	21°	30.2°
SN-GoGn	32°	41.4°
Maxillary incisor to SN	105°	97.4°
Mandibular incisor to GoGn	95°	85.5°
Soft tissue		
Lower lip to E-plane	−2 mm	+0.4 mm
Upper lip to E-plane	−1.6 mm	−3.5 mm

SNA, sella-nasion-A point; SNB, sella-nasion-B point; ANB, A point-nasion-B point; WITS appraisal, Witwatersrand appraisal; FMA, Frankfort horizontal-mandibular plane; SN-GoGn, sella nasion-gonion gnathion.

Table 3.2 The patient's problem list in three dimensions

	Transverse	Sagittal	Vertical
Soft tissue	Narrow and asymmetric	Straight profile; obtuse nasolabial angle	Hyperdivergent
Dental	Moderate space deficiency; posterior crossbite	Early mixed dentition; Class I with anterior crossbites of lateral incisors	1 mm overbite
Skeletal	Narrow and asymmetric	Class III	Hyperdivergent

Treatment Objectives

The patient's clinical problems will be addressed by correction of the posterior and anterior crossbites and alignment of the anterior dentition. The use of a rapid palatal expander would further allow the maxilla to move forward and correct for a developing Class III malocclusion. The implementation of a protraction face mask at this age would also augment maxillary movement, but lack of compliance is anticipated and may present a problem.

Treatment Options

The options presented to the parent and child were three-fold:

1) No treatment – this was not chosen since the crossbites would not self-correct and would interfere with normal growth if not treated.
2) Expansion with a rapid palatal expander (Hyrax) and anterior alignment with a fixed appliance.
3) The treatment of choice was to incorporate the use of a protraction face mask with option 2 and to stress compliance with this form of therapy (Figures 3.11 and 3.12).

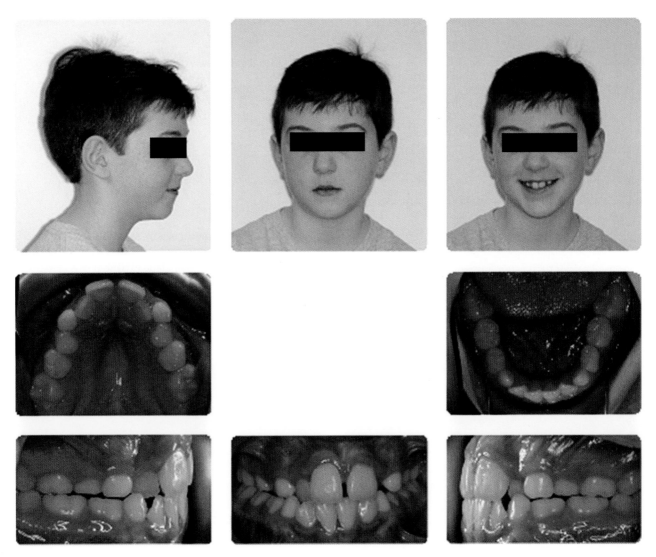

Figure 3.11 Pre-treatment extraoral and intraoral composite photograph of the patient.

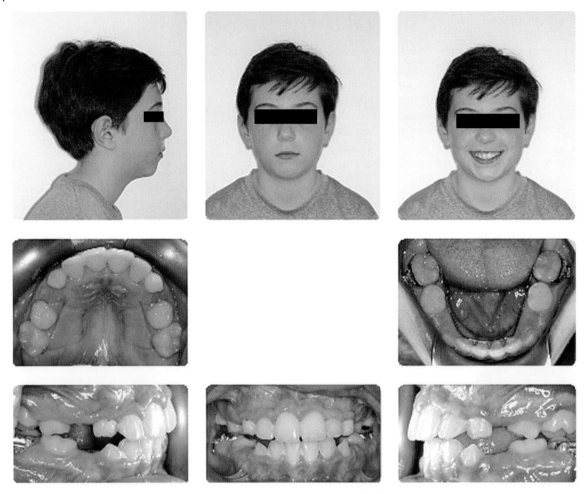

Figure 3.12 End of phase 1 extraoral and intraoral composite photograph of the patient.

First Active Appointment

Four weeks prior to the appointment, an iTero scan (Align Technology, Inc, San Jose, CA, USA) was performed for fabrication of a rapid palatal expander with soldered hooks for elastics placement for face mask therapy. One week prior to the appointment, elastic separators were placed. On the day of the appointment, the maxillary incisors were bonded and the rapid palatal expander was cemented with glass ionomer (Figures 3.13–3.17). The expander was initially turned twice in the office with instructions to turn the palatal screw once daily for 2 weeks.

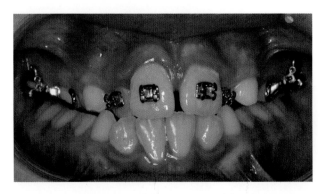

Figure 3.13 Anterior view of the dentition with bonded brackets and cemented palatal expander.

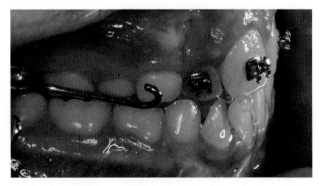

Figure 3.14 Right buccal view of the dentition with the cemented appliance.

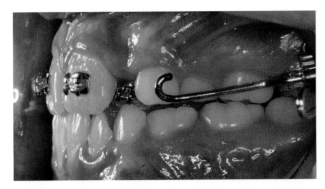

Figure 3.15 Left buccal view of the dentition with the cemented appliance.

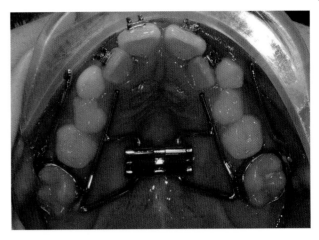

Figure 3.16 Occlusal view of the maxillary arch with the cemented appliance prior to activation.

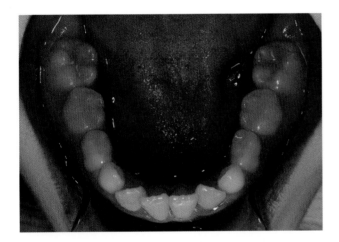

Figure 3.17 Occlusal view of the mandibular arch prior to maxillary appliance activation.

Second Active Appointment

Two weeks later, the patient returned with a bracket missing from the maxillary right lateral incisor. Expansion was considered complete. A .016 nickel-titanium wire was inserted and an elastomeric chain was ligated to the central incisors for diastema closure (Figures 3.18–3.21) Note that the chain is only attached to the mesial wings of the central incisor brackets to prevent the rotation of the incisors during space closure. The rotation would be a side-effect of the force operating distal to the centers of rotation of these teeth during translation.

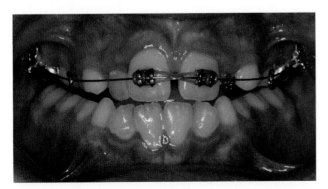

Figure 3.18 Anterior view of the dentition after the insertion of .016 nickel-titanium wire and elastomeric chain between the central incisors.

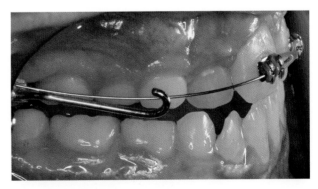

Figure 3.19 Right buccal view of the dentition after 2 weeks of expansion of the maxilla.

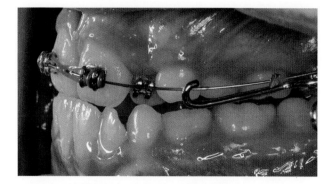

Figure 3.20 Left buccal view of the dentition after 2 weeks of expansion of the maxilla.

Third Active Appointment

Three weeks later, the maxillary primary canines and right lateral incisor were bonded and the .016 nickel-titanium arch wire was ligated. The midline diastema was closed at this point (Figures 3.22–3.25).

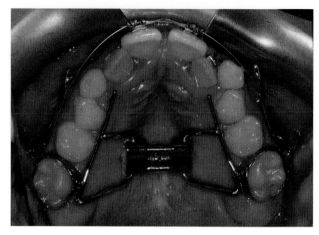

Figure 3.21 Occlusal view of the maxillary arch after 2 weeks of activation.

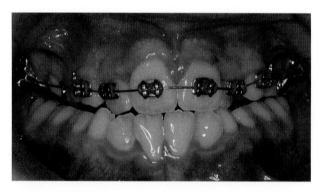

Figure 3.22 Anterior view of the dentition indicating that the maxillary primary canines have been bracketed for arch wire stabilization. Note that the diastema has closed.

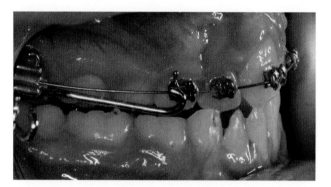

Figure 3.23 Right buccal view of the dentition after bonding of the primary canine.

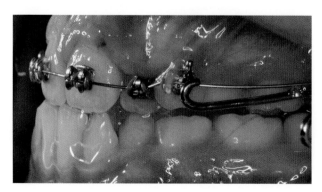

Figure 3.24 Left buccal view of the dentition after bonding of the primary canine.

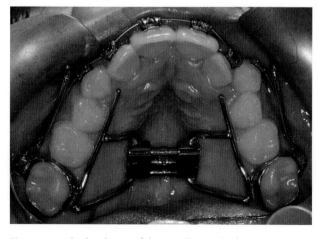

Figure 3.25 Occlusal view of the maxillary arch after expansion was completed and the primary canines have been bracketed.

Fourth Active Appointment

Six weeks later, the protraction face mask was delivered and instructions to wear for 14 hours/day were given (Whale elastics ½"; 14 oz.). Instructions for the rapid palatal expander to be turned one time a day for one additional week for expansion and suture mobilization were also given (Figures 3.26–3.31).

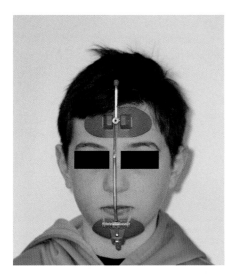

Figure 3.26 Facial view of the patient with the protraction face mask in place.

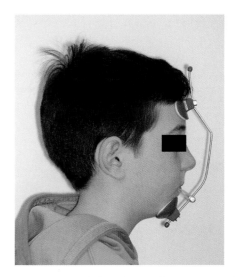

Figure 3.27 Right lateral view of the patient with the protraction face mask indicating the downward vector of elastic traction for maxillary protraction.

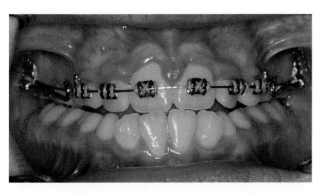

Figure 3.28 Anterior view of the dentition with aligned maxillary teeth.

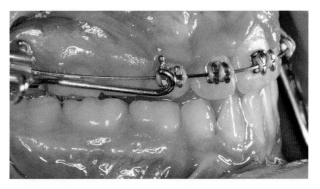

Figure 3.29 Right buccal view of the dentition with aligned maxillary teeth on the day the face mask was delivered.

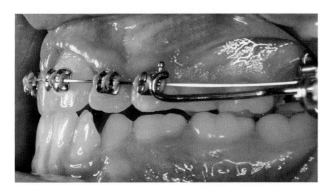

Figure 3.30 Left buccal view of the dentition with aligned maxillary teeth on the day the face mask was delivered.

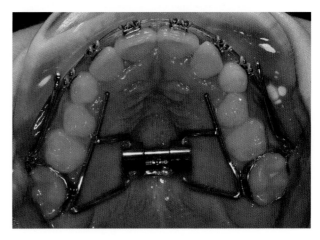

Figure 3.31 Occlusal view of the maxillary arch on the day the face mask was delivered.

Fifth Active Appointment

Four weeks later, the arch wire was changed to .016 × .022 nickel-titanium and the elastomeric chain was ligated from canine to canine for space closure as a result of the continued palatal expansion. The face mask was being worn only 8 hours per day and the patient and parent were advised that it needs to be worn at least 14 hours per day (Figures 3.32–3.35).

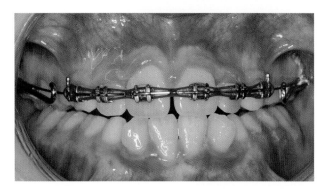

Figure 3.32 Anterior view of the dentition with a .016 × .022 arch wire in place and improved overjet and overbite. Elastomeric chain has been placed due to opening of the diastema.

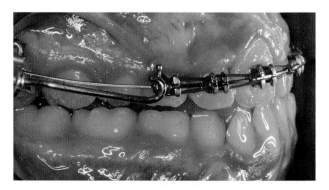

Figure 3.33 Right buccal view of the dentition with a .016 × .022 arch wire in place.

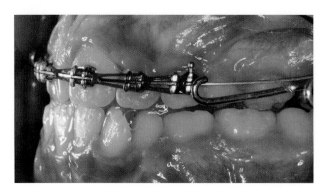

Figure 3.34 Left buccal view of the dentition with a .016 × .022 arch wire in place.

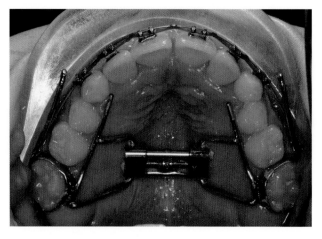

Figure 3.35 Occlusal view of the maxillary arch with an aligned and expanded maxillary arch.

Sixth Active Appointment

Four weeks later, the .016 × .022 nickel-titanium arch wire was retied with elastomeric chain from primary canine to primary canine for space consolidation (Figures 3.36 and 3.37). A further explanation for the use of the protraction face mask was given in relation to growth modification as the parent still did not fully comprehend its use because it was also extremely obtrusive. A new packet of extraoral elastics (Whale; ½"; 14 oz.) were given.

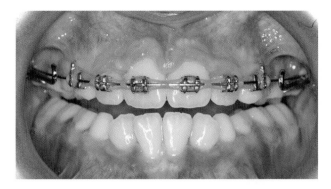

Figure 3.36 Anterior view of the dentition with maxillary expansion. Note that the overbite has opened due to the contact of the palatal cusps of the maxillary first molars with the mandibular molars.

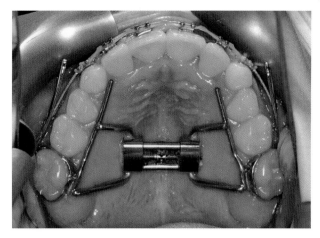

Figure 3.37 Occlusal view of maxillary arch with expansion 4 weeks after delivery of the protraction face mask.

Seventh and Eighth Active Appointments

Five weeks later, elastic separators were placed prior to the construction of a lingual holding arch. The maxillary and mandibular first primary molars were extracted and an iTero scan was done for the lingual arch construction.

Two weeks later, the lingual holding arch was cemented with glass ionomer and the mandibular incisors were bonded with .018 brackets (Figures 3.38–3.42). No arch wire was placed during this visit. The elastomeric chain was replaced on the maxillary arch. The patient did not bring in the protraction face mask and was advised again to wear this appliance 14 hours a day.

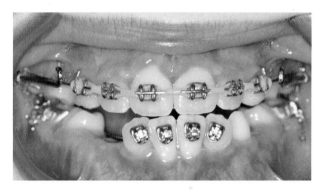

Figure 3.38 Anterior view of the dentition with elastomeric chain for space closure. The mandibular primary first molars have been extracted.

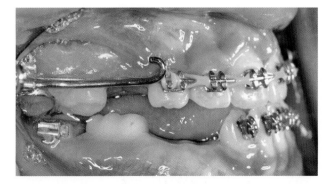

Figure 3.39 Right buccal view of the dentition displaying the overexpanded maxillary arch and extraction site of the mandibular right primary first molar.

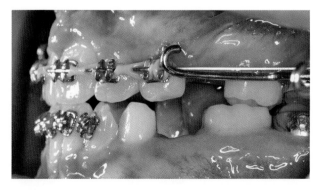

Figure 3.40 Left buccal view of the dentition displaying an over-corrected maxillary arch and extraction site of the mandibular left primary first molar.

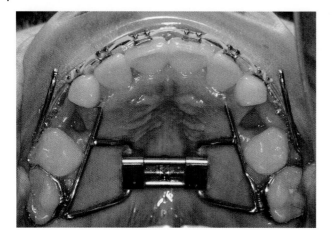

Figure 3.41 Occlusal view of the over-corrected maxillary arch on the day the primary first molars were extracted.

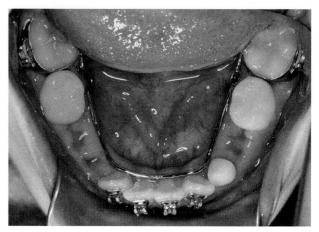

Figure 3.42 Occlusal view of the mandible when the lingual holding arch was placed.

Ninth and 10th Active Appointments

Four weeks later, a .016 nickel-titanium arch wire was ligated to the mandibular arch and the elastomeric chain was continued on the maxilla. The patient's parent said that the protraction face mask was being worn 10 hours a day, and we advised that 14 hours a day was necessary to achieve our goal of growth modification. The rapid palatal expander was unturned four turns chairside due to the buccal crossbite that developed due to overexpansion. The elastomeric chain was continued on the maxillary arch (Figures 3.43 and 3.45).

Four weeks later, the rapid palatal expander was again unturned four times to reduce the buccal crossbite.

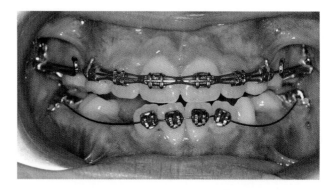

Figure 3.43 Anterior view of the dentition displaying initial alignment of the mandibular arch with .016 nickel-titanium.

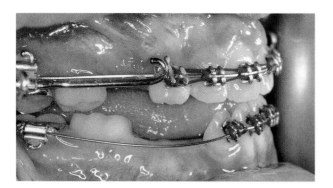

Figure 3.44 Right buccal view of the dentition with initial alignment of the mandibular incisors.

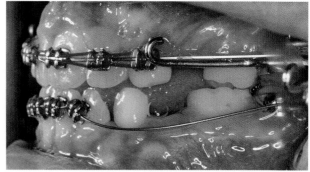

Figure 3.45 Left buccal view of the dentition with initial alignment of the mandibular incisors.

Eleventh Active Appointment

Six weeks later, the mandibular arch wire was changed to .016 × .022. A progress panoramic radiograph was taken, which indicated that alignment of the mandibular incisors progressed and that the primary second molars were closer to exfoliation. The anterior arms of the rapid palatal expander were removed due to palatal impingement and the expander was further unturned six times due to the buccal crossbite. The elastomeric chain was replaced on the maxillary arch (Figures 3.46–3.49).

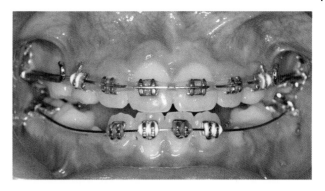

Figure 3.46 Anterior view of the dentition with insertion of a .016 × .022 nickel-titanium mandibular arch wire. Note the alignment of the four mandibular incisors since the original arch wire insertion.

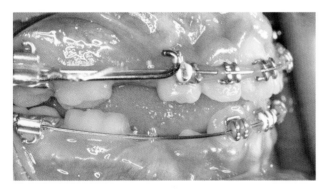

Figure 3.47 Right buccal view of the dentition with insertion of a .016 × .022 nickel-titanium arch wire.

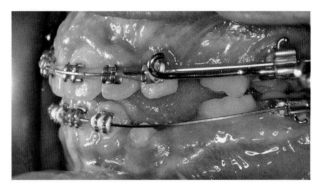

Figure 3.48 Left buccal view of the dentition with insertion of a .016 × .022 nickel-titanium arch wire.

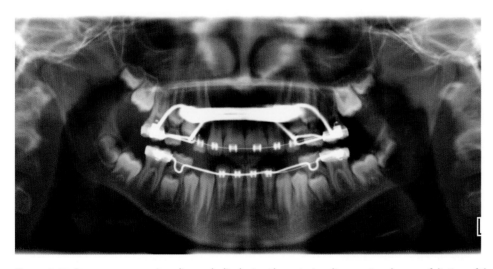

Figure 3.49 Progress panoramic radiograph displaying the anterior alignment and near exfoliation of the remaining primary dentition.

Twelfth Active Appointment

Seven weeks later, the buccal crossbite of the molars was corrected and elastomeric chain was ligated to the maxillary incisors only, as the primary canines were extremely mobile (Figures 3.50–3.54). It was decided that at the next visit an iTero scan would be done for fabrication of a maxillary Hawley retainer and that all of the appliances would be removed, except for the mandibular lingual holding arch. Inadequate use of the protraction face mask, but adequate overjet relationship provided by the arch wire, led to this decision for the completion of phase I treatment.

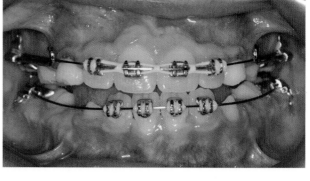

Figure 3.50 Anterior view of the dentition with aligned anterior teeth and over-corrected maxillary arch in the process of relapse to corrected width.

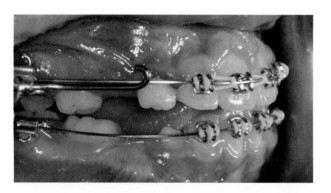

Figure 3.51 Right buccal view of the dentition with acceptable over-corrected expansion of the maxillary arch.

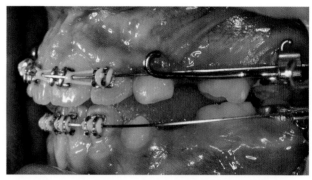

Figure 3.52 Left buccal view of the dentition with acceptable over-corrected expansion of the maxillary arch.

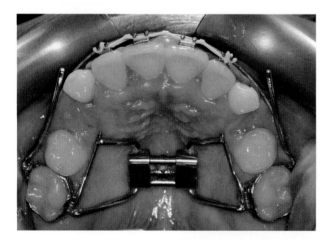

Figure 3.53 Occlusal view of the maxillary arch with aligned anterior teeth and the lateral arms of the rapid palatal expander removed.

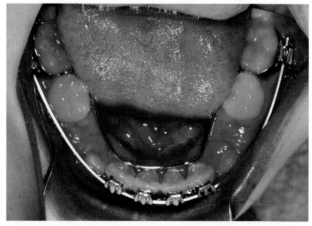

Figure 3.54 Occlusal view of mandibular arch with aligned anterior teeth and lingual arch in place.

Thirteenth Appointment

The appliances were removed except for the lingual holding arch, and a progress cephalometric radiograph was taken. The Hawley retainer was delivered and the lingual acrylic was slightly removed to allow for further relapse of the maxillary molars. The patient was to be seen again in 1 month for observation and on a 3-month recall to check the mandibular lingual holding arch and for the timing of extraction of the primary second molars.

The molar relationship is end-on Class II with a 3 mm overjet due to the over-correction of the skeletal Class III tendency. The lingual holding arch will maintain adequate space for the erupting mandibular dentition (Figures 3.55–3.62). Comprehensive orthodontic care

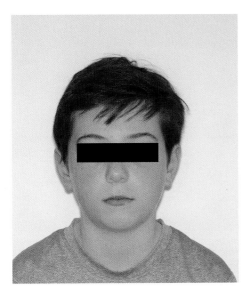

Figure 3.55 Full-face view at the end of phase 1 displaying a symmetric, ovoid face.

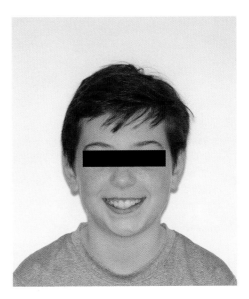

Figure 3.56 Full face with smile at the end of phase 1.

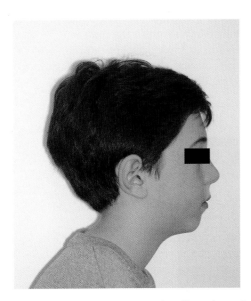

Figure 3.57 Right lateral view of profile at the end of phase 1 exhibiting a convex profile.

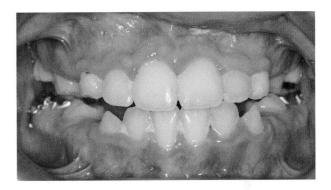

Figure 3.58 Anterior view of the dentition at the end of phase 1 displaying a corrected posterior crossbite and normal overjet and overbite with space closure.

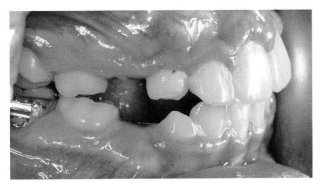

Figure 3.59 Right buccal view of the dentition at the end of phase 1 displaying a corrected posterior crossbite.

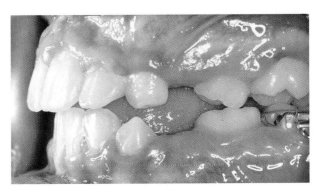

Figure 3.60 Left buccal view of the dentition at the end of phase 1 displaying a corrected posterior crossbite.

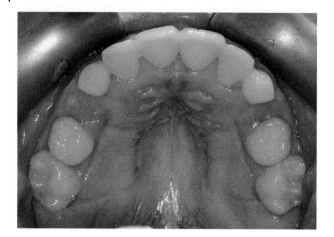

Figure 3.61 Occlusal view of the maxillary arch displaying a broad, U-shaped arch form.

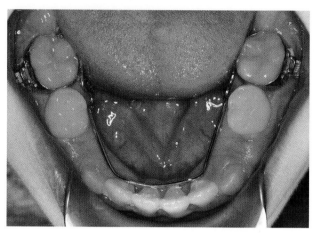

Figure 3.62 Occlusal view of the mandibular arch with lingual holding arch in place.

will begin once the remaining primary teeth are exfoliated. Treatment time for the phase I part of treatment was 13 months. The cephalometric measurements and the overall superimposition indicated that minimal growth had occurred during this period of treatment (Figures 3.63–3.64 – initial, black; progress, green), but the maxilla moved slightly forward as the result of face mask therapy coupled with flaring of the central incisors, which created a more convex profile. Regional superimposition indicated that anchorage of the posterior dentition was maintained as a result of the rigid rapid palatal expander and lingual holding arch. The minimal maxillary incisor retraction was the result of the elastomeric chain consolidating the anterior teeth.

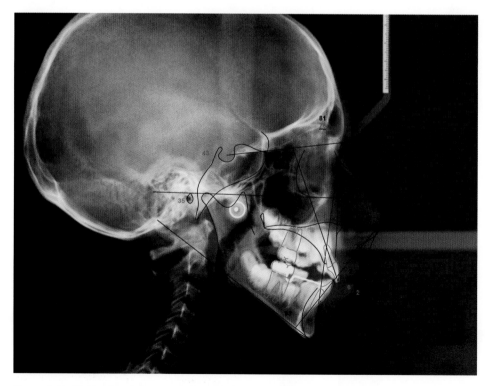

Figure 3.63 Digitized cephalogram at the end of phase 1 exhibiting a normal overjet and overbite, improved skeletal relationship of the maxilla and mandible, improved angulation of the incisors, and a convex profile.

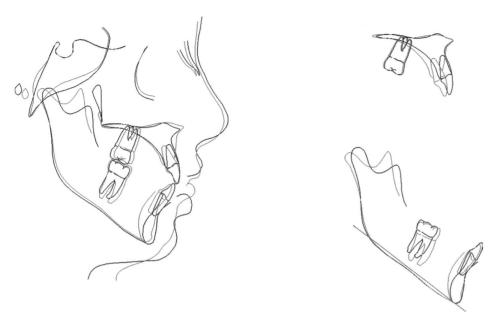

Figure 3.64 The overall superimposition tracings (pre-treatment, black; interim, green) reveal minimal growth, but anterior movement of the maxilla as a result of the protraction face mask. The regional superimposition tracings reveal a slight retraction of both the maxillary and mandibular incisors as a result of elastomeric traction during alignment and space closure.

Commentary

As the phase I treatment was completed with an over-corrected relationship in the anteroposterior dimension, no need for retention was provided. Anecdotally, it has been the practice of many clinicians to retain developing Class III patients with a functional-type retainer, such as a Frankel III, which may aid in the over-all treatment of patients who are mid-face-deficient (Table 3.3).

Table 3.3 Significant pre-treatment and post-treatment cephalometric values

	Norm	Pre-treatment	Post-treatment
SNA	82°	76°	81°
SNB	80°	76°	76°
ANB	2°	0°	5°
WITS appraisal	−1 to +1 mm	−6.4 mm	−3.5 mm
FMA	21°	29.4°	33.1°
SN-GoGn	32°	40.6°	42.9°
Maxillary incisor To SN	105°	97.0°	105.8°
Mandibular incisor to GoGn	95°	88°	92°
Soft tissue			
Lower lip to E-plane	−2.0 mm	+0.4 mm	+1.7 mm
Upper lip to E-plane	−1.6 mm	−3.5 mm	0.7 mm

SNA, sella-nasion-A point; SNB, sella-nasion-B point; ANB, A point-nasion-B point; WITS appraisal, Witwatersrand appraisal; FMA, Frankfort horizontal-mandibular plane; SN-GoGn, sella nasion-gonion gnathion.

Review Questions

1   The rapid palatal expander served two functions in this case. What are they?

2   What process caused the mandibular shift to the right in this patient?

3   How was the anterior crossbite corrected?

Suggested References

Bacetti T, Franchi L, McNamara JA. Treatment and post-treatment craniofacial changes after rapid maxillary expansion and facemask therapy. Am J Orthod Dentofac Orthop 118: 404–413, 2000.

Brennan MM, Gianelly AA. The use of the lingual arch in the mixed dentition to resolve incisor crowding. Am J Orthod Denofac Orthop 117: 81–85, 2000.

Da Silva Andrade A, Gameiro G, DeRossi M, Gaviao M. Posterior crossbite and functional change. Angle Orthod 79(2): 380–386, 2009.

DeClerck HJ, Cornelis MA, Cevidanes LH et al. Orthopedic traction of the maxilla with miniplates: a new perspective for treatment of midface deficiency. J Oral Maxillofac Surg 67(10): 2123–2129, 2009.

Gianelly AA. Leeway space and the resolution of crowding in the mixed dentition. Semin Orthod 1: 188–194, 1995.

Sonis A, Ackerman M. E-space preservation: Is there a relationship to mandibular second molar impaction? Angle Orthod 81(6): 1045–1049, 2011.

4

Class I Skeletal and Class I Dental with Blocked-Out Maxillary Canine: Non-Extraction

Interview Data

This 10-year-old pubescent female presented with the chief complaint of "needing orthodontics because of crowding."

- Development: pubescent 10-year-old female
- Motivation: good
- Medical history: non-contributory
- Dental history: seen for routine care in a pediatrics clinic
- Family history: no immediate family members, including the older sister, required orthodontic care
- Habits: none
- Limitations: none

- Facial form: mesoprosopic, ovoid face
- Facial proportions: normal lower facial height

Clinical Examination

- Incisor-stomion (Figures 4.1 and 4.2):
  - At rest: 1 mm
  - Smiling: 8 mm
- Breathing: nasal
- Lips: together at rest
- Soft tissue profile: straight (Figure 4.3)
- Nasolabial angle: obtuse
- Normal mandibular plane angle

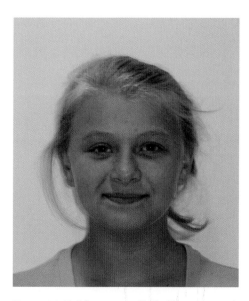

Figure 4.1 Full face at rest displaying a symmetric, ovoid form.

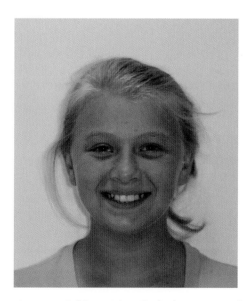

Figure 4.2 Full face with smile displaying 1 mm of gingiva.

Atlas of Orthodontic Case Reviews, First Edition. Marjan Askari and Stanley A. Alexander.
© 2017 John Wiley & Sons, Inc. Published 2017 by John Wiley & Sons, Inc.

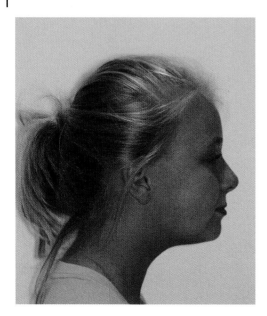

Figure 4.3 Right lateral view of profile displaying a straight profile and normal mandibular plane angle.

Dentition (Figure 4.4)

- Teeth present clinically:

654321	12456
654321	123456

- Overjet: 3 mm
- Overbite: 3 mm
- Midlines: maxillary midline is 3 mm left of face; mandibular midline is coincident with the face

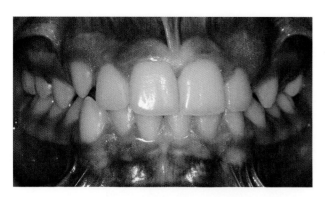

Figure 4.4 Anterior view of the dentition displaying a maxillary midline shift to the left of the patient's face and mandibular midline coincident with the facial midline.

Right Buccal View

The right buccal view can be seen in Figure 4.5.

- Right molar: Class I
- Right canine: end-on
- Curve of Spee: flat
- Crossbite: none
- Caries: none

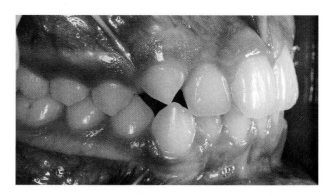

Figure 4.5 Right buccal of the dentition view displaying a Class I molar relationship and an end-on canine relationship.

Left Buccal View

The left buccal view can be seen in Figure 4.6.

- Left molar: Class I
- Left canine: non-determined
- Curve of Spee: flat
- Crossbite: none
- Caries: none

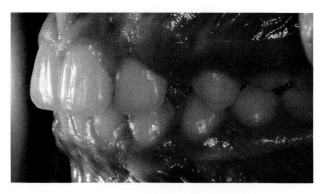

Figure 4.6 Left buccal view of the dentition displaying a Class I molar reltionship. The canine relationship is undetermined.

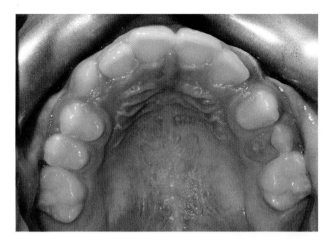

Figure 4.7 Occlusal view of the maxillary arch displaying a broad, U-shaped, asymmetric arch form due to the blocked-out maxillary left canine.

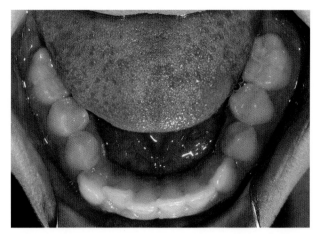

Figure 4.8 Occlusal view of the mandibular arch displaying a U-shaped arch form with minor crowding.

Maxillary Arch (Figure 4.7)

- Asymmetric, broad, U-shaped arch form with blocked out left canine
- No caries

Mandibular Arch (Figure 4.8)

- U-shaped arch form with minor crowding
- No caries

Function

- Normal range of motion with maximum opening at 42 mm; 8 mm right excursive; 10 mm left excursive; 8 mm protrusive
- Centric relation-centric occlusion: coincident
- Temporomandibular joint palpation: normal
- Full adult dentition with impacted maxillary left canine; all four third molars are developing
- Root lengths and periodontium appear normal
- Condyles appear normal (Figure 4.9)

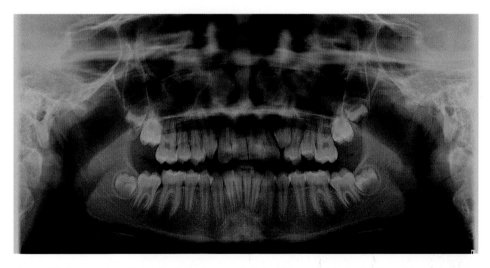

Figure 4.9 Panoramic radiograph displaying an adult dentition with blocked-out maxillary left canine and developing third molars.

Diagnosis and Treatment Plan

The patient presents with a Class I skeletal and Class I dental pattern with an impacted maxillary left canine, non-coincident maxillary midline with a dental shift to the left, and minimally crowded mandibular dentition (Figures 4.10 and 4.11). The treatment will consist of bringing the canine into the arch and correction of the

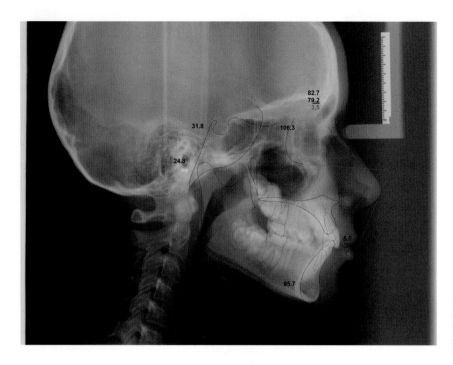

Figure 4.10 Cephalogram displaying a Class I skeletal relationship, normal vertical relationships, and normal incisor angulations.

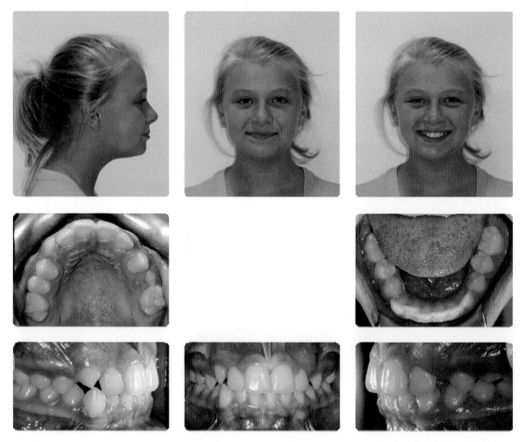

Figure 4.11 Composite photograph of the pre-treatment extraoral and intraoral relationship of the patient.

Table 4.1 Significant cephalometric values

	Norm	Patient pre-treatment
SNA	80°	82.7°
SNB	78°	79.2°
ANB	2°	+3.5°
WITS appraisal	−1 to +1 mm	+1.5 mm
FMA	21°	24.7°
SN-GoGn	32°	31.7°
Maxillary incisor to SN	105°	106.3°
Mandibular incisor to GoGn	95°	95.8°
Soft tissue		
Lower lip to E-plane	−2 mm	0.0 mm
Upper lip to E-plane	−1.6 mm	−2.5 mm

SNA, sella-nasion-A point; SNB, sella-nasion-B point; ANB, A point-nasion-B point; WITS appraisal, Witwatersrand appraisal; FMA, Frankfort horizontal-mandibular plane; SN-GoGn, sella nasion-gonion gnathion.

Table 4.2 The patient's problem list in three dimensions

	Transverse	Sagittal	Vertical
Soft tissue	Normal	Straight profile; obtuse nasolabial angle	Normodivergent
Dental	Space deficiency; mild crowding of mandible; severe crowding with impacted left canine of maxilla	Early adult dentition; Class I molar relationship with blocked out maxillary canine	3 mm overbite
Skeletal	Normal	Class I	Normodivergent

midline discrepancy with minor expansion of the arch and flaring of the anterior teeth. The mandibular arch will be aligned with minimal flaring as well. The patient's esthetics will not be compromised (Tables 4.1 and 4.2).

Treatment Objectives

The primary objective in this case was to align the dentition and to create room for the impacted maxillary canine. The patient's growth which was nearing completion would not be modified.

Treatment Options

1) No treatment – this choice is unacceptable as the maxillary canine was impacted, and if it was capable of eruption it would appear outside of the dental arch.

2) Non-extraction treatment – the creation of room for the impacted canine would be accomplished by shifting of the midline and with mild flaring of the anterior dentition that would not affect the esthetics or stability of the case.

3) Extraction of one or multiple teeth – extraction of a single maxillary premolar would not address the midline problem, but would allow for eruption of the canine. Selective reproximation of the opposite arch would be required to correct the midline problem. The extraction of all four premolars would maintain the Class I relationship and allow for both the midline correction and eruption of the canine. However, based upon the patient's esthetics, this form of treatment would be excessive.

Both the parent and patient indicated that they wanted option 2, which would be carried out with a bi-dimensional appliance to create space for the canine eruption (Figures 4.11 and 4.12) through minimal expansion and flaring of the incisors.

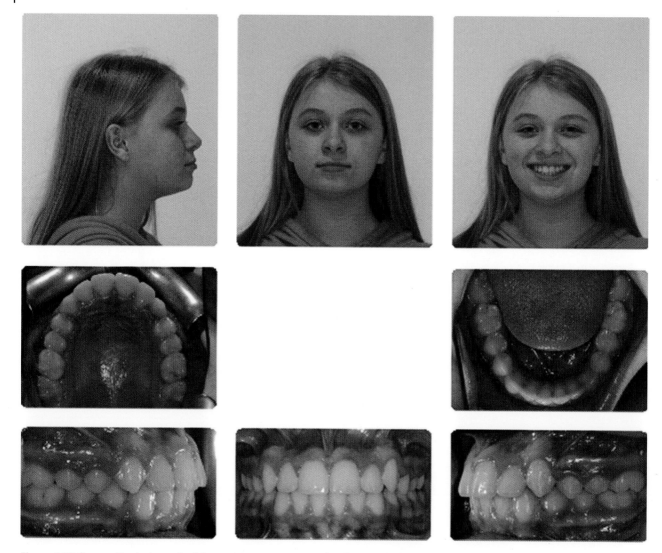

Figure 4.12 Composite photograph of the post-treatment extraoral and intraoral relationship of the patient.

First Active Appointment

Six months passed since the initial records were taken and the maxillary left canine erupted buccally out of the arch. A decision was made to fully bond both arches with brackets and tubes to save space that molar bands would normally occupy during treatment. In the event, the molar tubes debonded during the two weeks of treatment, separators were placed to allow banding if it proved necessary (Figures 4.13–4.17). Maxillary and mandibular .016 nickel- titanium arch wires were ligated to level and align the dentition and an open coil spring was placed between the maxillary left lateral incisor and first premolar to aid in shifting the midline and to create space for the blocked-out canine.

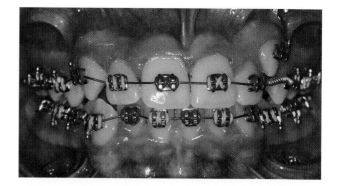

Figure 4.13 Anterior view of the dentition with the initial placement of the appliance and ligated with .016 nickel-titanium wires.

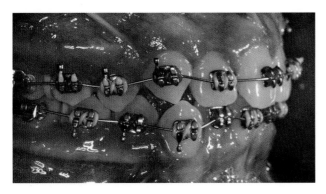

Figure 4.14 Right buccal view of the dentition with the initial insertion of the appliance.

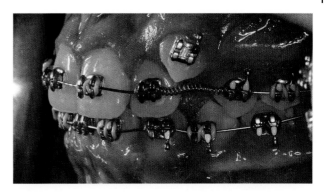

Figure 4.15 Left buccal view of the dentition with initial insertion of the appliance. Note the placement of an open coil spring between the lateral incisor and first premolar to create room for the blocked-out maxillary canine.

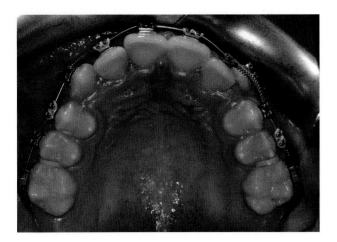

Figure 4.16 Occlusal view of the maxillary arch with appliance insertion. Note the placement of elastic separators between the first molars and second premolars in anticipation of the tubes being debonded by the patient prior to the next visit and the need to position molar bands in their place.

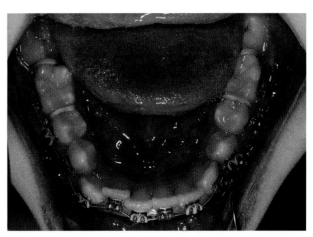

Figure 4.17 Occlusal view of the mandibular arch with appliance insertion. Note the placement of elastic separators between the first and second molars and second premolars in anticipation of the tubes being debonded by the patient prior to the next visit and the need to position molar bands in their place.

Second Active Appointment

Two weeks later the appointment was cancelled. The patient was seen again 8 weeks after the initial appointment and all separators were lost at this time; however, the appliance remained intact. The maxillary arch wire was changed to .016 × .022 nickel-titanium with a .014 nickel-titanium overlay to engage the displaced maxillary left canine. The length of the open coil spring between the maxillary left lateral incisor and first premolar was increased as the initial spring became inactive over the previous 8 weeks. The mandibular arch wire was changed to .018 nickel-titanium. The patient was instructed to wear triangle elastics (3/16", 4.5 oz.) daily from the maxillary right canine to the mandibular right canine and first premolar, and from the maxillary left first premolar to the mandibular left first and second premolars. These elastics would offset the intrusive forces placed on the maxillary left premolar as the displaced canine is brought occlusally into the arch. The use of the triangle elastic on the right side of the arch would maintain symmetric force levels (Figures 4.18–4.22).

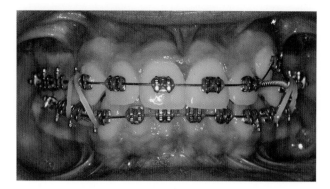

Figure 4.18 Anterior view of the dentition 8 weeks after appliance insertion. The maxillary base arch wire has been changed to .016×.022 nickel-titanium with a .014 nickel-titanium overlay wire to engage the maxillary left canine. The mandibular wire has been changed to .018 nickel-titanium.

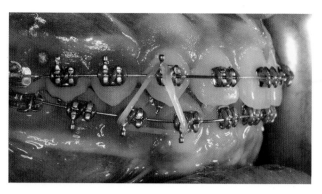

Figure 4.19 Right buccal view of the dentition 8 weeks after appliance insertion with triangle elastics worn by the patient to maintain the occlusal intercuspation and to balance the triangle elastic of the left side of the patient.

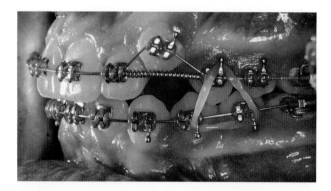

Figure 4.20 Left buccal view of the dentition 8 weeks after appliance insertion. Note the overlay wire to engage the maxillary canine and open coil spring to create space for the placement of the canine into the arch. The triangle elastic was being worn to prevent the premolar occlusion from opening as a side-effect of the canine extrusion.

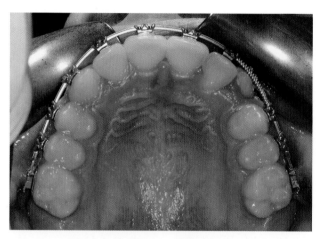

Figure 4.21 Occlusal view of the maxillary arch 8 weeks after appliance insertion. Note the improvement in arch form. The molar tubes remained in place and the elastic separators were lost during this time.

Third to Fifth Active Appointments

Four weeks later, the maxillary arch wires were replaced with a single .018 nickel-titanium wire as the left molar tube had debonded and was rebonded at this visit. The mandibular arch wire was changed to .016×.022 nickel-titanium. Minimal reproximation of the mandibular incisors was performed, followed by fluoride varnish. Triangle elastics were continued as previously instructed (Figures 4.23–4.25).

The patient was not seen for 5 months after the third appointment. At the fourth and fifth appointments, both maxillary and mandibular arch wires were changed to .017×.025 nickel-titanium to perfect the tip and torque of the dentition. The mandibular arch wire had a reverse curve of Spee to aid in bite opening. Triangle elastics were continued as instructed to settle the buccal occlusion.

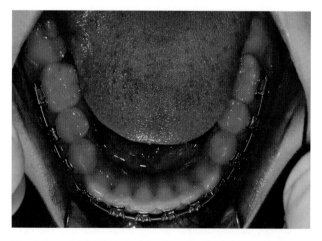

Figure 4.22 Occlusal view of the mandibular arch 8 weeks after appliance insertion. Note the improvement in arch form. The molar tubes remained in place and the elastic separators were lost during this time.

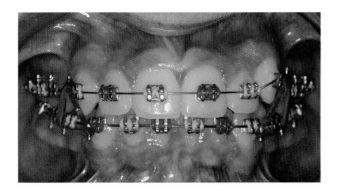

Figure 4.23 Anterior view of the dentition displaying an improved dental midline position. The maxillary arch wire was changed to .018 nickel-titanium and the mandibular arch wire to .016×.022 nickel-titanium.

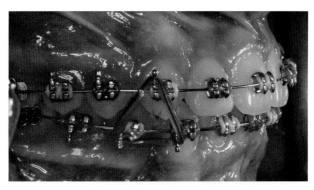

Figure 4.24 Right buccal view of the dentition indicating a well-maintained occlusal relationship and the continued wearing of triangular elastics by the patient.

Sixth Appointment

The patient was debonded and impressions were taken for immediate Essix retainers (DENTSPLY Raintree Essix, Sarasota, FL, USA). The occlusion was corrected to a Class I molar and canine relationship and the midlines were coincident. All root lengths appear normal and no iatrogenic effects were evident. Recommendations for third molar removal will be made an appropriate age. Photographs, an iTero scan (Align Technology, Inc, San Jose, CA, USA), and panoramic and cephalometric films were taken (Figures 4.26–4.35; Table 4.3). The patient was instructed to wear the retainers at night and during sleep. Retainer wear will be monitored periodically for the first year post-treatment. The patient was scheduled for retainer compliance 1 month after the appliances

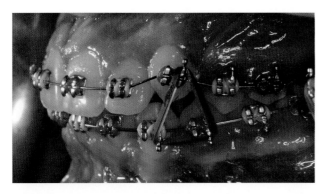

Figure 4.25 Left buccal view of the dentition indicating an improved position of the maxillary left canine as it erupts into the arch.

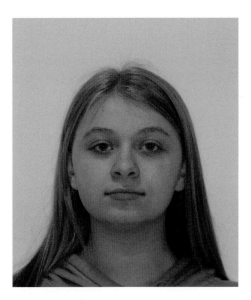

Figure 4.26 Full-face view of the patient at the time of appliance removal.

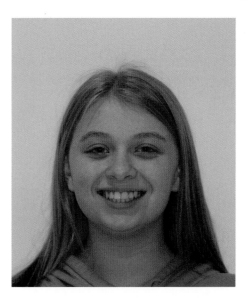

Figure 4.27 Full-face view with smile at the time of appliance removal.

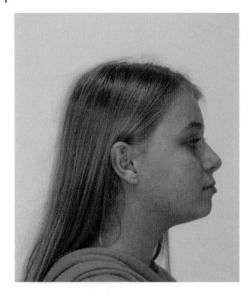

Figure 4.28 Lateral view of the patient at the time of appliance removal.

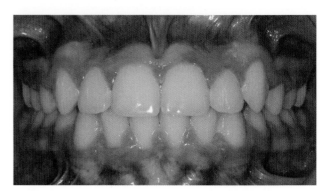

Figure 4.29 Anterior view of the dentition at the time of appliance removal. Note the improvement of the dental midlines.

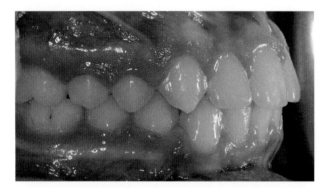

Figure 4.30 Right buccal view of the dentition at the time of appliance removal. Note the Class I molar and canine relationship.

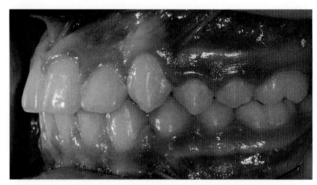

Figure 4.31 Left buccal view of the dentition at the time of appliance removal. Note the Class I molar and canine relationship.

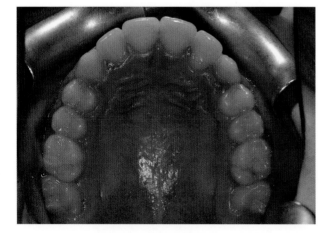

Figure 4.32 Occlusal view of the maxillary arch at the time of appliance removal. Note the symmetry of the arch as compared with pre-treatment.

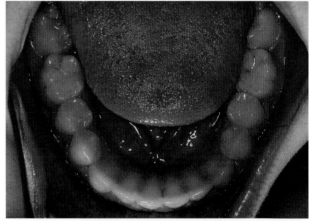

Figure 4.33 Occlusal view of the mandibular arch at the time of appliance removal displaying an aligned dentition.

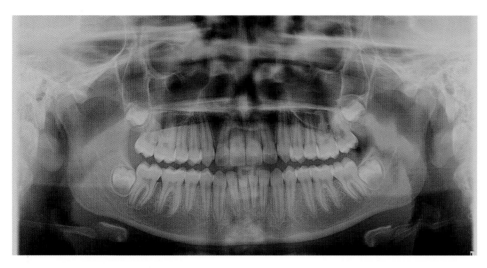

Figure 4.34 Panoramic radiograph at the time of appliance removal with a full adult dentition in place and developing third molars. The periodontium and all root lengths appear normal.

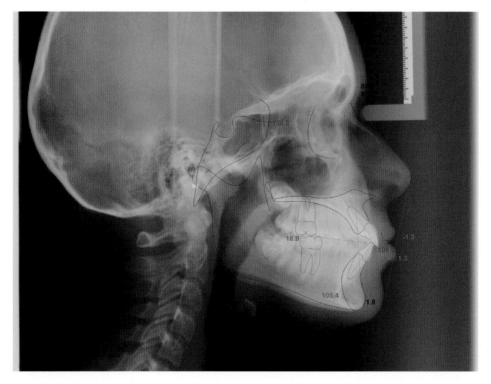

Figure 4.35 Digitized cephalogram at post-treatment indicating a normal skeletal relationship and normal angulations of the incisors.

Table 4.3 Significant pre-treatment and post-treatment cephalometric values

	Norm	Pre-treatment	Post-treatment
SNA	82°	82.7°	85.0°
SNB	80°	79.2°	81.3°
ANB	2°	+3.5°	+3.7°
WITS appraisal	−1 to +1 mm	+1.5 mm	−2.9 mm
FMA	21°	24.7°	21.4°
SN-GoGn	32°	31.7°	30.8°
Maxillary incisor To SN	105°	106.3°	114.8°
Mandibular incisor to GoGn	95°	95.8°	105.4°
Soft tissue			
Lower lip to E-plane	−2.0 mm	+0.0 mm	+1.3 mm
Upper lip to E-plane	−1.6 mm	−2.5 mm	−1.3 mm

SNA, sella-nasion-A point; SNB, sella-nasion-B point; ANB, A point-nasion-B point; WITS appraisal, Witwatersrand appraisal; FMA, Frankfort horizontal-mandibular plane; SN-GoGn, sella nasion-gonion gnathion.

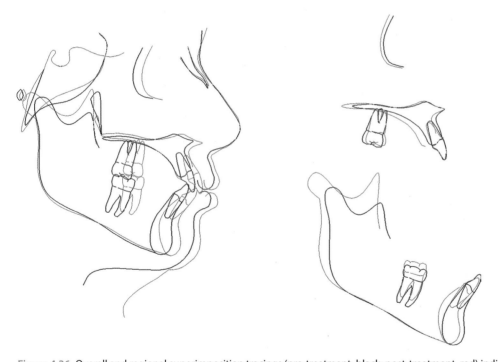

Figure 4.36 Overall and regional superimposition tracings (pre-treatment, black; post-treatment, red) indicating increased horizontal growth of the mandible and slightly flared incisor teeth as compared with the pre-treatment values.

were removed followed by evaluations every 3 months during the first year. The total treatment time was 14 months, which included the 5 months of non-appearance for treatment.

During the course of treatment (14 months), the predominant vector of growth was horizontal, resulting in a slightly more forward chin position which affected the WITS appraisal to a more Class III relationship. Upon regional superimposition, both the maxillary and mandibular incisors assumed a more flared position, while the lower lip became more prominent (Figure 4.36).

Commentary

As a result of the non-extraction mode of therapy, the lower lip appears to be slightly full, but the relaxed face and smile are esthetic. With the mandibular incisor angulated at 105.4° to the mandibular plane, the patient was advised that long-term retention or permanent retention of the treatment result was recommended. After the discussion with the patient and parents regarding the oral hygiene requirements of permanent or fixed retention, the patient and parents opted for removable retainers where oral hygiene would not be a major deterrent to maintenance for a teenage female.

Review Questions

1 What mechanical process allowed for the correction of the maxillary midline and space for the eruption of the maxillary left canine?

2 What was the purpose of triangle elastic placement during the early course of canine eruption with the overlay nickel-titanium wire?

Suggested References

Bishara SE. Impacted maxillary canines. Am J Orthod Dentofac Orthop 101: 159–171, 1992.

Dean, JA, Jones, JE, Vinson LAW. Managing the Developing Dentition. In: McDonald and Avery's Dentistry for the Child and Adolescent, 10th edn. Elsevier, 2016; pp.473–476.

Ericson S, Kurol J. Resorption of incisors after ectopic eruption of maxillary canines: a CT study. Angle Orthod 70: 415–423, 2000.

Ngan P, Alkire RG, Fields HW Jr. Management of space problems in the primary and mixed dentitions. J Am Dent Assoc 130(9): 1330–1339, 1999.

5

Class I Skeletal and Class I Dental with a Deep Bite

Interview Data

The mother's chief complaint was that her daughter's teeth were coming in wrong. She wanted to do something about it.

- Development: pre-pubescent
- Motivation: good
- Medical history: surgical correction for a "lazy" eye at 7 months of age
- Dental history: seen by a local dentist periodically
- Family history: older brother was treated for a malocclusion; twin brother was being treated concurrently and required maxillary first premolar extractions (Chapter 7)
- Habits: chews gum and tops of erasers and pens

- Facial form: symmetric, mesoprosopic, ovoid facial form
- Facial proportions: normal

Clinical Examination

- Incisor-stomion (Figures 5.1 and 5.2):
  - At rest: 5 mm
  - Smiling: 9 mm
- Breathing: nasal
- Lips: 2 mm apart at rest; tense circumoral muscle tone
- Soft tissue profile: straight to slightly concave (Figure 5.3)
- Nasolabial angle: obtuse
- Normal to slightly high, mandibular plane angle; strong chin projection

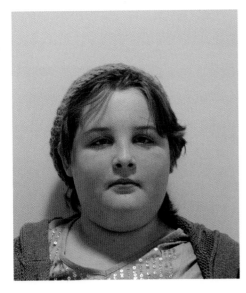

Figure 5.1 Full face at rest displaying a symmetric, ovoid form.

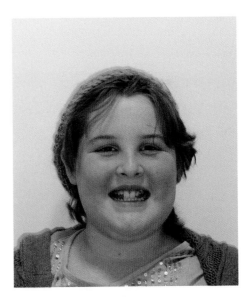

Figure 5.2 Full face with smile displaying 3 mm of gingiva.

Atlas of Orthodontic Case Reviews, First Edition. Marjan Askari and Stanley A. Alexander.
© 2017 John Wiley & Sons, Inc. Published 2017 by John Wiley & Sons, Inc.

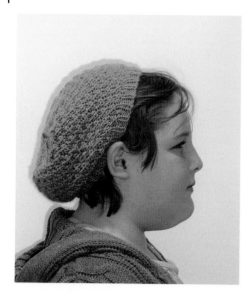

Figure 5.3 Right lateral view of profile displaying a straight to mildly concave form.

Dentition (Figure 5.4)

- Teeth clinically present:

	3
654321	12c456
7654321	124567

- Overjet: 4 mm
- Overbite: 8 mm, deep and impinging on palate
- Midlines: maxillary midline is coincident with the face; mandibular midline is 3 mm to the left of the maxillary midline

Right Buccal View

The right buccal view can be seen in Figure 5.5.

- Molar: weak Class I
- Canine: Class I
- Curve of Spee: deep
- Caries: none

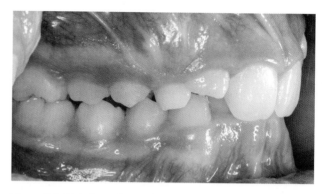

Figure 5.5 Right buccal view of the dentition displaying a weak Class I molar relationship and deep curve of Spee.

Left Buccal View

The left buccal view can be seen in Figure 5.6.

- Molar: Class I
- Canine: undetermined
- Curve of Spee: deep
- Caries none

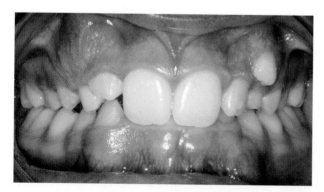

Figure 5.4 Anterior view of the dentition displaying a deep bite and mandibular midline 3 mm to the patient's left of facial midline.

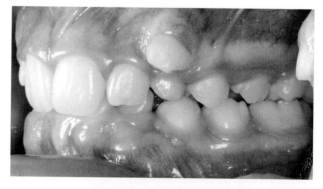

Figure 5.6 Left buccal view of the dentition displaying a Class I molar relationship and deep curve of Spee.

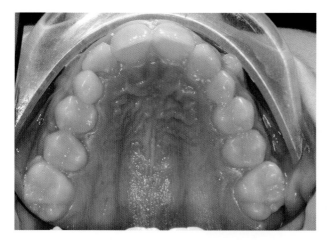

Figure 5.7 Occlusal view of the maxillary arch displaying a tapered, U-shaped arch form and labially placed left canine.

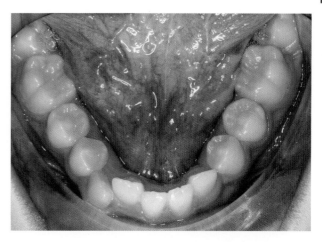

Figure 5.8 Occlusal view of the mandibular arch displaying a tapered, U-shaped arch form and severe crowding.

Maxillary Arch (Figure 5.7)
- Tapered, U-shaped, symmetric arch form with labial erupting left canine
- No caries

Mandibular Arch (Figure 5.8)
- Tapered, U-shaped arch form with severe anterior crowding and blocked-out left canine
- No caries

Function

- Maximum opening: 35 mm
- Centric relation-centric occlusion: coincident
- Maximum excursive movements: right = 8 mm; left = 7 mm; protrusive = 4 mm

- Temporomandibular joint palpation: tenderness noted in joint areas and masseter areas
- Late mixed dentition with blocked-out mandibular left canine and erupting maxillary canines; all third molars are developing
- Root length and periodontium appear normal
- Condyles appear normal (Figure 5.9)

The patient presents with a Class I malocclusion, blocked-out canines and a deep and impinging overbite. The mandibular plane angle is slightly high and the maxillary and mandibular incisors are extremely upright, thus contributing to the deep bite and crowded dentition (Figure 5.10; Tables 5.1 and 5.2). The treatment plan consists of bite opening and aligning of the dentition via non-extraction, while maintaining the facial esthetics.

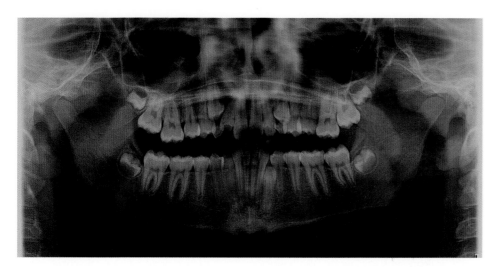

Figure 5.9 Panoramic view indicating a late mixed dentition, blocked-out mandibular left canine, and developing third molars.

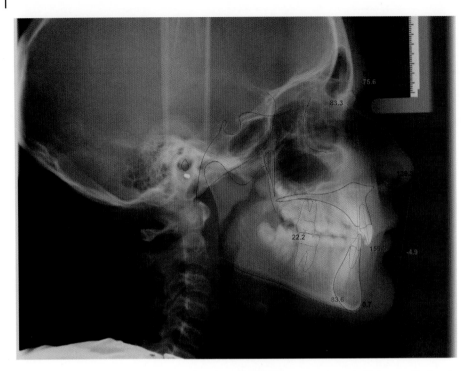

Figure 5.10 Digitized cephalogram indicating a Class I skeleton, moderately high mandibular plane angle, and upright maxillary and mandibular incisors.

Table 5.1 Significant cephalometric values

	Norm	Patient pre-treatment
SNA	80°	80.2°
SNB	78°	75.6°
ANB	2°	+4.6°
WITS appraisal	−1 to +1 mm	−0.1 mm
FMA	21°	24.2°
SN-GoGn	32°	38.1°
Maxillary incisor to SN	105°	83.3°
Mandibular incisor to GoGn	95°	83.6°
Soft tissue		
Lower lip to E-plane	−2 mm	−4.9 mm
Upper lip to E-plane	−1.6 mm	−4.4 mm

SNA, sella-nasion-A point; SNB, sella-nasion-B point; ANB, A point-nasion-B point; WITS appraisal, Witwatersrand appraisal; FMA, Frankfort horizontal-mandibular plane; SN-GoGn, sella nasion-gonion gnathion.

Table 5.2 The patient's problem list in three dimensions

	Transverse	Sagittal	Vertical
Soft tissue	Normal	Straight to slightly concave profile; obtuse nasolabial angle; prominent chin projection	Slightly hyperdivergent, but soft tissues mask the form
Dental	Crowded dentition	Late mixed dentition; Class I molar; labially erupting maxillary canines; blocked-out mandibular left canine	8 mm overbite with palatal impingement
Skeletal	Normal	Class I	Slightly hyperdivergent

Treatment Objectives

As the skeleton and dentition presented a Class I relationship, it was decided to maintain the full dentition as a treatment goal. Bite opening would be accomplished through posterior extrusion, while the deep bite relationship would be improved by flaring the teeth, which would in turn create room for the blocked-out canines. As the soft tissue profile of the patient bordered on concave, facial esthetics would be maintained if non-extraction treatment was successful.

Treatment Options

1) No treatment – this would not be a viable option because of the positioning of the maxillary canines and blocked-out mandibular left canine.

2) Extraction of the four first premolars or second premolars as the patient has a Class I malocclusion – this extraction pattern would create room for the blocked-out canine and labial positioned maxillary canines, but soft tissue esthetics would be compromised due to the concave profile. Bite opening would also become more difficult with an extraction pattern.

3) Non-extraction – this was the treatment of choice that would include dental expansion and interproximal reduction as necessary because it would maintain the facial esthetics, open the bite, and align the dentition. During the first 6 months of treatment, the success of this mode of therapy was to be evaluated (Figures 5.11 and 5.12).

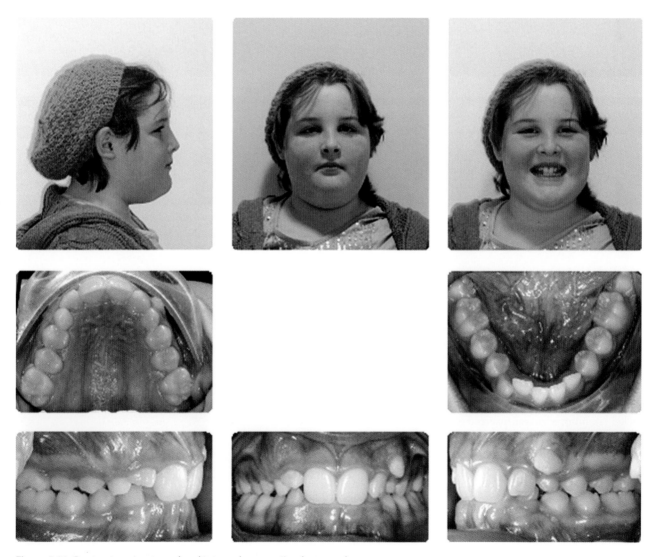

Figure 5.11 Pre-treatment extraoral and intraoral composite photograph.

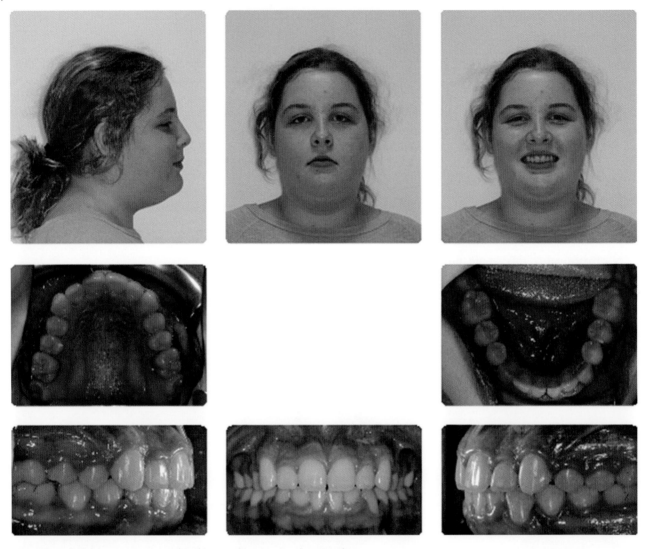

Figure 5.12 Post-treatment extraoral and intraoral composite photograph.

First and Second Active Appointments

One week prior to this appointment, elastic separators were placed. At the appointment, bands were fitted and an impression was taken for a quad-helix appliance. The mandibular bands were cemented with glass ionomer. Two weeks later, the quad-helix was activated and cemented. The maxillary premolars and central incisors were bonded with bi-dimensional brackets and a .016 nickel-titanium wire was inserted with closed coil springs between the first premolars and incisors. The mandibular teeth were bonded with bi-dimensional brackets and a .016 nickel-titanium wire was ligated with a closed coil spring placed between the mandibular left lateral incisor and first premolar (Figures 5.13–5.17).

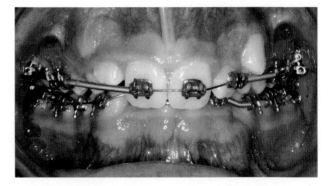

Figure 5.13 Anterior view of the dentition on the day of appliance insertion.

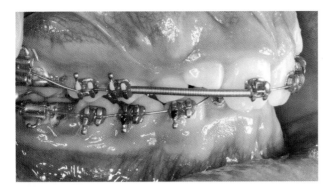

Figure 5.14 Right buccal view of the dentition on the day of appliance insertion. Note the inactive, closed coil spring to maintain space between the central incisor and first premolar.

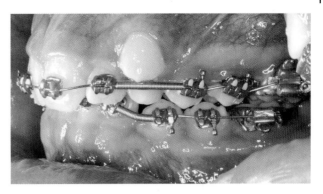

Figure 5.15 Left buccal view of the dentition on the day of appliance insertion. Note the inactive, closed coil spring to hold space between the lateral incisor and the first premolar.

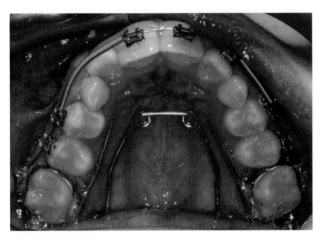

Figure 5.16 Occlusal view of the maxillary arch with the cemented quad-helix appliance.

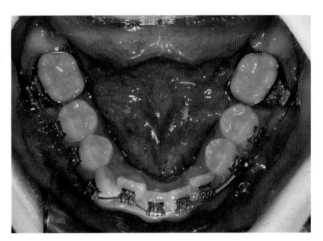

Figure 5.17 Occlusal view of the mandibular arch on the day of appliance insertion. A closed coil spring is in place between the mandibular left lateral incisor and the first premolar.

Third Active Appointment

Four weeks later, both the maxillary and mandibular arch wires were changed to .016 × .022 nickel-titanium. The primary canines were removed. An open coil spring was placed between the mandibular left lateral incisor and the first premolar to create space for the impacted canine. Closed coil springs remained in place on the maxillary arch wire to maintain space (Figures 5.18–5.22).

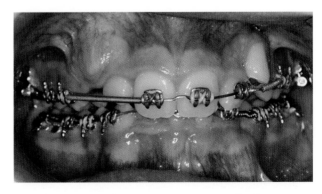

Figure 5.18 Anterior view of the dentition 4 weeks after appliance insertion. Note the activated open coil spring between the mandibular left lateral incisor and the first premolar to create room for the canine and to shift the midline to the right.

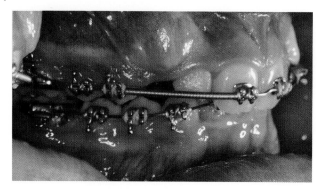

Figure 5.19 Right buccal view of the dentition 4 weeks after the insertion of the appliance.

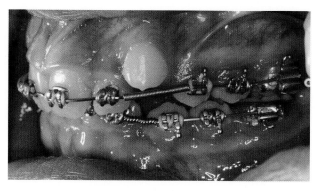

Figure 5.20 Left buccal view of the dentition 4 weeks after the insertion of the appliance. Note the tension of the active open coil spring between the mandibular lateral incisor and the first premolar.

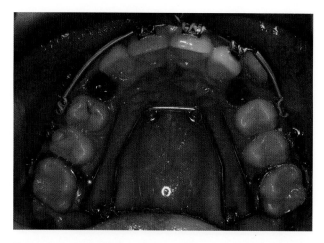

Figure 5.21 Occlusal view of the maxillary arch 4 weeks after the initial insertion. Note the moderate change in arch form as a result of the active quad-helix.

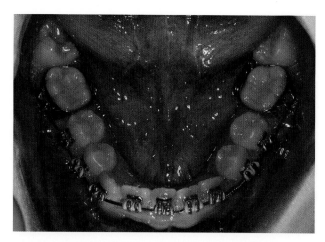

Figure 5.22 Occlusal view of the mandibular arch 4 weeks after appliance insertion. Note the improvement in alignment.

Fourth Active appointment

Five weeks later, the maxillary lateral incisors and left canine were bonded and a .016 nickel-titanium wire was ligated. An open coil spring was placed between the maxillary right lateral incisor and the first premolar to create room for the erupting canine. The mandibular arch was re-ligated. Triangle elastics (3/16"; 4.5 oz.) were placed bilaterally on the maxillary second premolars and the mandibular first molars and second premolars to bring them into occlusion and to prevent intrusive side-effects from the erupting maxillary left canine (Figures 5.23–5.27).

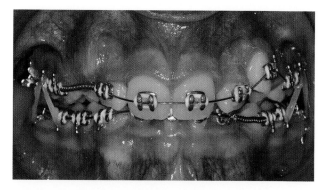

Figure 5.23 Anterior view of the dentition 5 weeks later with the maxillary left canine engaged with the wire.

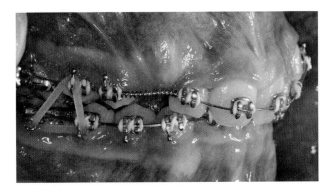

Figure 5.24 Right buccal view of the dentition 5 weeks later with an active, open coil spring to create room for the canine. The triangle elastics are being worn to maintain intercuspation.

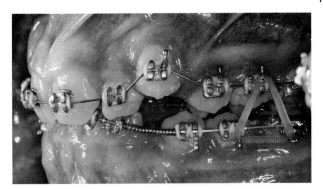

Figure 5.25 Left buccal view of the dentition 5 weeks later with the maxillary canine engaged with the wire and triangular elastics being worn to maintain intercuspation and balance the intrusive side-effects due to the eruption (extrusion) of the maxillary canine.

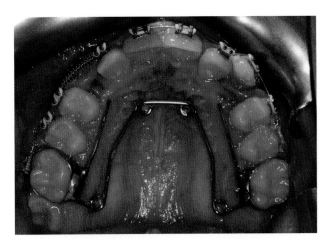

Figure 5.26 Occlusal view of the maxillary arch 5 weeks later showing an improved arch form.

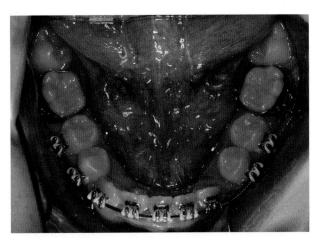

Figure 5.27 Occlusal view of the mandibular arch 5 weeks later displaying improved alignment and space creation for the blocked-out left canine.

Fifth Active Appointment

Eight weeks later both the maxillary and mandibular arch wires were changed to .017 × .025 nickel-titanium. The maxillary open coil spring and the mandibular open coil spring were replaced with closed coil springs to maintain the space. The triangle elastics were discontinued (Figures 5.28–5.32). Note the amount of space created for the eruption of the mandibular left canine over this time period (Figure 5.32).

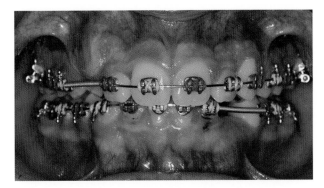

Figure 5.28 Anterior view of the dentition 8 weeks after the previous appointment. Note the improvement in the overbite relationship.

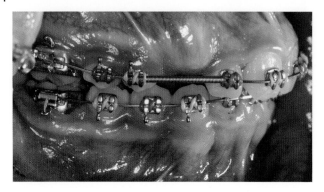

Figure 5.29 Right buccal view of the dentition 8 weeks after the previous appointment.

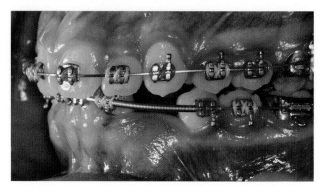

Figure 5.30 Left buccal view of the dentition 8 weeks after the previous appointment. Note the space that was created with the open coil spring for the mandibular left canine.

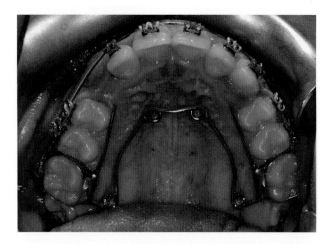

Figure 5.31 Occlusal view of the maxillary arch 8 weeks after the previous appointment. Note the space created for the eruption of the right canine.

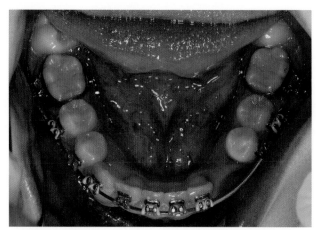

Figure 5.32 Occlusal view of the mandibular arch 8 weeks after the previous appointment. Note the space that was created with the open coil spring for the eruption of the left canine.

Sixth Active Appointment

Four weeks later, the quad-helix was removed, as it placed the maxillary molars and premolars molars into a buccal crossbite. To correct the situation the patient was instructed to wear cross elastics (3/16"; 4.5 oz.) from the buccal of the maxillary molars to the lingual of the mandibular first molars (Figure 5.33). These were to be changed daily. No other changes were implemented (Figures 5.33–5.38).

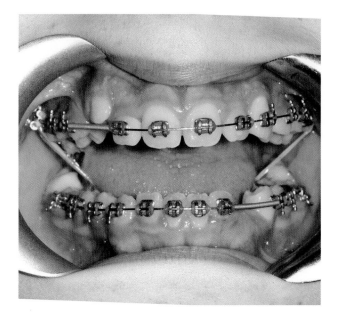

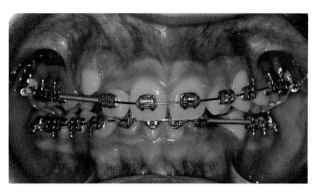

Figure 5.34 Anterior view of the dentition at the sixth appointment displaying the buccal crossbite that was created as a result of over-expansion of the quad-helix.

Figure 5.33 At the sixth active appointment, the buccal crossbite is being corrected with cross elastics attached from the buccal hooks of the maxillary first molars to the lingual buttons of the mandibular first molars.

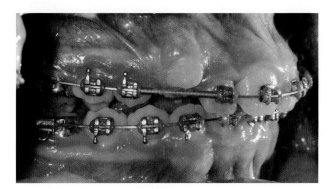

Figure 5.35 Right buccal view of the dentition at the sixth appointment indicating the creation of a buccal crossbite.

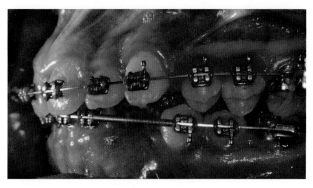

Figure 5.36 Left buccal view of the dentition at the sixth appointment indicating the buccal crossbite.

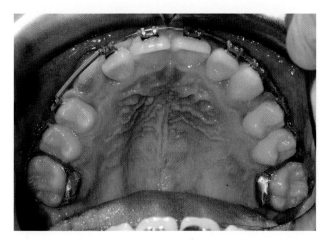

Figure 5.37 Occlusal view of the maxillary arch displaying the over-expansion created by the Quad-Helix which has now been removed.

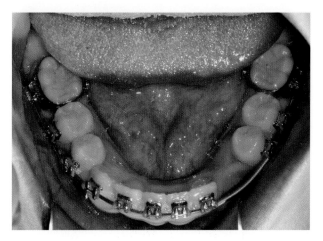

Figure 5.38 Occlusal view of the mandibular arch displaying the space that was created with the open coil spring for the eruption of the left canine.

Seventh Active Appointment

Five weeks later the buccal crossbite was corrected. A bracket was bonded to the maxillary right canine and an overlay wire (.014 nickel-titanium) was ligated with the same base arch wire as in the previous appointment. The closed coil spring remained in the mandibular left canine area. Triangle elastics (3/16″; 4.5 oz.) were placed on the maxillary first premolars and the mandibular first and second premolars to offset the side effects of erupting the maxillary right canine (Figures 5.39–5.43).

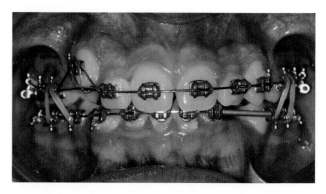

Figure 5.39 Anterior view of the dentition at 5 weeks after the previous appointment, exhibiting the correction of the buccal crossbite as a result of relapse and engagement of the maxillary right canine with an overlay nickel-titanium wire.

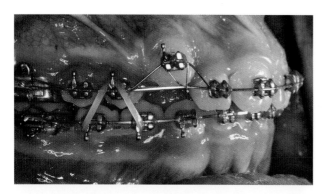

Figure 5.40 Right buccal view of the dentition 5 weeks after the previous appointment, exhibiting the ligation of the canine with an overlay wire. The triangle elastics are being worn to offset the intrusive side-effects of the canine eruption and to maintain the intercuspation.

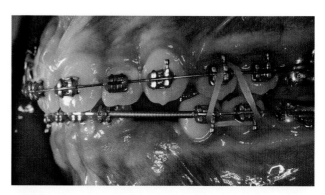

Figure 5.41 Left buccal view of the dentition 5 weeks after the previous appointment with triangle elastics to maintain intercuspation and to balance the elastic force of the right side.

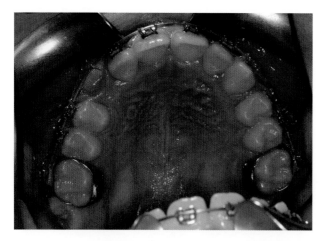

Figure 5.42 Occlusal view of the maxillary arch 5 weeks after the previous appointment, indicating the corrected over-expansion of the arch.

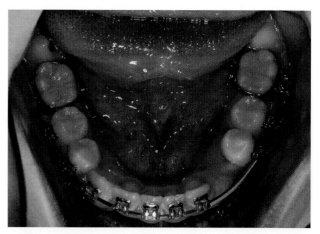

Figure 5.43 Occlusal view of the mandibular arch 5 weeks after the previous appointment, indicating alignment and room for the left canine for eruption.

Eighth and Ninth Active Appointments

Four weeks later, the maxillary arch wire was changed to .018 nickel-titanium to engage the right canine. Triangle elastics (3/16"; 4.5 oz.) were placed on the maxillary canines and the mandibular first and second premolars to settle the occlusion (Figures 5.44–5.48).

Four weeks after the eighth appointment, the maxillary arch wire was changed to .016 × .022 nickel-titanium. The same triangle elastic pattern was used and the patient was told to replace the elastics daily.

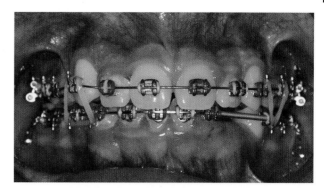

Figure 5.44 Anterior view of the dentition 5 weeks later, displaying an improved overbite relationship. The maxillary arch wire has been changed to .018 nickel-titanium to engage the right maxillary canine.

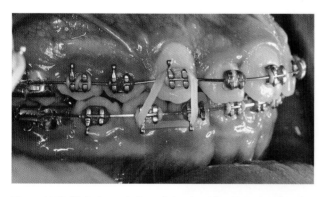

Figure 5.45 Right buccal view of the dentition 5 weeks after the previous appointment with triangle elastics to aid in canine eruption.

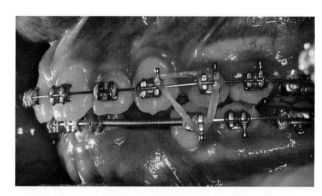

Figure 5.46 Left buccal view of the dentition 5 weeks after the previous appointment. Note that the triangle elastic has been inverted to erupt the first premolar and to gain better intercuspation.

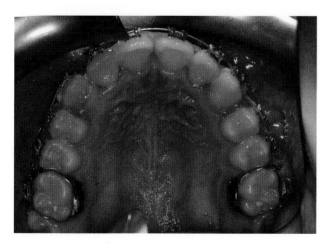

Figure 5.47 Occlusal view of the maxillary arch indicating an improved arch form.

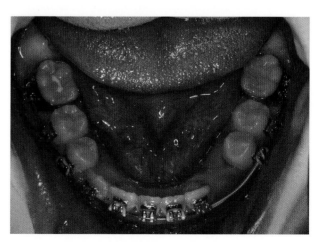

Figure 5.48 Occlusal view of the mandibular arch in alignment and waiting for canine eruption.

Tenth Active Appointment

Six weeks later a progress panoramic radiograph was taken to evaluate root positions and the eruption status of the mandibular left canine (Figure 5.49). The mandibular second molars were bonded with tubes and occlusal build-up of the palatal cusps of the maxillary first molars was performed with glass ionomer. This procedure was performed to allow for clearance of the mandibular tubes. The maxillary arch wire was changed to .017 × .025 nickel-titanium and a .016 nickel-titanium arch wire was ligated to the mandibular teeth. The closed coil spring was replaced to hold space for the erupting left canine (Figures 5.50–5.54).

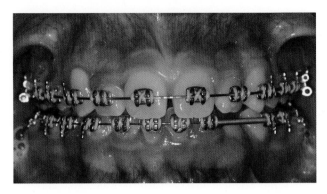

Figure 5.50 Anterior view of the dentition 5 weeks after the previous appointment with a .017 × .025 nickel-titanium wire ligated to the maxillary arch.

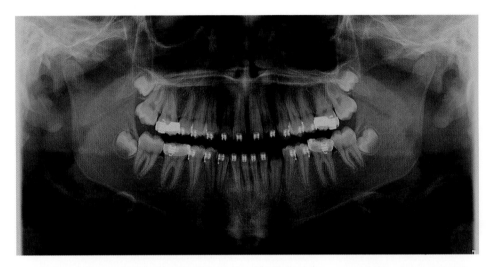

Figure 5.49 A progress panoramic radiograph 5 weeks after the previous appointment to evaluate root positions and eruption status of the mandibular left canine.

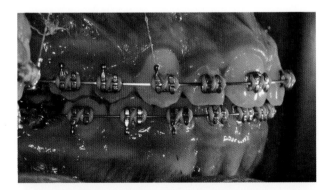

Figure 5.51 Right buccal view 5 weeks after the previous appointment indicating an improved position of the maxillary canine.

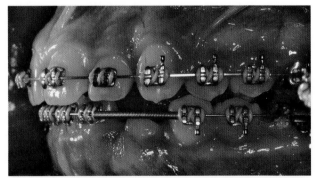

Figure 5.52 Left buccal view of the dentition 5 weeks after the previous appointment indicating the eruption of the mandibular canine.

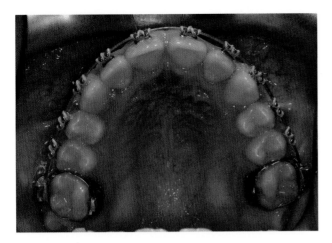

Figure 5.53 Occlusal view of the maxillary arch with glass ionomer bite blocks bonded to the palatal cusps of the first molars. These blocks were placed to allow for the bonding of tubes to the mandibular second molars and to prevent their interference from initial occlusion.

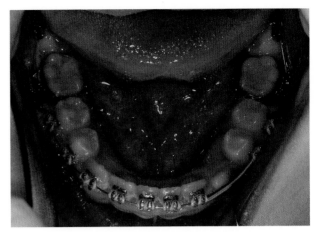

Figure 5.54 Occlusal view of the mandibular arch displaying the bonded tubes to the second molars.

Thirteenth Active Appointment

Five weeks later, the mandibular left lateral incisor bracket was repositioned. The mandibular arch wire was changed to .017 × .025 nickel-titanium. Class II vector triangle elastics (3/16"; 4.5 oz.) were placed on the maxillary canines and the mandibular first molars and second premolars to perfect the overjet and help settle the occlusion (Figures 5.55–5.59).

Eleventh and 12th Active Appointments

Seven weeks later, the mandibular left canine was bonded and the occlusal build-up on the maxillary first molars was removed. An elastomeric chain was placed on the maxillary arch for space consolidation. The mandibular arch wire was changed to .018 nickel-titanium. Triangle elastics (3/16"; 4.5 oz.) were continued bilaterally from the maxillary canines to the mandibular first and second premolars.

Six weeks after the 11th appointment, the mandibular canine brackets were repositioned. The four mandibular incisor brackets were turned upside down to express labial crown torque. Elastomeric chain was ligated to the maxillary arch and triangle elastics were continued as per the previous appointment.

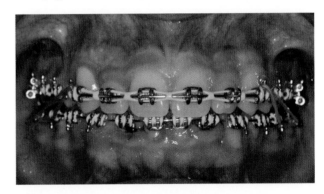

Figure 5.55 Anterior view of the dentition at the 13th appointment. Elastomeric chain has been continued to close anterior spacing.

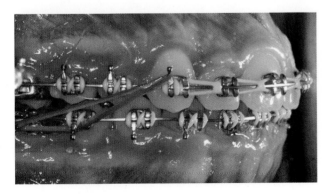

Figure 5.56 Right buccal view of the dentition at the 13th appointment. Class II triangular vector elastics were being used to perfect the intercuspation.

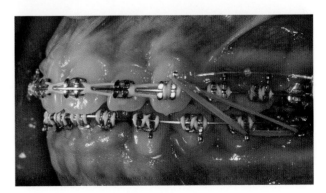

Figure 5.57 Left buccal view of the dentition at the 13th appointment. Class II triangular vector elastics were being used to perfect the intercuspation.

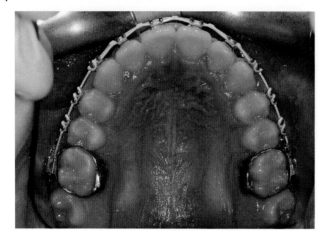

Figure 5.58 Occlusal view of the maxillary arch at the 13th appointment, with elastomeric chain engaged from canine to canine.

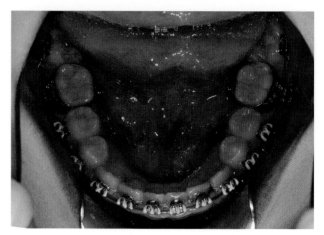

Figure 5.59 Occlusal view of the mandibular arch at the 13th appointment.

Fourteenth Active Appointment

Five weeks later, the maxillary arch wire was sectioned distal to the lateral incisors and an elastomeric chain was placed from lateral incisor to lateral incisor. Settling elastics (3/8"; 4.5 oz.) were to be worn daily (Figures 5.60–5.62).

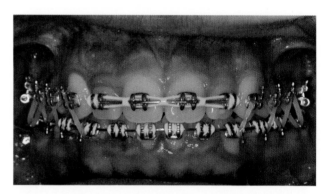

Figure 5.60 Anterior view of the dentition 5 weeks later at the 14th appointment with elastomeric chain engaged from maxillary lateral incisor to lateral incisor. Note the improvement in the overbite relationship and midline positions.

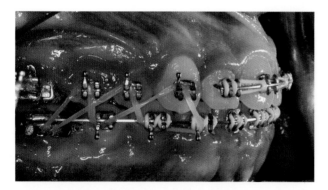

Figure 5.61 Right buccal view of the dentition at the 14th appointment with settling elastics to perfect the intercuspation.

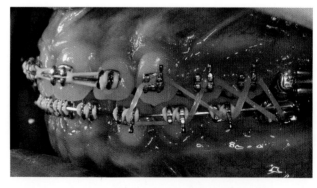

Figure 5.62 Left buccal view of the dentition at the 14th appointment with settling elastics to perfect the occlusion.

Fifteenth Appointment

Eight weeks later, the patient was debonded and impressions were taken for immediate Essix retainers (DENTSPLY Raintree Essix, Sarasota, FL, USA), which are to be worn every evening and during sleep. Final photographs, cephalogram, and panoramic radiographs were taken. An iTero scan (Align Technology, Inc, San Jose, CA, USA) was scheduled for the following retainer appointment. The occlusion would be examined following the first month after debonding and then quarterly for the first year.

The molar and canine occlusion was Class I and the overbite had been improved. The arch forms were symmetric and U-shaped. The soft tissues were balanced and the profile remained slightly concave due to the prominent chin projection. The panoramic radiograph indicated that root morphology remained normal and root parallelism was maintained for stability. The parent was advised of the recommendation that the third molars be removed in future (Figures 5.63–5.71). Treatment time was 19 months.

The overall superimposition indicated that the patient actively grew equally in the vertical and horizontal

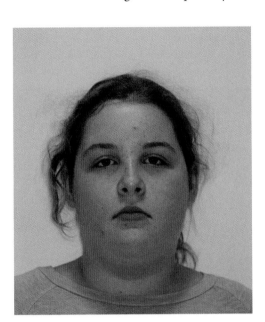

Figure 5.63 Full-face view at the time of debonding and delivery of retainers.

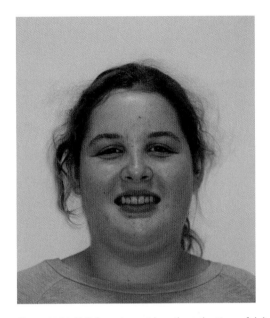

Figure 5.64 Full-face view with smile at the time of debonding and delivery of retainers.

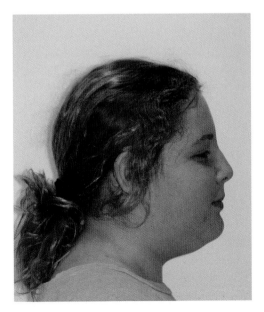

Figure 5.65 Right lateral view of the profile at the time of debonding.

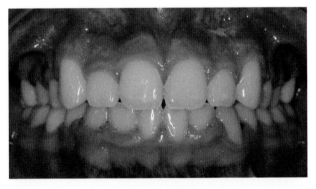

Figure 5.66 Anterior view of the dentition at the time of debonding. Note the improved overbite and midline relationships.

vectors during treatment which augmented bite opening. Regional superimposition indicated that bite opening was achieved through molar extrusion and by flaring of the incisors into a more favorable angular position. Molar anchorage was maintained, except for the extrusive effect of the mechanics (Figures 5.72 and 5.73; Table 5.3).

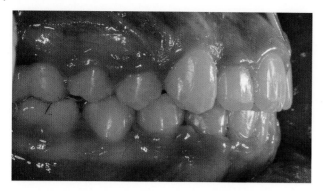

Figure 5.67 Right buccal view of the dentition at the time of debonding. Note the Class I molar and canine relationships.

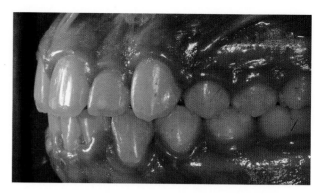

Figure 5.68 Left buccal view of the dentition at the time of debonding. Note the Class I molar and canine relationships.

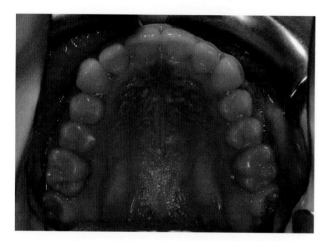

Figure 5.69 Occlusal view of the maxillary arch at the time of debonding.

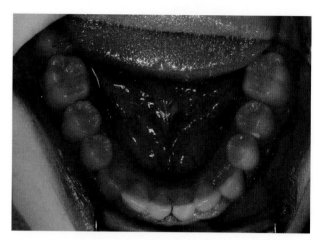

Figure 5.70 Occlusal view of the mandibular arch at the time of debonding.

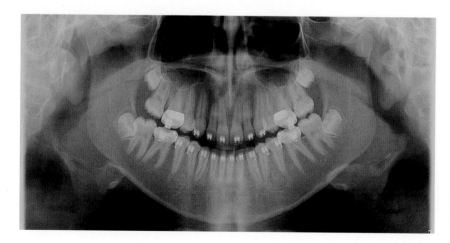

Figure 5.71 Panoramic radiograph at the day of debonding indicating normal root lengths and periodontium. The third molars have been recommended for extraction.

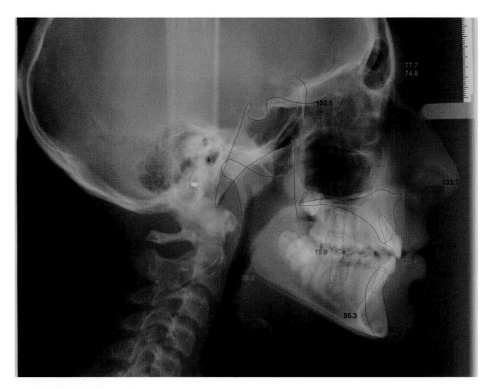

Figure 5.72 Digitized cephalogram at the time of debonding indicating an improved maxillary and mandibular incisor position and balanced soft tissues.

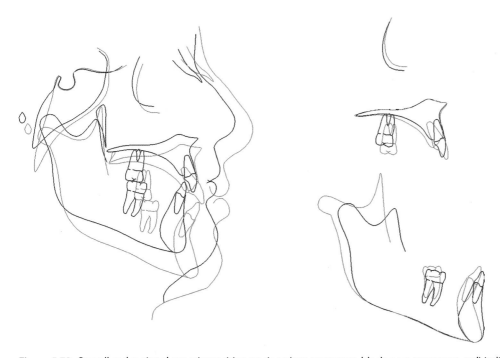

Figure 5.73 Overall and regional superimposition tracings (pre-treatment, black; post-treatment, red) indicating that growth occurred both horizontally and vertically, which aided in the overbite correction, and that increases in the angulations of the incisor teeth contributed to the improved overbite relationship.

Table 5.3 Significant pre-treatment and post-treatment cephalometric values

	Norm	Pre-treatment	Post-treatment
SNA	82°	80.2°	77.7°
SNB	80°	75.6°	74.6°
ANB	2°	+4.6°	+3.1°
WITS Appraisal	−1 to +1 mm	−0.1 mm	+0.9 mm
FMA	21°	24.2°	27.9°
SN-GoGn	32°	38.1°	39.8°
Maxillary incisor To SN	105°	83.3°	102.5°
Mandibular incisor to GoGn	95°	83.6°	95.3°
Soft tissue			
Lower lip to E-plane	−2.0 mm	−4.9 mm	−2.0 mm
Upper lip to E-plane	−1.6 mm	−4.4 mm	−5.4 mm

SNA, sella-nasion-A point; SNB, sella-nasion-B point; ANB, A point-nasion-B point; WITS appraisal, Witwatersrand appraisal; FMA, Frankfort horizontal-mandibular plane; SN-GoGn, sella nasion-gonion gnathion.

Commentary

The extreme upright position of the maxillary and mandibular incisors and the concave profile for the patient at the beginning of treatment heavily influenced the decision for the non-extraction mode of therapy. The profile at the completion of treatment still remained concave due to the strong chin button, and had the decision to extract teeth been implemented the soft tissue result would have been extremely unesthetic.

Review Questions

1   What purpose did the quad-helix have in this case?

2   What methods were used to improve the deep over-bite relationship?

3   Near the end of treatment, what was the purpose of the occlusal build-up of the palatal cusps of the first molars?

4   List the purposes of the triangle elastics used in this case.

Suggested References

Bishara SE. Impacted maxillary canines. Am J Orthod Dentfac Orthop 101: 159–171, 1992.

Upadhyay M, Nanda R. Etiology, diagnosis, and treatment of deep overbite. In: Nanda R, Kapila S, eds. Current Therapy in Orthodontics. St Louis, MO: Mosby Elsevier; pp. 186–198, 2010.

6

Class I Skeletal and Class I Dental with Asymmetry: Non-Extraction

---

LEARNING OBJECTIVES

- Shifting of dental midlines with elastomeric chain and asymmetric elastics
- Partial camouflaging of a skeletal asymmetry with dental midline correction

---

Interview Data

The parent's chief complaint was that her canine sticks out "like a fang" and her teeth tilt.

- Development: pubescent 14-year-old female
- Motivation: good
- Medical history: asthma
- Dental history: routine care by a local dentist
- Family history: the stepsister was treated for a malocclusion
- Habits: chews on blankets
- Facial form: ovoid, mesoprosopic asymmetric face with mandible to the right
- Facial proportions: normal

Clinical Examination

- Incisor-stomion (Figures 6.1 and 6.2):
  - At rest: 3 mm
  - Smiling: 10 mm
- Breathing: nasal
- Lips: together at rest
- Mild to moderate crowding
- Soft tissue profile: mildly convex (Figure 6.3)
- Nasolabial angle: normal
- Normal mandibular plane

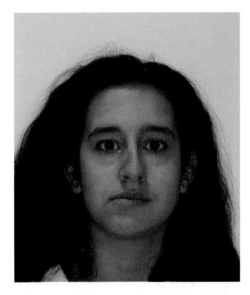

Figure 6.1 Full face at rest showing mandibular asymmetry with the mandible to the right of the patient's midline.

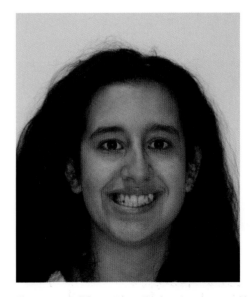

Figure 6.2 Full face with smile showing the mandibular asymmetry with 1 mm of gingival show.

Atlas of Orthodontic Case Reviews, First Edition. Marjan Askari and Stanley A. Alexander.
© 2017 John Wiley & Sons, Inc. Published 2017 by John Wiley & Sons, Inc.

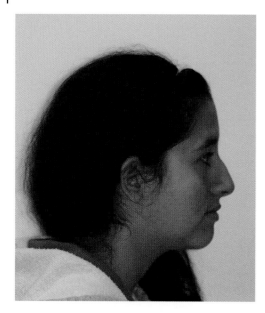

Figure 6.3 Lateral view of right profile exhibiting a slightly convex face with a normal nasolabial angle.

Dentition (Figure 6.4)

- Teeth clinically present:

7654321	1234567
7654321	1234567

- Overjet: 1 mm
- Overbite: 1 mm
- Midlines: the maxillary midline is 2 mm to the left of the facial midline. The mandibular midline is 2 mm to the right of the facial midline

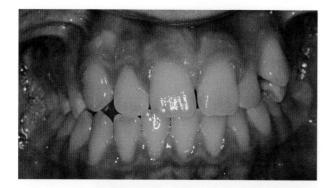

Figure 6.4 Anterior view of the dentition indicating the maxillary midline 2 mm to the left of the facial midline and the mandibular midline 2 mm to the right of the facial midline.

Right Buccal View (Figure 6.5)

- Molar: Class I
- Canine: Class II end-on
- Curve of Spee: moderate
- Caries: none

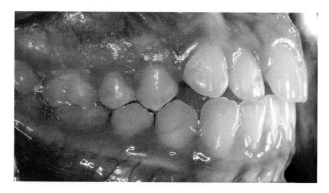

Figure 6.5 Right buccal view of the dentition indicating a Class I molar and a Class II end-on canine relationship.

Left Buccal View (Figure 6.6)

- Molar: Class III (3 mm)
- Canine: Class III
- Curve of Spee: moderate
- Caries: none

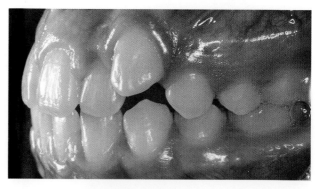

Figure 6.6 Left buccal view of the dentition indicating a Class III molar and a Class III canine relationship.

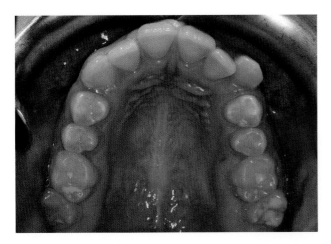

Figure 6.7 Occlusal view of the maxillary arch indicating a U-shaped, asymmetric arch form with labially displaced left canine.

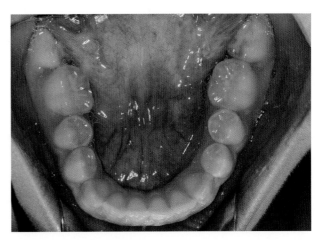

Figure 6.8 Occlusal view of the mandibular arch indicating a U-shaped, symmetric arch form.

Maxillary Arch (Figure 6.7)

- U-shaped asymmetric arch form with buccally displaced left canine
- No caries

Mandibular Arch (Figure 6.8)

- U-shaped, symmetric arch form
- No caries

Function

- Maximum opening = 40 mm
- Centric relation-centric occlusion: coincident
- Maximum excursive movements: right = 5 mm; left = 7 mm; protrusive = 7 mm
- Temporomandibular joint palpation: popping of both joints and occasional pain on the right side; no pain upon palpation
- Adult dentition with third molars developing (Figure 6.9)
- Root length and periodontium appear normal
- Condyles appear asymmetric with the left condyle longer, thereby shifting the lower midline to the right

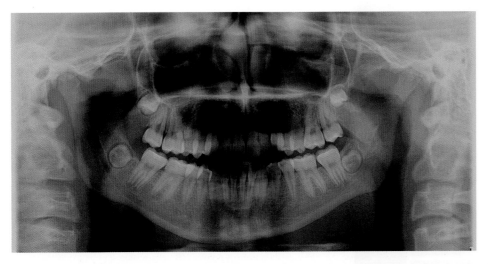

Figure 6.9 Panoramic radiograph indicating a full adult dentition with the development of third molars. The condyles are asymmetric, with the left condyle longer than the right condyle, thereby causing the mandible to shift to the patient's right.

Diagnosis and Treatment Plan

The patient is a 14-year-old female with a Class I skeletal malocclusion and asymmetry of the mandible with minimal dental crowding (Figures 6.9–6.11). The treatment plan was to address the midline discrepancy, the minor crowding, and to camouflage the mandibular asymmetry. The manner of treatment would be non-extraction based upon the facial esthetics, skeletal pattern, and the parent's wishes to avoid any surgical procedures (Tables 6.1 and 6.2).

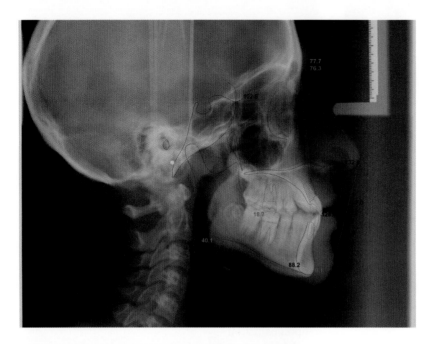

Figure 6.10 Digitized cephalogram indicating a Class I skeletal and dental pattern, high mandibular plane angle, and upright mandibular incisors.

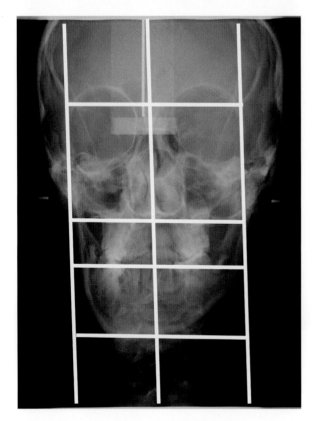

Figure 6.11 Posteroanterior (PA) cephalogram with grid indicating skeletal asymmetry due to the mandible.

Table 6.1 Significant cephalometric values

	Norm	Patient pre-treatment
SNA	80°	77.7°
SNB	78°	76.3°
ANB	2°	+1.4°
WITS appraisal	−1 to +1 mm	−1.1 mm
FMA	21°	22.3°
SN-GoGn	32°	40.1°
Maxillary incisor to SN	105°	102.8°
Mandibular incisor to GoGn	95°	89.2°
Soft tissue		
Lower lip to E-plane	−2 mm	−3.0 mm
Upper lip to E-plane	−1.6 mm	−7.0 mm

SNA, sella-nasion-A point; SNB, sella-nasion-B point; ANB, A point-nasion-B point; WITS appraisal, Witwatersrand appraisal; FMA, Frankfort horizontal-mandibular plane; SN-GoGn, sella nasion-gonion gnathion.

Table 6.2 The patient's problem list in three dimensions

	Transverse	Sagittal	Vertical
Soft tissue	Asymmetric chin to the right	Mildly convex profile; normal nasolabial angle; prominent chin	Hyperdivergent
Dental	Slightly narrow maxillary arch	Adult dentition; Class I molar and canine right and Class III molar and canine left	1 mm overbite
Skeletal	Asymmetric mandible with shift to the right	Class I	Hyperdivergent

Treatment Objectives

The treatment objectives were to create a bilateral Class I occlusion with coincident midlines, alleviate the crowding, and to camouflage the mandibular asymmetry without any surgical intervention.

Treatment Options

1) No treatment – but this was not recommended due to the dental crowding, asymmetric presentation of the maxillary and mandibular midlines, and the skeletal asymmetry.

2) Alignment of the dentition and with the creation of coincident midlines and improvement of the mandibular asymmetry without surgery – this was the parent's treatment of choice, although it was stressed that full correction of the asymmetry would not be possible with this option (Figures 6.12 and 6.13). A request was made for the mother to bring facial photographs in to the office to determine whether the facial asymmetry was always present or whether it was a recent development.

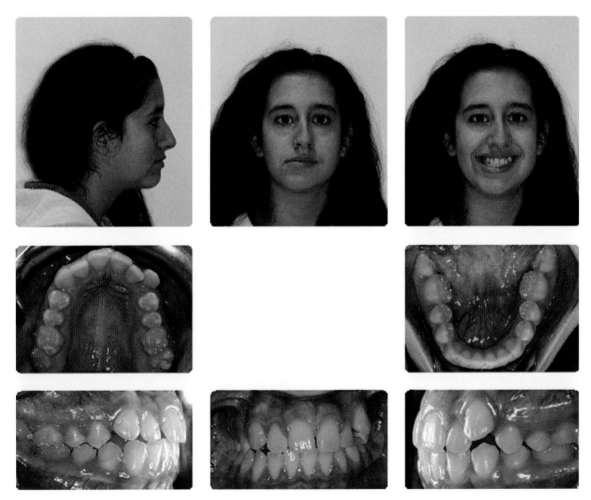

Figure 6.12 Pre-treatment extraoral and intraoral composite photograph.

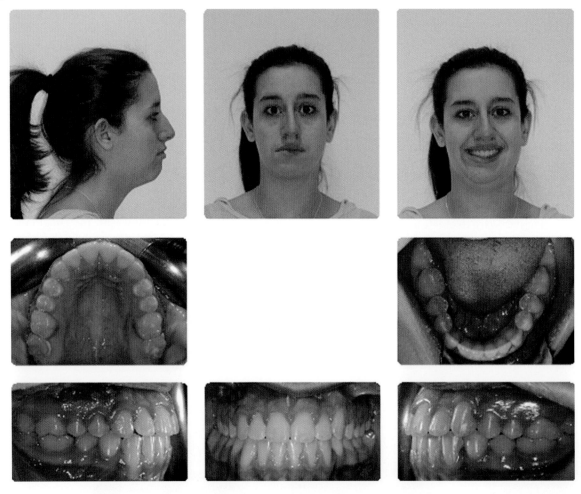

Figure 6.13 Post-treatment extraoral and intraoral composite photograph.

3) Alignment of the dentition followed with orthognathic surgery to correct the mandibular asymmetry and chin deviation – this choice was not acceptable to the parents.
4) Alignment of the dentition followed with a genioplasty to camouflage the skeletal asymmetry – the parents would make this decision after conventional orthodontic treatment was performed.

First Active Appointment

One week prior to the appointment, elastic separators were placed. At the scheduled appointment, all first molars were banded and bi-dimensional brackets were placed from second premolar to second premolar. Nickel-titanium wires (.016) were placed on both arches. The patient was instructed to wear triangle elastics (3/16"; 4.5 oz.) from the maxillary canine to the mandibular first premolar and canine, which were

to be changed daily. Fluoride varnish was applied. Homecare, diet, and adverse outcomes were discussed (Figures 6.14–6.18).

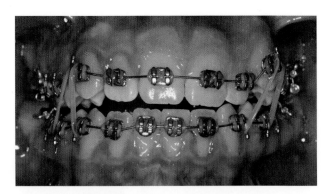

Figure 6.14 Anterior view of the dentition on the day of appliance placement. Maxillary and mandibular .016 nickel-titanium arch wires have been ligated and the triangle elastics are being worn for improvement in the intercuspation.

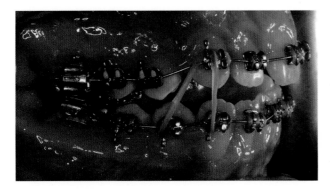

Figure 6.15 Right buccal view of the dentition on the day of appliance placement. The triangle elastic is being worn to gain better intercuspation.

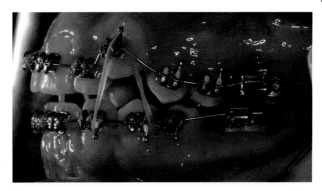

Figure 6.16 Left buccal view of the dentition on the day of appliance placement. The triangle elastic is being worn to gain better intercuspation.

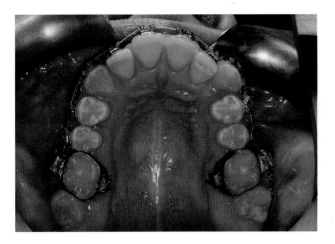

Figure 6.17 Occlusal view of the maxillary arch on the day of appliance placement.

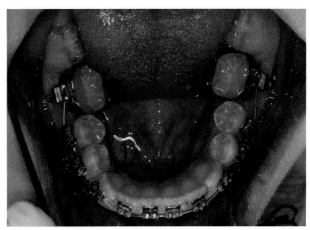

Figure 6.18 Occlusal view of the mandibular arch on the day of appliance placement.

Second Active Appointment

Five weeks later, the mandibular wire was changed to .016 × .022 nickel-titanium and elastomeric chain was continuously ligated from the maxillary right first molar to the maxillary left lateral incisor. Triangle elastics were continued, but changed on the right side in a Class II vector to be attached from the maxillary canine to the mandibular first and second premolars. This change would aid in the correction of the patient's midline discrepancy (Figures 6.19–6.23).

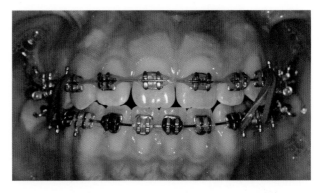

Figure 6.19 Anterior view of the dentition 5 weeks later. The mandibular arch wire was changed to .016 × .022 nickel-titanium and elastomeric chain was ligated to the maxillary arch.

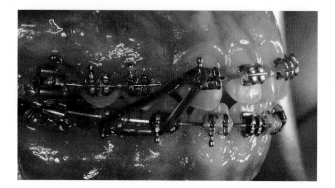

Figure 6.20 Right buccal view of the dentition 5 weeks after the first appointment. The triangle elastic has a Class II vector to aid in shifting the mandibular midline to the patient's left.

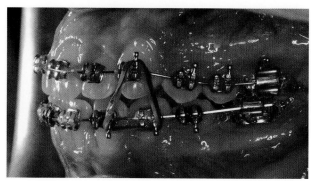

Figure 6.21 Left buccal view of the dentition 5 weeks after the first appointment. The triangle elastic is still being used to settle the occlusion.

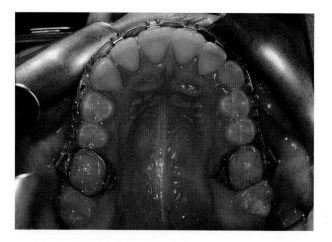

Figure 6.22 Occlusal view of the maxillary arch 5 weeks after the initial placement of the appliance.

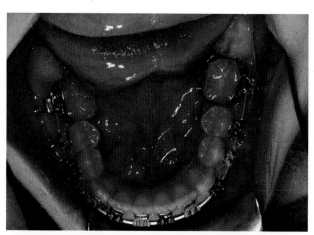

Figure 6.23 Occlusal view of the mandibular arch 5 weeks after the initial placement of the appliance.

Third Active Appointment

Five weeks later, both arch wires were changed to .017 × .025 nickel-titanium. Elastomeric chain was placed from the maxillary right first molar to the maxillary left first molar and from the mandibular left first molar to the mandibular right canine. A triangle elastic was placed from the maxillary right canine to the mandibular right canine and first premolar and a Class III elastic (3/16"; 6 oz.) from the mandibular left canine to the maxillary left first molar for the midline correction (Figures 6.24–6.28).

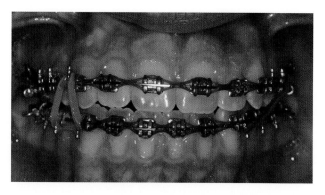

Figure 6.24 Anterior view of the dentition 5 weeks later with .017 × .025 nickel-titanium arch wires placed on the maxillary and mandibular arches. Elastomeric chain is being used to consolidate space.

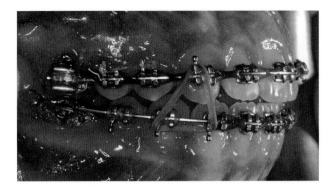

Figure 6.25 Right buccal view of the dentition 5 weeks later. The triangle elastic is being used for intercuspation of the arches.

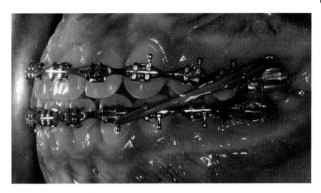

Figure 6.26 Left buccal view of the dentition 5 weeks later. The long Class III elastic is being used to shift the mandibular dentition to the left and the maxillary dentition slightly to the right.

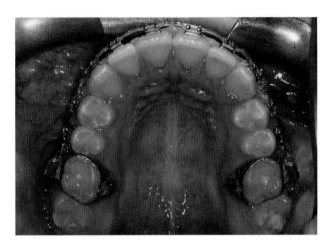

Figure 6.27 Occlusal view of the maxillary arch 5 weeks later. Note the improvement in arch form.

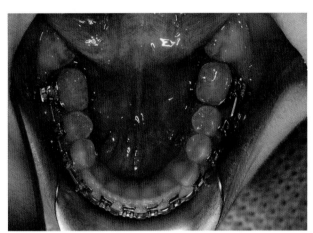

Figure 6.28 Occlusal view of the mandibular arch 5 weeks later. Note the improvement in arch form and further uprighting of the first molars.

Fourth Active Appointment

Four weeks later, elastomeric chain was continued on the maxillary arch and mandibular arches from first molar to first molar. The arch wires and the elastic wear pattern remained the same (Figures 6.29–6.33).

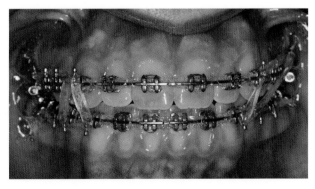

Figure 6.29 Anterior view of the dentition 4 weeks later with an improved overbite and overjet relationship.

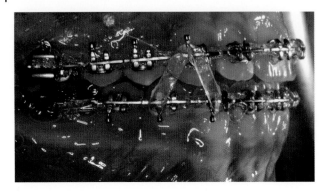

Figure 6.30 Right buccal view of the dentition 4 weeks later. The patient continues the wear of the triangle elastic.

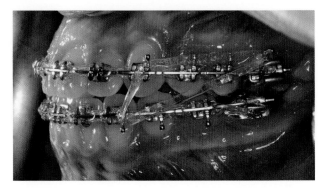

Figure 6.31 Left buccal view of the dentition 4 weeks later. The triangle elastic has a Class III vector to improve the midline and to improve intercuspation.

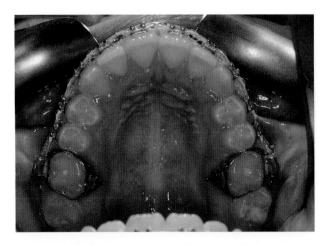

Figure 6.32 Occlusal view of the maxillary arch with elastomeric chain in place for space consolidation.

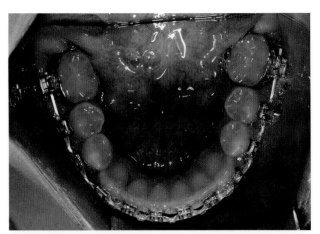

Figure 6.33 Occlusal view of the mandibular arch. Note the improved arch form and elastomeric chain for space consolidation.

Fifth Active Appointment

Five weeks later, elastomeric chain was continued on both arches. A Class II elastic was placed on the maxillary right canine to the mandibular right first molar and a Class III elastic was placed on the mandibular left canine and the maxillary first molar (3/16"; 6 oz.). These elastics were to be changed daily and used to correct the midline discrepancy and to create a bilateral Class I occlusion (Figures 6.34–6.36).

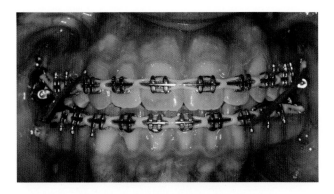

Figure 6.34 Anterior view of the dentition 5 weeks later. Elastomeric chain has been continued with a Class II elastic used on the patient's right and a Class III elastic used on the patient's left for a midline correction and creation of a bilateral Class I occlusion.

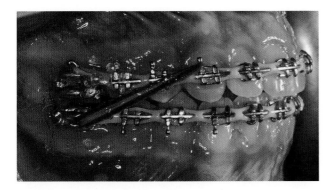

Figure 6.35 Right buccal view of the dentition 5 weeks later with a Class II elastic being worn.

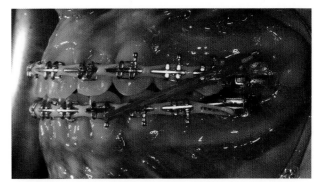

Figure 6.36 Left buccal view of the dentition 5 weeks later with a Class III elastic being worn.

Sixth and Seventh Active Appointments

Seven weeks later, it was determined that both the patient's cooperation with elastic wear and her oral hygiene declined. The importance of compliance and maintenance of good oral hygiene was stressed. Elastomeric chain was replaced and elastic wear was to be continued as per the previous appointment.

Six weeks later at appointment seven, elastic wear and oral hygiene improved. Elasomeric chain was continued on the maxillary arch.

Eighth Active Appointment

Eight weeks later, the same nickel-titanium arch wires were in place and elastomeric chain was continued on the maxillary arch. A trangle elastic (3/16"; 6 oz.) was to be worn from the maxillary left canine to the mandibular left first and second premolars and a Class II elastic from the maxillary right canine to the mandibular right first molar (Figures 6.37–6.41).

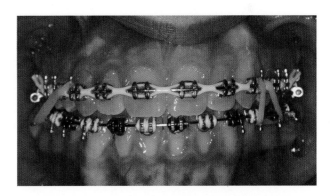

Figure 6.37 Anterior view of the dentition 8 weeks later with an improved midline position of the maxillary and mandibular arches.

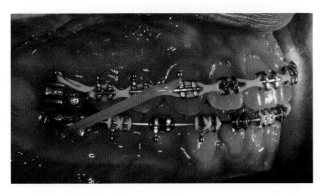

Figure 6.38 Right buccal view of the dentition 8 weeks later with the patient wearing a Class II elastic to perfect the intercuspation.

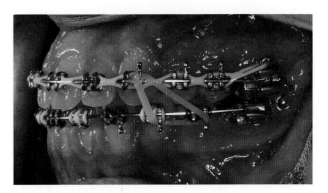

Figure 6.39 Left buccal view of the dentition 8 weeks later with the patient wearing a triangle elastic with a Class II vector to improve intercuspation.

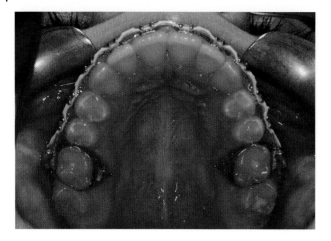

Figure 6.40 Occlusal view of the maxillary arch 8 weeks later.

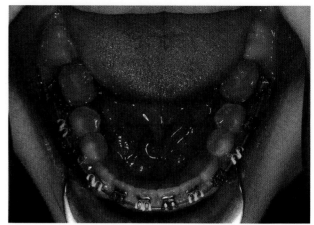

Figure 6.41 Occlusal view of the mandibular arch 8 weeks later.

Ninth Appointment

Six weeks later, the appliances were removed and impressions were taken for Essix retainers (DENTSPLY Raintree Essix, Sarasota, FL, USA). The retainers were to be worn every night and during sleep. The patient would return in 1 month for observation and for quarterly appointments during the first year after completion of treatment. The patient's occlusion was Class I molar and canine with the mandibular midline 1.5 mm to the right due to the skeletal asymmetry. Both arches were broad and U-shaped. The panoramic radiograph indicated that the roots were parallel and no resorption was evident. The condyles displayed the same asymmetric image as in the pre-treatment stage.

The patient was referred for removal of the third molars. The soft tissues were balanced, but the mandibular asymmetry was still apparent though this was acceptable to both the patient and the mother as they understood at the initiation of treatment that a surgical correction would be necessary to alleviate the asymmetry (Figures 6.42–6.51). The overall treatment time was 12 months. The overall superimposition indicated slight horizontal growth with minimal, if any, vertical components. The occlusal plane rotated in a counterclockwise direction which increased the WITS appraisal to a more Class II skeletal relationship. Regional superimposition indicated slight retraction of the incisors due to the elastomeric chain and minimal extrusive effects (Figure 6.52, Table 6.3).

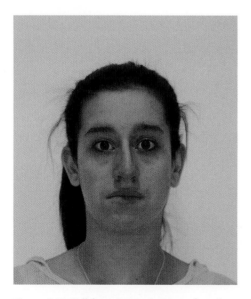

Figure 6.42 Full-face view at the time of appliance removal. The mandiblular position is improved but the chin is asymmetric to the right.

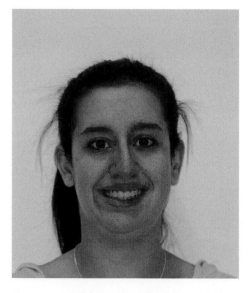

Figure 6.43 Full face with smile at the time of appliance removal.

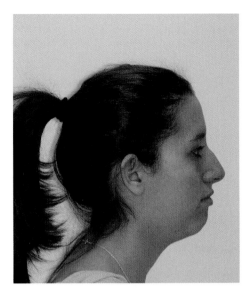

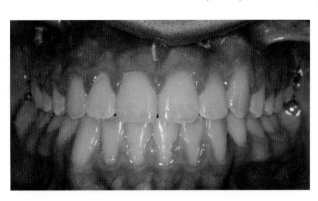

Figure 6.45 Anterior view of the dentition at the time of appliance removal. Note the improved overbite and overjet relationship and midline position.

Figure 6.44 Lateral view of the right profile indicating a convex form.

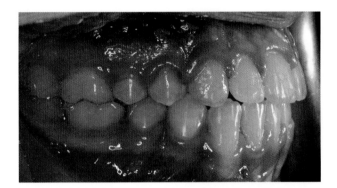

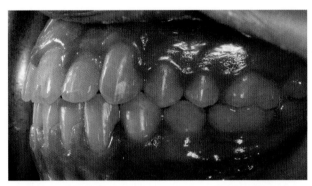

Figure 6.46 Right buccal view of the dentition at the time of appliance removal. Note the Class I molar and canine relationships.

Figure 6.47 Left buccal view of the dentition at the time of appliance removal. Note the Class I molar and canine relationships.

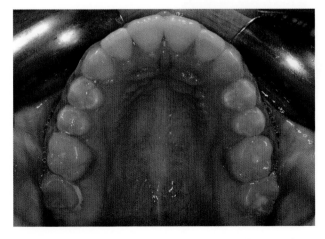

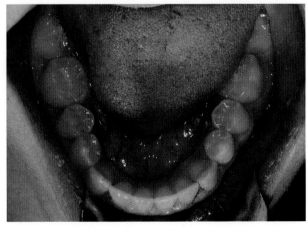

Figure 6.48 Occlusal view of the maxillary arch at the time of appliance removal.

Figure 6.49 Occlusal view of the mandibular arch at the time of appliance removal.

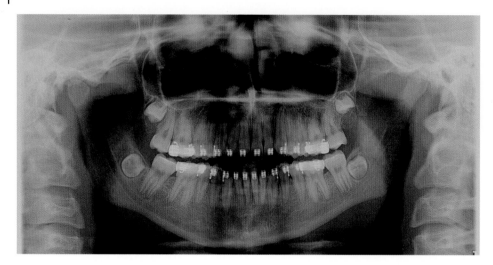

Figure 6.50 Panoramic radiograph prior to the removal of attachments. All root lengths are normal and no iatrogenic side-effects are apparent.

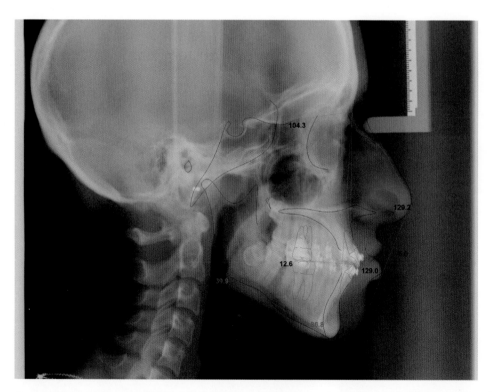

Figure 6.51 Post-treatment digitized cephalogram indicating the maintenance of the skeletal and dental relationships.

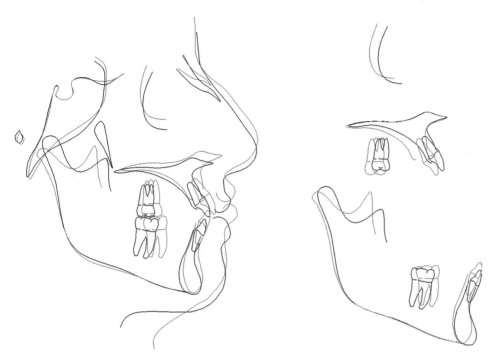

Figure 6.52 Overall and regional superimpositions (pre-treatment, black; post-treatment, red) indicating minimal growth effects and slight retraction of the incisors due to space consolidation with the elastomeric chain.

Table 6.3 Significant pre-treatment and post-treatment cephalometric values

	Norm	Pre-treatment	Post treatment
SNA	82°	77.7°	80.7°
SNB	80°	76.3°	77.6°
ANB	2°	+1.6°	+3.1°
WITS appraisal	−1 to +1 mm	−1.1 mm	+1.8 mm
FMA	21°	22.3°	27.8°
SN-GoGn	32°	40.1°	39.9°
Maxillary incisor to SN	105°	102.8°	104.3°
Mandibular incisor to GoGn	95°	89.6°	86.8°
Soft tissue			
Lower lip to E-plane	−2.0 mm	−3.0 mm	−0.8 mm
Upper lip to E-plane	−1.6 mm	−7.0 mm	−5.0 mm

SNA, sella-nasion-A point; SNB, sella-nasion-B point; ANB, A point-nasion-B point; WITS appraisal, Witwatersrand appraisal; FMA, Frankfort horizontal-mandibular plane; SN-GoGn, sella nasion-gonion gnathion.

Commentary

Although the treatment of this patient concentrated on the dentition, the significant feature of this case was the skeletal asymmetry. The alignment of the arches and the creation of a functional occlusion helped to camouflage a case that may have required extensive surgery as an option in conjunction with conventional orthodontics. The further masking of the asymmetry with a genioplasty once growth is complete may avoid the need for further elaborate surgical procedures in the future.

Review Questions

1 How were the dental midlines improved in this case?

2 How could facial esthetics be improved in this case?

Suggested References

Faustini MM, Hale C, Cisneros GC. Mesh diagram analysis: Developing a norm for African Americans. Angle Orthod 67: 121–128, 1997.

Janakiraman N, Feinberg M, Vishwanath M et al. Integration of 3-dimensional surgical technologies with orthognathic "surgery-first" approach in the management of unilateral condylar hyperplasia. Am J Orthod Dentofac Orthop 148: 1054–1066, 2015.

Severt TR, Proffit WR. The prevalence of facial asymmetry in the dentofacial deformities population at the University of North Carolina. Int J Adult Orthogn Sur 12: 171–176, 1997.

7

Class II Skeletal and Class II Dental: Extraction of Maxillary First Premolars

---

LEARNING OBJECTIVES

- When to extract only two premolars in the maxilla
- Anchorage requirements required for a single arch extraction pattern

---

Interview Data

The parents' and patient's chief concern was the continuation of orthodontic care because the initial orthodontist retired from practice during the early phase of treatment.

- Development: 12-year-old male, pre-pubescent
- Motivation: good
- Medical history: non-contributory
- Dental history: routine dental examinations
- Family history: older twin sister required orthodontic treatment; malocclusion was unspecified
- Habits: none
- Limitations: none
- Facial form: mesoprosopic and ovoid
- Facial proportions: long lower facial height

Clinical Examination

- Incisor-stomion (Figures 7.1 and 7.2):
  - At rest: 5 mm
  - Smiling: 7 mm
- Breathing: nasal
- Lips: together at rest
- Soft tissue profile: straight (Figure 7.3)
- Nasolabial angle: obtuse
- High mandibular plane angle
- Chin projection: retrusive
- Mentalis activity: normal

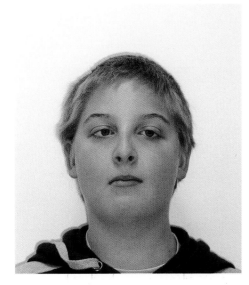

Figure 7.1 Full face at rest displaying an ovoid, symmetric form.

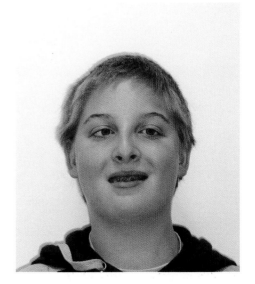

Figure 7.2 Full face with smile displaying minimal gingiva.

Atlas of Orthodontic Case Reviews, First Edition. Marjan Askari and Stanley A. Alexander.
© 2017 John Wiley & Sons, Inc. Published 2017 by John Wiley & Sons, Inc.

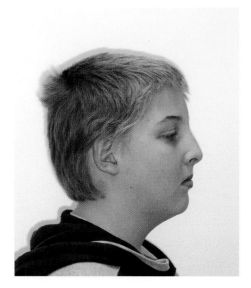

Figure 7.3 Right lateral view of profile patient indicating a straight form and obtuse nasolabial angle.

Dentition (Figure 7.4)

654c21	12456
654321	123456

- Overjet: 2 mm
- Overbite: 2 mm
- Midlines: maxillary midline is 2 mm to right of patient's facial midline; mandibular midline is 2 mm right of patient's facial midline.
- Molar, right: end-on Class II
- Molar, left: full cusp Class II
- Canines: undetermined
- Curve of Spee: moderate

- Crossbite: none
- Caries: none

Right Buccal View (Figure 7.5)

- Molar: end-on
- Canine: undetermined
- Curve of Spee: moderate
- Crossbite: none
- Caries: none, but gross plaque deposits

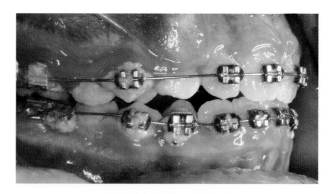

Figure 7.5 Right buccal view of appliances in place from previous orthodontist with the presence of gross plaque around the appliance.

Left Buccal View (Figure 7.6)

- Molar: Class II
- Canine: undetermined
- Curve of Spee: moderate
- Crossbite: none
- Caries: none

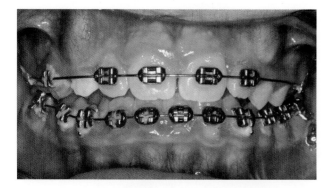

Figure 7.4 Anterior view of the dentition with appliances in place from previous orthodontist.

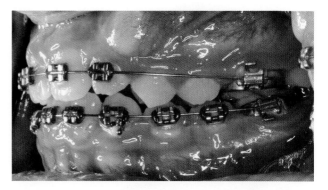

Figure 7.6 Left buccal view of appliances in place from previous orthodontist.

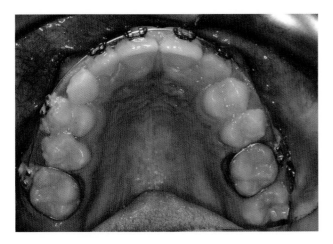

Figure 7.7 Occlusal view of the maxillary arch with appliances in place and blocked-out left canine.

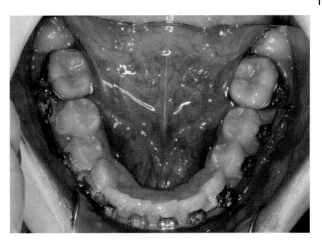

Figure 7.8 Occlusal view of the mandibular arch with appliances in place from previous orthodontist.

Maxillary Arch (Figure 7.7)

- U-shaped, asymmetric arch with blocked-out left canine
- No caries

Mandibular Arch (Figure 7.8)

- Tapered, U-shaped arch form
- Slight crowding

Function

- Maximum opening: 35 mm
- Centric relation-centric occlusion: coincident
- Maximum excursive movements: right = 10 mm; left = 11 mm; protrusive = 5 mm
- Temporomandibular joint palpation: no tenderness or pain
- Right and left masseter: within normal limits
- Habits: none
- Speech: normal
- Late mixed dentition with blocked-out maxillary left canine with all 32 teeth present or developing (Figure 7.9)
- Root length and periodontium appear normal
- Condyles appear normal

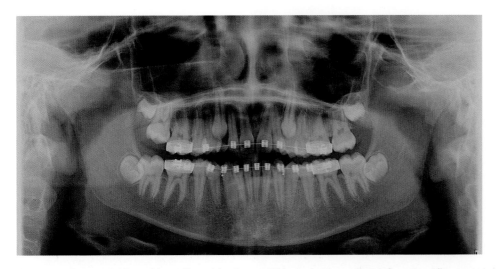

Figure 7.9 Panoramic view with appliances in place and blocked-out maxillary left canine. All permanent teeth are present with developing third molars. Root lengths and periodontium are normal.

Diagnosis and Treatment Plan

The patient presents with a Class II dental and skeletal pattern, a completely blocked-out maxillary left canine, and a retrusive mandible and is hyperdivergent. The mandible, however, displays a non-crowded dentition (Tables 7.1 and 7.2; Figures 7.9 and 7.10).

Maxilla and mandible – due to the Class II dental and skeletal problems and the blocked-out canine, it was recommended that the maxillary first premolars be extracted and the mandible treated on a non-extraction basis.

Table 7.1 Significant cephalometric values

	Norm	Patient pre-treatment
SNA	80°	79.7°
SNB	78°	74.4°
ANB	2°	+5.3°
WITS appraisal	−1 to +1 mm	+3.9 mm
FMA	21°	28°
SN-GoGn	32°	40.3°
Maxillary incisor to SN	105°	103.6°
Mandibular incisor to GoGn	95°	89.3°
Soft tissue		
Lower lip to E-plane	−2 mm	−2.2 mm
Upper lip to E-plane	−1.6 mm	−5.3 mm

SNA, sella-nasion-A point; SNB, sella-nasion-B point; ANB, A point-nasion-B point; WITS appraisal, Witwatersrand appraisal; FMA, Frankfort horizontal-mandibular plane; SN-GoGn, sella nasion-gonion gnathion.

Table 7.2 The patient's problem list in three dimensions

	Transverse	Sagittal	Vertical
Soft tissue	Normal	Straight profile; obtuse nasolabial angle	Hyperdivergent
Dental	Space deficiency	Late mixed dentition; Class II molar relationship with blocked-out canine	2 mm overbite
Skeletal	Normal	Class II	Hyperdivergent

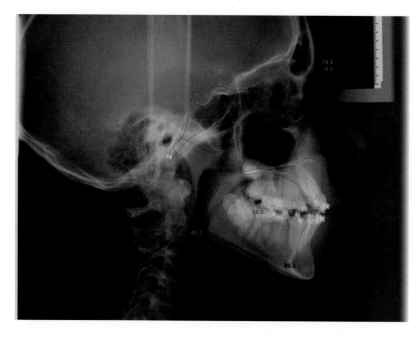

Figure 7.10 Digitized cephalogram exhibiting a Class II skeletal relationship and high mandibular plane angle.

Treatment Objectives

With a single arch extraction of maxillary first premolars to relieve the crowding, the final result would create a Class II molar and Class I canine relationship that was both functional and esthetic. Non-extraction treatment of the lower arch, which was both non-crowded and retrusive, is also preferable for esthetic reasons (Figures 7.11 and 7.12).

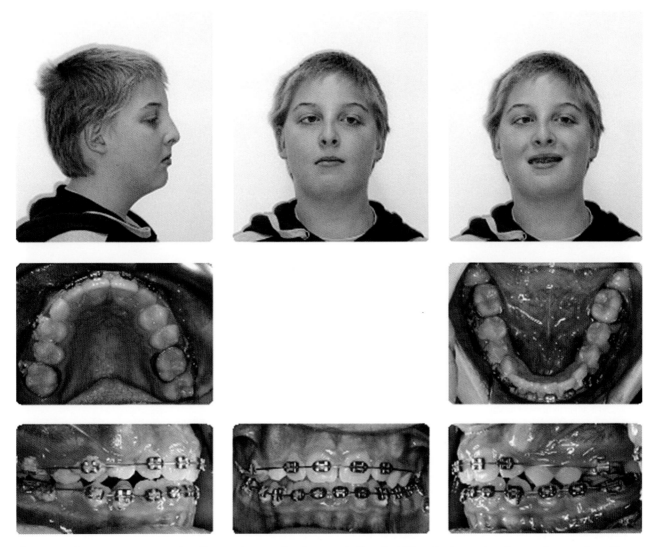

Figure 7.11 Pre-treatment extraoral and intraoral composite photograph. Note that this patient was a transfer case from another office and was therefore wearing appliances. These appliances would be removed and new appliances placed once the treatment plan was accepted.

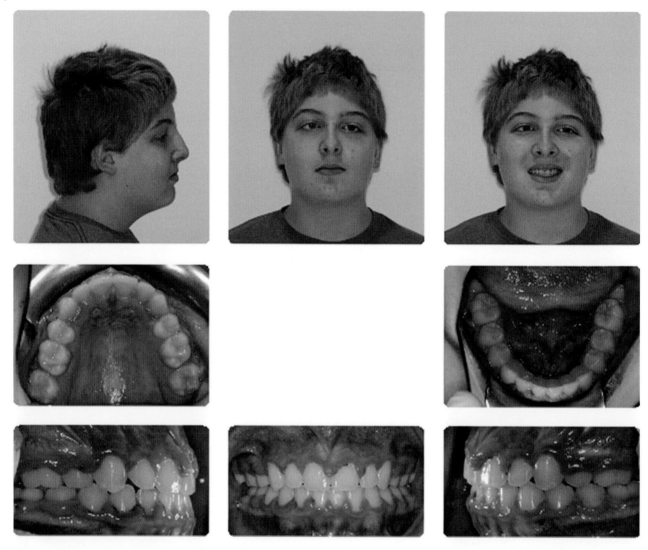

Figure 7.12 Post-treatment extraoral and intraoral composite photograph.

Treatment Options

1) No treatment.
2) Extraction of maxillary first premolars.
3) Extraction of maxillary first premolars and mandibular second premolars
4) Non-extraction – expansion of the maxilla in an attempt to make room for the blocked-out canine. This choice was presented, but was given a poor prognosis due to the level of crowding and the vertical growth pattern of the patient that would add to its lack of stability.

The parents chose option 2 as each treatment option was given its respective positive and negative features.

First Active Appointment

Prior to the placement of new appliances, the previous appliances were removed and separators were placed for banding the following week. Bands were fitted and an iTero scan (Align Technology, Inc, San Jose, CA, USA) was taken for fabrication of a Nance appliance for maxillary anchorage. The mandibular bands were cemented with glass ionomer. On the following visit, the Nance appliance was cemented. The maxillary second premolars and incisors were bonded with bi-dimensional brackets. The maxillary first premolars and right primary canine were extracted. The mandibular incisors, left canine and right and left first premolars were bonded with bi-dimensional brackets. Nickel-titanium wires (.016) were placed in both arches and cinched. An open coil spring was placed between the mandibular right lateral incisor and first premolar to open space for the right canine and to shift the mandibular midline to the left (Figures 7.13–7.17).

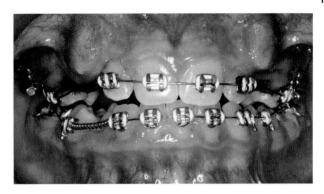

Figure 7.13 Anterior view of the dentition with new appliances in place and .016 nickel-titanium wires ligated to the brackets.

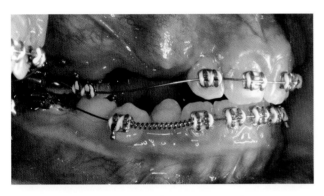

Figure 7.14 Right buccal view of the dentition with new appliances in place. An open coil spring was placed on the mandibular arch to shift the midline to the patient's left and to open space for the malaligned right canine.

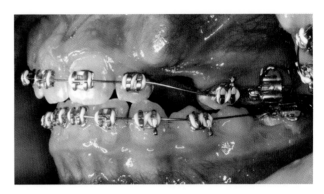

Figure 7.15 Left buccal view of the dentition with new appliances in place.

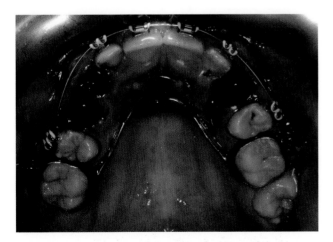

Figure 7.16 Occlusal view of the maxillary arch exhibiting a Nance appliance for anchorage enhancement. Note the current extraction sites on the day of appliance placement.

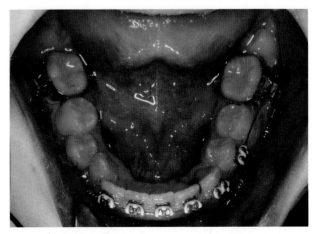

Figure 7.17 Occlusal view of the mandibular arch with the new appliance in place.

Second Active Appointment

Four weeks later, the maxillary arch wire was changed to .017 × .025 nickel-titanium. The mandibular arch wire remained the same and was re-ligated. The maxillary canines began eruption into the arch (Figures 7.18–7.22). Oral hygiene was in need of improvement and was re-enforced.

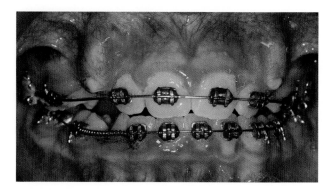

Figure 7.18 Anterior view of the dentition 4 weeks later. The maxillary arch wire was changed to .017 × .025 nickel-titanium.

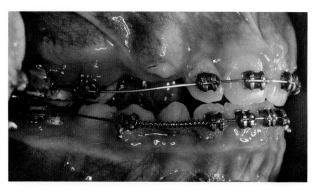

Figure 7.19 Right buccal view of the dentition after 4 weeks. Note the beginning of eruption of the maxillary canine and the space created on the mandibular arch for the canine.

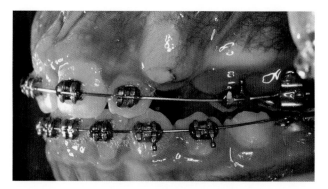

Figure 7.20 Left buccal view of the dentition after 4 weeks. Note the beginning of the eruption of the maxillary canine.

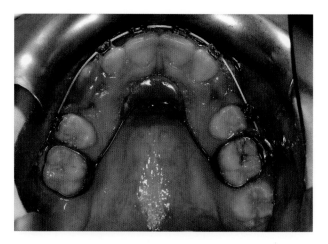

Figure 7.21 Occlusal view of the maxillary arch 4 weeks later.

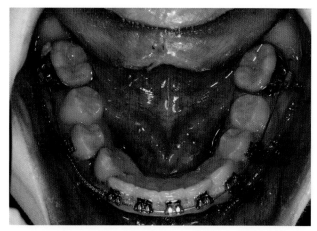

Figure 7.22 Occlusal view of the mandibular arch 4 weeks later.

Third Active Appointment

At 5 weeks, the mandibular right canine was bonded and ligated into the arch with the .016 nickel-titanium arch wire. The maxillary canines had erupted further (Figures 7.23–7.27). Oral hygiene was poor and again re-enforced.

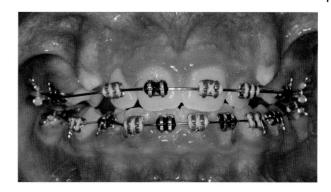

Figure 7.23 Anterior view of the dentition 5 weeks later. Note the improvement of the mandibular midline.

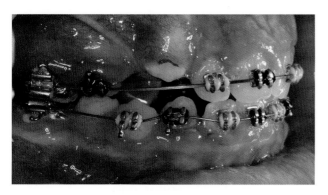

Figure 7.24 Right buccal view of the dentition 5 weeks later.

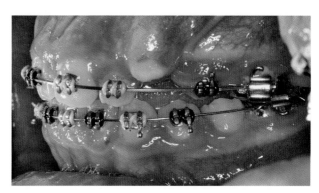

Figure 7.25 Left buccal view of the dentition 5 weeks later.

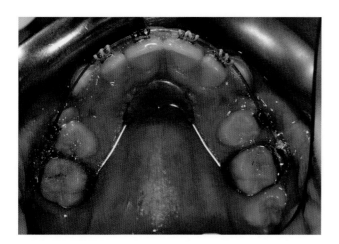

Figure 7.26 Occlusal view of the maxillary arch 5 weeks later.

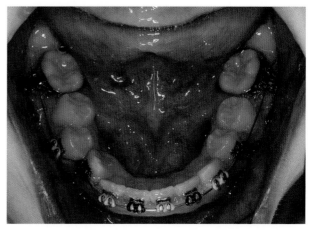

Figure 7.27 Occlusal view of the mandibular arch 5 weeks later.

Fourth Active Appointment

Thirteen weeks later the remaining premolars and canines were bonded. The maxillary rectangular nickel-titanium wire was replaced with a .016 nickel-titanium wire for flexibility to engage the maxillary canines. Triangle elastics (3/16″, 4.5 oz.) were to be worn from the maxillary canines to the mandibular canines and first premolars to further erupt the canines and to offset any intrusive side-effects on the maxillary lateral incisors and second premolars as a result of forced canine eruption through extrusive mechanics (Figures 7.28–7.32).

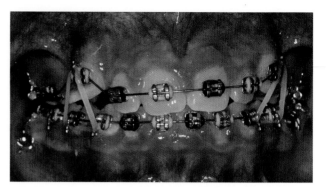

Figure 7.28 Anterior view of the dentition 13 weeks later. The remaining teeth have been bonded with brackets.

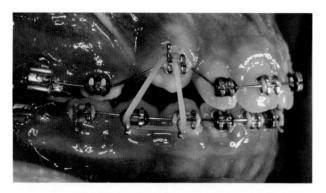

Figure 7.29 Right buccal view of the dentition 13 weeks later. A triangle elastic was used to augment the extrusive force on the canine.

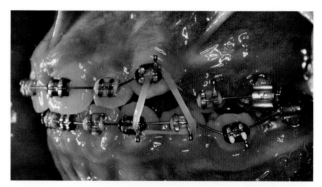

Figure 7.30 Left buccal view of the dentition 13 weeks later. A triangle elastic was used to augment the extrusive force on the canine.

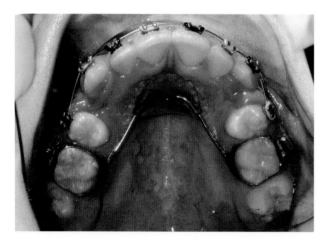

Figure 7.31 Occlusal view of the maxillary arch 13 weeks later.

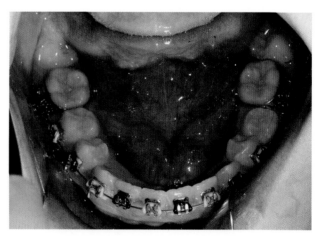

Figure 7.32 Occlusal view of the mandibular arch 13 weeks later.

Fifth Active Appointment

Five weeks later, both maxillary and mandibular wires were replaced with .016 × .022 rectangular nickel-titanium arch wires (Figure 7.33). The maxillary arch wire was placed gingival for both the second premolar brackets to aid in eruption (Figures 7.34 and 7.35). An elastomeric chain was placed in the maxilla from first molar to first molar to aid in space consolidation. Both the maxillary and mandibular arch forms begin coordination taking on a U-shaped appearance (Figures 7.36 and 7.37). Triangle elastics (3/16", 4.5 oz.) were continued on a daily basis extending from the maxillary right canine to the mandibular first and second premolars to perfect a Class I canine position and from the maxillary second premolars to the mandibular first and second premolars to augment the extrusion of the maxillary left second premolar. Oral hygiene continued to be a problem and this was again re-emphasized.

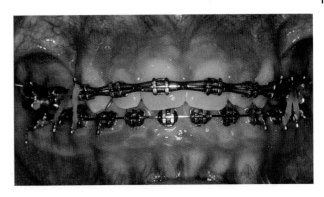

Figure 7.33 Anterior view of the dentition 5 weeks later; the maxillary and mandibular arch wires were replaced with .016 × .022 nickel-titanium. Elastomeric chain was placed on the maxillary arch for space consolidation.

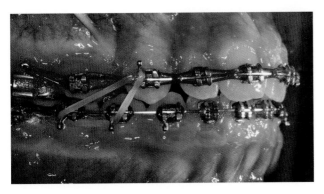

Figure 7.34 Right buccal view of the dentition 5 weeks later. The triangle elastic had a Class II vector to improve the intercuspation. Note the placement of the maxillary arch wire gingival to the second premolar bracket for extrusive effects.

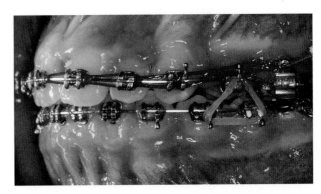

Figure 7.35 Left buccal view of the dentition 5 weeks later. The triangle elastic was worn to improve intercuspation of the left segment. Note the placement of the maxillary arch wire gingival to the second premolar bracket for extrusive effects.

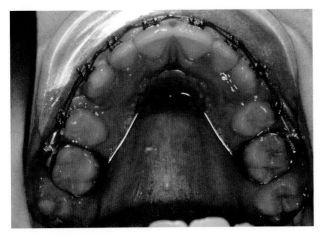

Figure 7.36 Occlusal view of the maxillary arch 5 weeks later. Note the improvement in arch form.

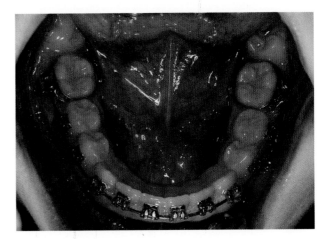

Figure 7.37 Occlusal view of the mandibular arch 5 weeks later. Note the improvement in arch form.

Sixth and Seventh Active Appointments

At the sixth appointment 5 weeks later, the Nance appliance was removed. Maxillary and mandibular .017 × .025 nickel-titanium arch wires were placed.

Elastic wear was discontinued. At the seventh appointment 6 weeks later, a progress panoramic radiograph was taken to examine the angulation of the dentition and to monitor for root resorption (Figure 7.38). It was noted that a buccal crossbite of the right second molars had developed during eruption. The maxillary first

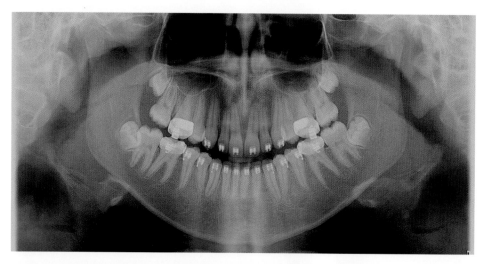

Figure 7.38 Progress panoramic radiograph exhibiting normal root morphology.

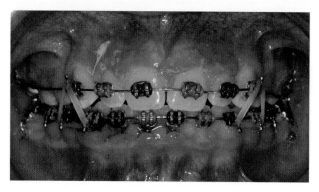

Figure 7.39 Anterior view of the dentition 5 weeks later. The mandibular brackets were removed and replaced upside down to reverse the torque expression and improve the overjet.

molar bands and second premolar brackets were removed due to gingival inflammation as a result of poor oral hygiene. This procedure also aided in the mechanics for the correction of the right second molars, which were banded, cemented with glass ionomer, and ligated to a .016 × .022 nickel-titanium arch wire. The mandibular incisor brackets were re-bonded and inverted to produce labial crown torque to perfect the overjet relationship. Triangle elastics (3/16", 4.5 oz.) were placed on the maxillary canines and the mandibular canines and second premolars and changed daily (Figures 7.39–7.43).

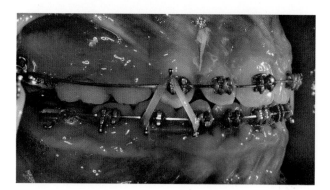

Figure 7.40 Right buccal view of the dentition 5 weeks later. The maxillary molar band and second premolar bracket were removed due to hygiene problems.

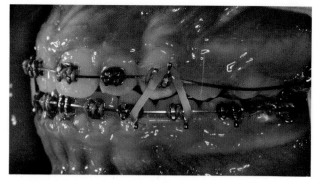

Figure 7.41 Left buccal view of the dentition 5 weeks later. The maxillary molar band and second premolar bracket were removed due to hygiene problems.

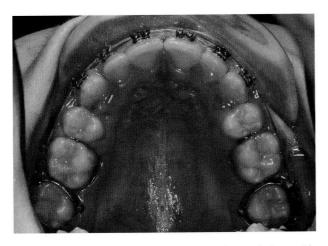

Figure 7.42 Occlusal view of the maxillary arch 5 weeks later with the first molar bands and second premolar brackets removed due to poor hygiene.

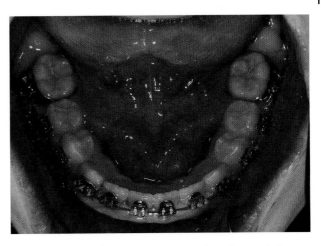

Figure 7.43 Occlusal view of the mandibular arch 5 weeks later.

Eighth Active Appointment

Six weeks later the maxillary first molars and second premolars were bonded with tubes and brackets, respectively. A .017 × .025 nickel-titanium wire was placed. The patient continued to wear triangle elastics (3/16", 4.5 oz.) from the maxillary canines to the mandibular canines and first premolars. An elastomeric chain was attached to the maxillary canine to canine to consolidate space (Figures 7.44–7.48). The chain was ligated to the mesial wings of the canine brackets to prevent canine mesial rotation.

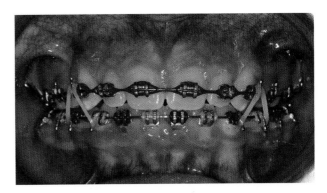

Figure 7.44 Anterior view of the dentition 6 weeks later with elastomeric chain in place for space closure.

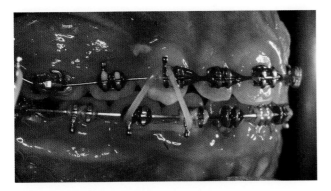

Figure 7.45 Right buccal view of the dentition 6 weeks later. Note the bonded first molar tube in place of the molar band. The elastomeric chain was ligated to the mesial wing of the canine to prevent rotation and the triangle elastic was being worn for improved intercuspation.

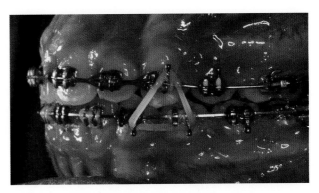

Figure 7.46 Left buccal view of the dentition 6 weeks later. Note the bonded first molar tube in place of the molar band. The elastomeric chain was ligated to the mesial wing of the canine to prevent rotation and the triangle elastic was being worn for improved intercuspation.

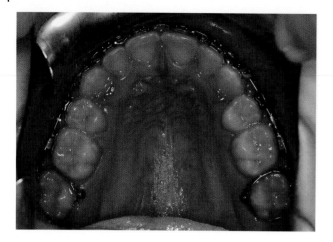

Figure 7.47 Occlusal view of the maxillary arch 6 weeks later with bonded first molar tubes in place.

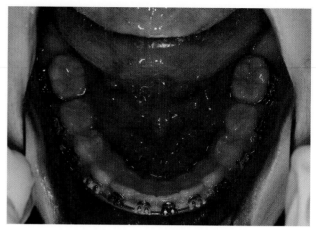

Figure 7.48 Occlusal view of the mandibular arch 6 weeks later.

Ninth and 10th Active Appointments

For 10 weeks the patient wore triangle elastics while the arches leveled and the crossbite of the right second molars corrected. The maxillary arch wire was sectioned distal to the lateral incisors, while the mandibular arch wire was sectioned distal to the canines (Figure 7.49). Note that no arch wire was present distal to the maxillary incisors and mandibular canines. Elastomeric chain was attached to the maxillary incisors to maintain space closure. Settling elastics (3/8", 4.5 oz.) extending from the mandibular first molar to the maxillary and mandibular canines in an up-and-down configuration were to be worn daily for 1 month for intercuspation (Figures 7.50 and 7.51).

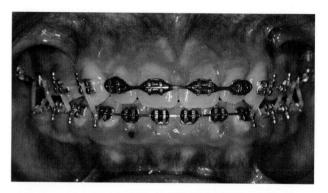

Figure 7.49 Anterior view of the dentition 10 weeks later. The maxillary arch wire was sectioned distal to the lateral incisors, and elastomeric chain was placed from lateral incisor to lateral incisor. The mandibular arch wire was sectioned distal to the canines.

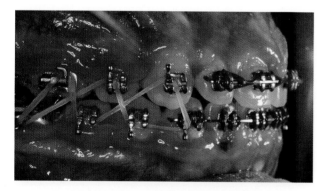

Figure 7.50 Right buccal of the dentition view 10 weeks later. Note the settling elastics placed to improve intercuspation.

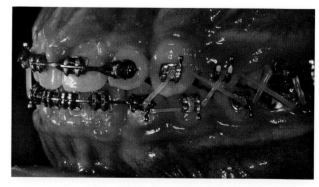

Figure 7.51 Left buccal view of the dentition 10 weeks later. Note the settling elastics placed to improve intercuspation.

Eleventh and 12th Active Appointments

Three weeks later, it was observed that a 0.5 mm midline discrepancy was present. For correction, an anterior diagonal elastic (3/8", 4.5 oz.) was to be worn from the maxillary left canine to the mandibular right canine each evening to aid in the correction (Figure 7.52). The settling elastics continued to be worn. For the next 4 weeks, the patient wore the settling elastics and anterior diagonal elastic intermittently; the occlusion, however, settled

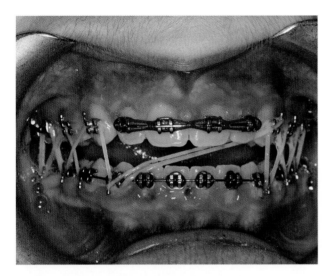

Figure 7.52 Anterior view of the dentition 3 weeks later. It was noted that a midline discrepancy had occurred and the patient was instructed to wear a diagonal elastic for its correction.

and the mild midline discrepancy was acceptable, and the patient was debonded at the following visit, 2 weeks after the 12th appointment.

Thirteenth Appointment (Debond and Retainer Delivery)

The patient was debonded. Impressions were taken for immediate Essix retainers (DENTSPLY Raintree Essix, Sarasota, FL, USA). The patient was instructed to wear these retainers at night and during sleep only. An iTero scan, photographs, and a cephalogram were taken (Figures 7.53–7.62). The patient attained a Class II molar relationship and a Class I canine relationship due to the extraction of the maxillary first premolars. The overjet and overbite were normal. Arch forms were U-shaped. The patient was to return in 1 month for observation and to check for retainer comfort and was to be seen every 3 months thereafter to observe retainer compliance and to monitor the oral hygiene. The entire treatment time took 17 months.

Upon measurement, very little growth took place during the 17-month treatment time, with the mandible moving forward minimally (Figures 7.61 and 7.62; Table 7.3). Regional superimposition indicated that the majority of dental changes that occurred were a result of protraction of the maxillary first molar to a full Class II position due to the maxillary first premolar extractions and tipping of the mandibular incisors (Figure 7.62). The angulation of the mandibular incisors to the mandibular plane changed from 89.3° to 95.2° due to the inversion of the mandibular incisor brackets, thereby changing the torque prescription.

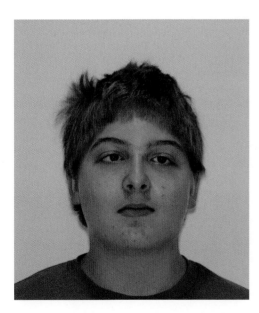

Figure 7.53 Full facial view at the time of appliance removal.

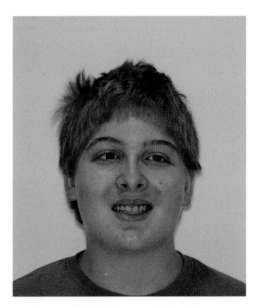

Figure 7.54 Full facial view with smile at the time of appliance removal.

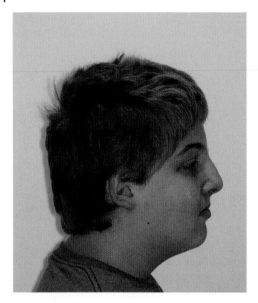

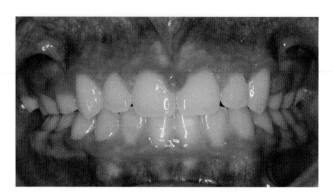

Figure 7.56 Anterior view of the dentition at the time of appliance removal. Note the improvement in the patient's midline.

Figure 7.55 Lateral view of right profile at the time of appliance removal exhibiting a straight form.

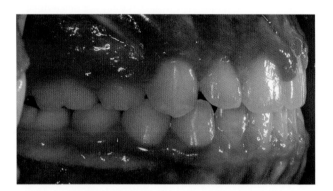

Figure 7.57 Right buccal view of the dentition at the time of appliance removal. Note the Class II molar relationship, the Class I canine relationship and improved overjet as a result of the extraction of the maxillary first premolar.

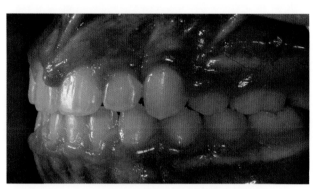

Figure 7.58 Left buccal view of the dentition at the time of appliance removal. Note the Class II molar relationship, the Class I canine relationship and improved overjet as a result of the extraction of the maxillary first premolar.

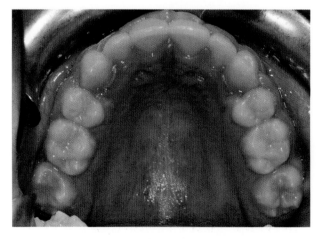

Figure 7.59 Occlusal view of the maxillary arch at the time of appliance removal. Note the improved arch form.

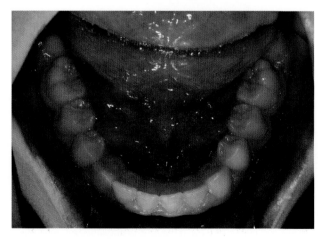

Figure 7.60 Occlusal view of the mandibular arch at the time of appliance removal.

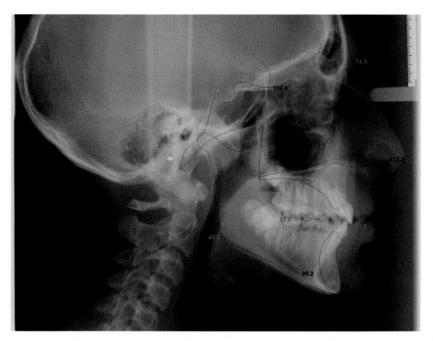

Figure 7.61 Digitized cephalogram at the time of appliance removal. Note the improvement of the skeletal relationship and incisor angulations for facial balance.

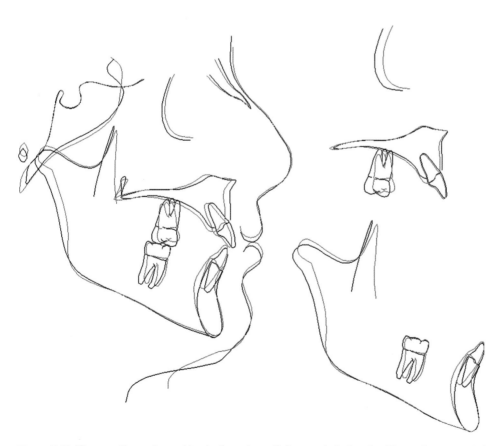

Figure 7.62 The overall superimposition indicated very little growth during the 17-month treatment time. Regional superimpositions indicate protraction of the maxillary molar and improved incisor angulations.

Table 7.3 Significant pre-treatment and post-treatment cephalometric values

	Norm	Pre-treatment	Post-treatment
SNA	82°	79.7°	78.6°
SNB	80°	74.4°	74.9°
ANB	2°	+5.3°	+3.7°
WITS appraisal	−1 to +1 mm	+3.9 mm	+2.0 mm
FMA	21°	28°	26.8°
SN-GoGn	32°	40.3°	40.2°
Maxillary incisor To SN	105°	103.6°	104.4°
Mandibular incisor to GoGn	95°	89.3°	95.2°
Soft tissue			
Lower lip to E-plane	−2.0 mm	−2.2 mm	−2.1 mm
Upper lip to E-plane	−1.6 mm	−5.3 mm	−5.9 mm

SNA, sella-nasion-A point; SNB, sella-nasion-B point; ANB, A point-nasion-B point; WITS appraisal, Witwatersrand appraisal; FMA, Frankfort horizontal-mandibular plane; SN-GoGn, sella nasion-gonion gnathion.

Commentary

Unlike his fraternal twin (Chapter 5), whose teeth were extremely upright and could be treated on a non-extraction basis, this patient required the extraction of maxillary premolars due to the relatively normal angulations of the maxillary incisors and extreme crowding that entirely blocked out a tooth from its normal eruptive position. As a result of treatment, the angulations of the maxillary central incisors remained approximately the same as they were pre-treatment, while the position of the mandibular incisors improved.

Review Questions

1   How was maxillary anchorage attained in this case?

2   The open coil spring used in the mandible achieved two goals. What were these goals in treatment?

3   What quality of bracket prescription is changed by inversion of mandibular incisor brackets in this case?

Suggested References

Proffit WR. Mechanical principles in orthodontic force control. In: Proffit WR, Fields H, Sarver D, eds. Contemporary Orthodontics, 5th edn. CV Mosby Co., 2013; pp. 314–318.

Proffit WR. The second stage of comprehensive treatment. In: Proffit WR, Fields H, Sarver D, eds. Contemporary Orthodontics, 5th edn. CV Mosby Co., 2013; pp. 556–581.

Sondhi A. The impact of bracket selection and bracket placement on expressed tooth movement and finishing details. In: Nanda R, Kapila S, eds. Current Therapy in Orthodontics. St Louis, MO: Mosby Elsevier, 2010; pp. 68–77.

Sondhi A. The implications of bracket selection and bracket placement on finishing details. Semin Orthod 9: 155–164, 2003.

Von Bremen J, Pancherz H. Efficiency of early and late Class II division 1 treatment. Am J Orthod Dentofac Orthop 121(1): 31–37, 2002.

8

Class II Skeletal and Class II Dental: Non-Compliant

Interview Data

The patient is an 11-year-old pre-pubescent male seen privately by a pediatric dentist and treated with a mandibular lingual holding arch to maintain space and a cervical headgear to correct the Class II malocclusion. Compliance with the appliance was poor. The parent's chief complaint was for their son to have a normal occlusion.

- Development: 11-year-old pre-pubertal male
- Motivation: poor to average
- Medical history: non-contributory
- Dental history: seen for routine care in a pediatrics clinic
- Family history: none
- Habits: none

- Facial form: ovoid, mesoprosopic face with prominent chin
- Facial proportions: normal facial ratios

Clinical Examination

- Incisor-stomion (Figures 8.1 and 8.2):
  - At rest: 1 mm
  - Smiling: 5 mm
- Breathing: nasal
- Lips: together at rest
- Mandibular lingual arch and maxillary molar bands in place prior to treatment
- Soft tissue profile: convex (Figure 8.3)
- Nasolabial angle: obtuse
- Normal mandibular plane angle

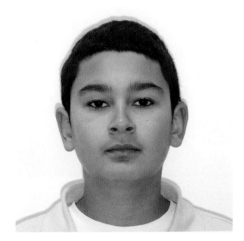

Figure 8.1 Full face at rest displaying an ovoid, symmetric form.

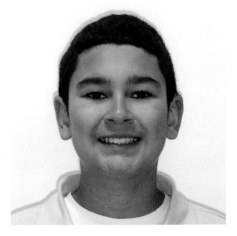

Figure 8.2 Full face with smile with minimal gingival display.

Atlas of Orthodontic Case Reviews, First Edition. Marjan Askari and Stanley A. Alexander.
© 2017 John Wiley & Sons, Inc. Published 2017 by John Wiley & Sons, Inc.

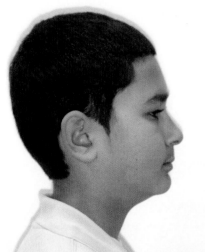

Figure 8.3 Lateral view of profile exhibiting a mild, convex form and obtuse nasolabial angle.

Dentition (Figure 8.4)

- Teeth present clinically:

64321	1234567
7654321	1234567

- Overjet: 4 mm
- Overbite: 5 mm
- Midlines: maxillary midline is 1 mm to the left of the face; the mandibular midline is 3 mm to the left of the maxillary midline

Right Buccal View (Figure 8.5)
- Molar: end-on Class II
- Canine: Class II end-on
- Curve of Spee: deep
- Crossbite: buccal crossbite of maxillary first premolar
- Caries: none

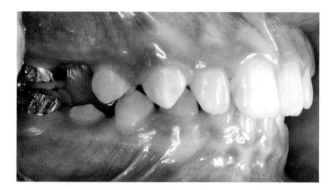

Figure 8.5 Right buccal view of the dentition exhibiting an end-on Class II molar relationship and deep curve of Spee.

Left Buccal View (Figure 8.6)
- Molar: Class II
- Canine: Class II
- Curve of Spee: deep
- Caries: none

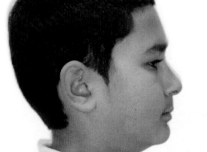

Figure 8.4 Anterior view of the dentition with the maxillary midline 1 mm to the left of the facial midline and the mandibular midline 3 mm to the left of the maxillary midline.

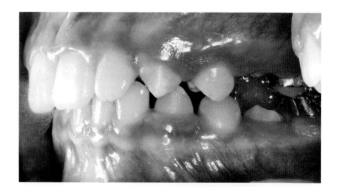

Figure 8.6 Left buccal view of the dentition exhibiting a full Class II molar relationship and deep curve of Spee.

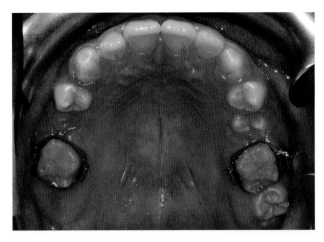

Figure 8.7 Occlusal view of the maxillary arch exhibiting a broad, U-shaped arch form and rotated first molars.

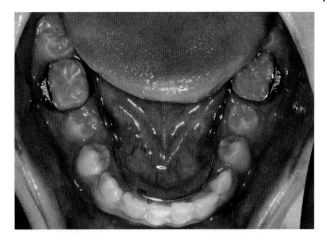

Figure 8.8 Occlusal view of the mandibular arch exhibiting a U-shaped arch form with a lingual holding arch in place.

Maxillary Arch (Figure 8.7)
- Broad, U-shaped symmetric arch form with rotated first molars
- No caries

Mandibular Arch (Figure 8.8)
- U-shaped arch form with lingual arch in place
- No caries

Function

- Maximum opening = 40 mm
- Centric relation-centric occlusion: coincident
- Maximum excursive movements: right = 7 mm; left = 8 mm; protrusive = 8 mm
- Temporomandibular joint palpation: normal without any popping, pain, or crepitus
- Early permanent dentition with the eruption of all four second premolars and maxillary right second molar; third molars are in early development
- Root lengths and periodontium appear normal
- Condyles appear normal (Figure 8.9)

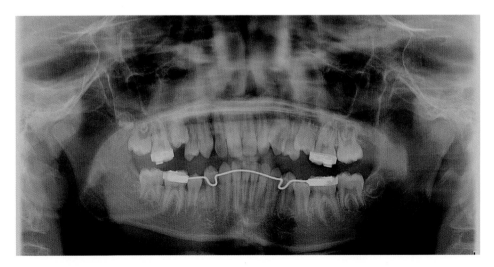

Figure 8.9 Panoramic radiograph of an early adult dentition with development of the third molars. All root lengths and periodontium appear normal.

Diagnosis and Treatment Plan

The patient presents with a mild Class II skeletal and Class II dental malocclusion, moderately deep bite, and moderate overjet with a history of non-compliance with an orthodontic appliance. The soft tissues appear bimaxillary protrusive, but are esthetic and balanced in appearance (Figures 8.9 and 8.10; Tables 8.1 and 8.2).

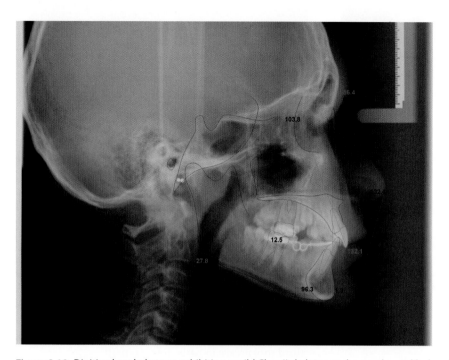

Figure 8.10 Digitized cephalogram exhibiting a mild Class II skeleton and normal mandibular plane angle and incisor angulations.

Table 8.1 Significant cephalometric values

	Norm	Patient pre-treatment
SNA	80°	86.4°
SNB	78°	82.7°
ANB	2°	+3.7°
WITS appraisal	−1 to +1 mm	+0.7 mm
FMA	21°	23.0°
SN-GoGn	32°	27.8°
Maxillary incisor to SN	105°	103.8°
Mandibular incisor to GoGn	95°	96.3°
Soft tissue		
Lower lip to E-plane	−2 mm	−3.1 mm
Upper lip to E-plane	−1.6 mm	−3.1 mm

SNA, sella-nasion-A point; SNB, sella-nasion-B point; ANB, A point-nasion-B point; WITS appraisal, Witwatersrand appraisal; FMA, Frankfort horizontal-mandibular plane; SN-GoGn, sella nasion-gonion gnathion.

Table 8.2 The patient's problem list in three dimensions

	Transverse	Sagittal	Vertical
Soft tissue	Normal	Bimaxillary protrusive profile; obtuse nasolabial angle; prominent chin	Normodivergent
Dental	Buccal posterior crossbite of right premolar	Early adult dentition; Class II molar and canines; moderate overjet	5 mm overbite
Skeletal	Normal	Class II	Normodivergent

Treatment Objectives

The goal of treatment is to create a Class I occlusion and to maintain the facial esthetics, while permitting the patient to grow normally. As treatment in the past was met with resistance, the use of an appliance that requires minimal cooperation was anticipated, although cervical headgear therapy would still be initiated in an attempt at growth modification.

Treatment Options

1) No treatment.
2) Extraction of the maxillary first premolars which would correct the overjet, but may have negative esthetic results due to the obtuse nasolabial angle and continued nasal growth.
3) Extraction of the maxillary second premolars which would have less of an impact on nasal balance with the face.
4) Non-extraction therapy with a fixed appliance and growth modification. This was the option of choice by the parents (Figures 8.11 and 8.12).

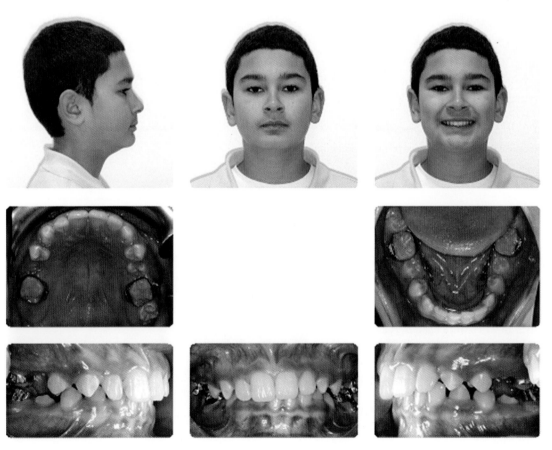

Figure 8.11 Pre-treatment extraoral and intraoral composite photograph.

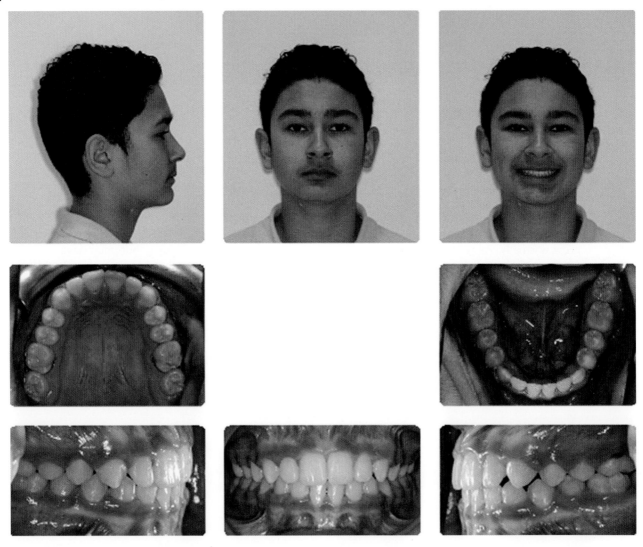

Figure 8.12 Post-treatment extraoral and intraoral composite photograph.

First Active Appointment

The current maxillary molar bands were removed. The mandibular bands and lingual arch were kept in place. New maxillary first molar bands were cemented with glass ionomer. The remaining dentition was bonded with bi-dimensional brackets. During the process of ligation the mandibular left second premolar debonded and a button was bonded in its place. Maxillary and mandibular .016 nickel-titanium arch wires were ligated. A closed coil spring was placed between the maxillary first molars and maxillary first premolars to hold space for the erupting second premolars. An elastomeric chain was attached to the mandibular left second premolar button and to the first molar hook to correct the rotation. The maintenance of the lingual arch prevented reciprocal rotation of the molar. The cervical headgear was adjusted and proper wear was stressed (Figures 8.13–8.17).

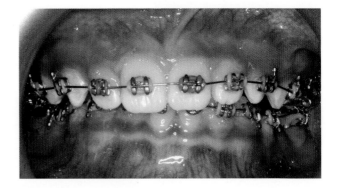

Figure 8.13 Anterior view of the dentition on the day of appliance placement.

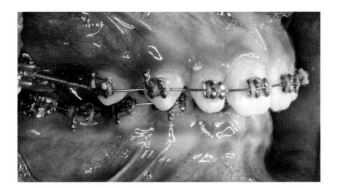

Figure 8.14 Right buccal view of the dentition on the day of appliance placement. Note the closed coil spring between the maxillary first molar and first premolar to preserve space.

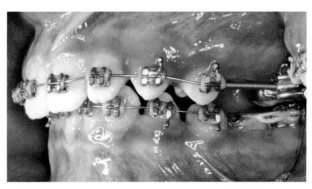

Figure 8.15 Left buccal view of the dentition on the day of appliance placement. Note the closed coil spring between the maxillary first molar and first premolar to preserve space and the elastic chain to the mandibular second premolar and first molar for rotation correction.

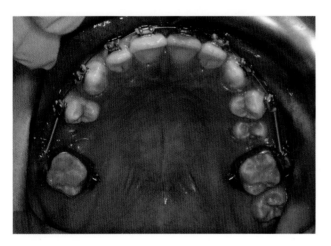

Figure 8.16 Occlusal view of the maxillary arch on the day of appliance placement exhibiting the closed coil springs for space preservation.

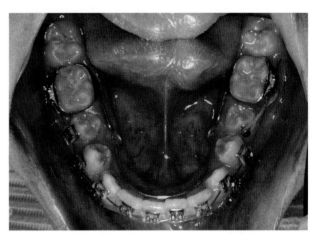

Figure 8.17 Occlusal view of the mandibular arch on the day of appliance placement exhibiting the lingual holding arch and elastic chain from the button of the left second premolar to the first molar for rotation correction.

Second and Third Active Appointments

Four weeks later, the maxillary arch wire was changed to .016 × .022 nickel-titanium and the closed coil springs were kept in place. The mandibular arch wire was passed under the right second premolar and the left canine to extrude them. An elastomeric chain was replaced on the mandibular second premolar for rotation.

Eight weeks later, the button on the mandibular left second premolar was replaced with a bracket. The same arch wires were in place (Figures 8.18–8.22).

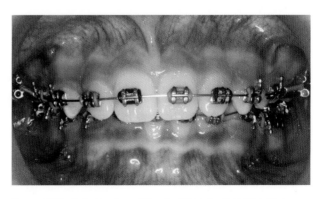

Figure 8.18 Anterior view of the dentition 4 weeks later. The maxillary arch wire was changed to .016 × .022.

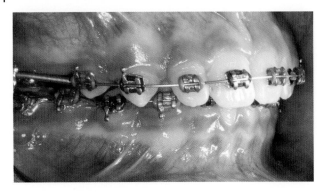

Figure 8.19 Right buccal view of the dentition 4 weeks later.

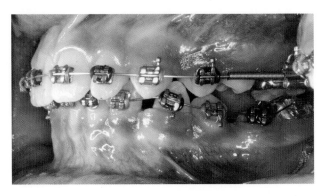

Figure 8.20 Left buccal view of the dentition 4 weeks later.

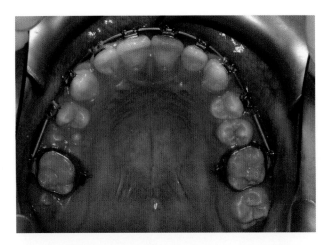

Figure 8.21 Occlusal view of the maxillary arch 4 weeks later. Note the improved rotation of the first molars as a result of the molar tube angulation prescription.

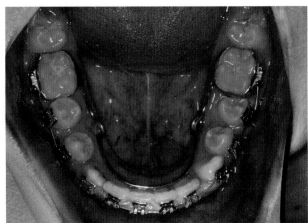

Figure 8.22 Occlusal view of the mandibular arch 4 weeks later. Note the improved rotation of the left second premolar.

Fourth and Fifth Active Appointments

Four weeks later the maxillary arch wire was changed to .017 × .025 stainless steel and cinched. The mandibular arch wire was changed to .016 × .022 nickel-titanium. The mandibular arch wire was passed under the second premolar brackets for extrusion. An elastomeric chain was placed between the first premolars for space consolidation. The patient was not wearing the cervical headgear as often as prescribed.

Four weeks later, the mandibular lingual arch was removed and new bands were cemented to the first molars with glass ionomer. The maxillary left second premolar was bonded. A .017 × .025 nickel-titanium was ligated to the maxillary arch and passed under the second premolar bracket for extrusion. Elastomeric chain was placed from maxillary canine to canine and from mandibular first premolar to first premolar for space consolidation (Figures 8.23–8.27). During this time

period, the cervical headgear was misplaced and not worn. The patient and parent were requested to discontinue the sporadic headgear use.

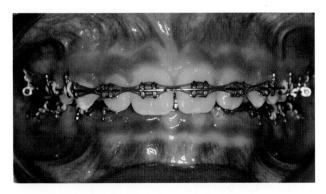

Figure 8.23 Anterior view of the dentition 8 weeks later. Elastomeric chain has been placed on the maxillary arch from canine to canine and from the mandibular first premolar to first premolar for space consolidation. The maxillary arch wire was changed to .017 × .025 nickel-titanium.

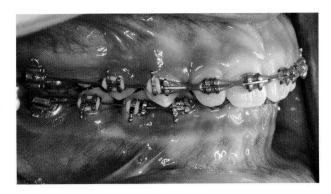

Figure 8.24 Right buccal view of the dentition 8 weeks later.

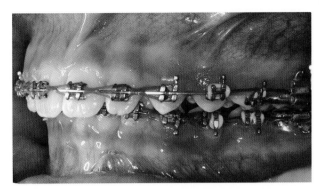

Figure 8.25 Left buccal view of the dentition 8 weeks later.

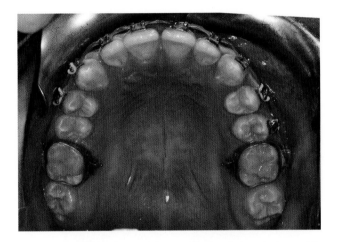

Figure 8.26 Occlusal view of the maxillary arch 8 weeks later with the eruption of the right second premolar.

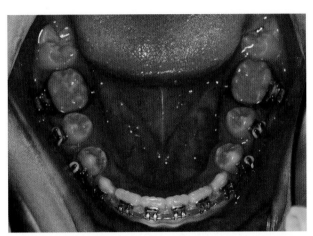

Figure 8.27 Occlusal view of the mandibular arch with the lingual holding arch removed.

Sixth Active Appointment

Four weeks later, the maxillary arch wire was changed to .017 × .025 stainless steel and passed under the left second premolar for extrusion. The mandibular arch wire was changed to .017 × .025 nickel-titanium. An elastomeric chain was placed between the maxillary canines for space consolidation. The patient was instructed to wear Class II elastics (1/4"; 4.5 oz.) from the maxillary canines to the mandibular first molars. These elastics were to be changed daily. Compliance would be monitored (Figures 8.28–8.32).

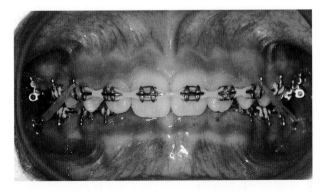

Figure 8.28 Anterior view of the dentition 4 weeks later. The maxillary arch wire was changed to .017 × .025 stainless steel and the mandibular arch wire was changed to .017 × .025 nickel-titanium. Elastomeric chain was continued from the maxillary canine to canine.

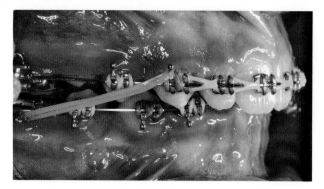

Figure 8.29 Right buccal view of the dentition 4 weeks later displaying the wear of Class II elastics.

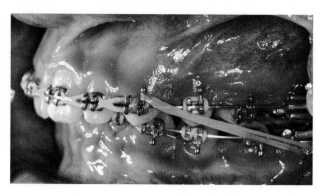

Figure 8.30 Left buccal view of the dentition 4 weeks later displaying the use of Class II elastics. Note the placement of the maxillary arch wire gingival to the second premolar bracket to aid in extrusion.

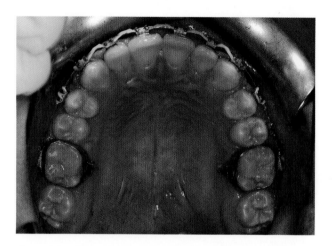

Figure 8.31 Occlusal view of the maxillary arch 4 weeks later.

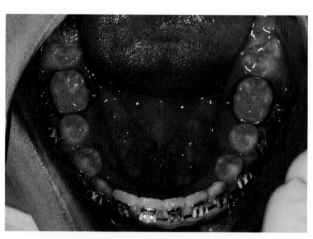

Figure 8.32 Occlusal view of the mandibular arch 4 weeks later. Note the completed rotation of the left second premolar.

Seventh and Eighth Active Appointments

Six weeks later, the mandibular arch wire was changed to .017 × .025 stainless steel. Elastomeric chain was continued between the maxillary canines. Class II elastics were continued, but compliance appeared to be poor.

Four weeks later, the maxillary left second premolar bracket was removed to allow for natural eruption. As both headgear and elastic appliance were poor, it was decided to place a Forsus appliance (3 M Unitek, Monrovia, CA, USA) that would require minimal cooperation in the correction of the Class II malocclusion. Rigid .017 × .025 stainless steel arch wires were placed in both arches. This would prevent arch distortion from the inter-arch spring mechanisms of the 29 mm Forsus spring (Figures 8.33–8.37).

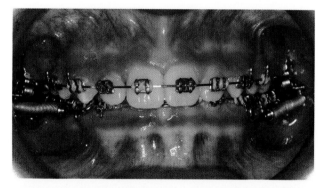

Figure 8.33 Anterior view of the dentition 4 weeks later. Both maxillary and mandibular arch wires are .017 × .025 stainless steel. The Forsus springs can be seen in the buccal quadrants.

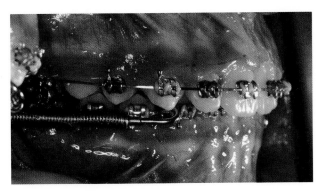

Figure 8.34 Right buccal view of the dentition 4 weeks later with the Forsus spring in place.

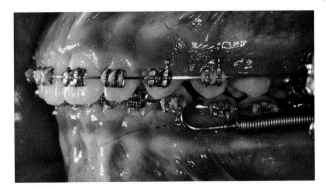

Figure 8.35 Left buccal view of the dentition 4 weeks later with the Forsus spring in place.

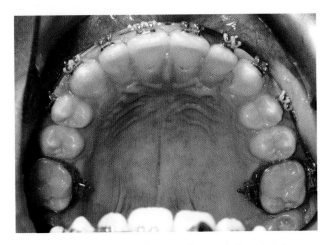

Figure 8.36 Occlusal view of the maxillary arch 4 weeks later.

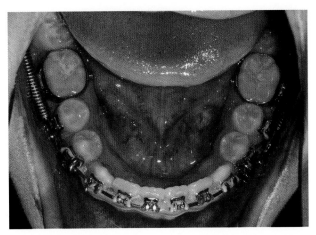

Figure 8.37 Occlusal view of the mandibular arch 4 weeks later.

Ninth to 12th Active Appointments

Four weeks later, the patient returned with the mandibular right canine bracket broken and the Forsus arm and spring missing. The bracket was rebonded and a new Forsus spring was placed on the right side.

Four weeks later, a 1 mm shim was added to both Forsus arms to increase the mandibular projection. An elastomeric chain was placed from the maxillary first molar to first molar and to right and left mandibular first molars to canines, respectively.

Four weeks later, an additional 1 mm shim was added to the patient's left side. Elastomeric chain was placed as per the prior appointment.

Four weeks later, the Forsus springs were removed as the overjet was over-corrected. The maxillary second premolars were bonded. A .018 nickel-titanium maxillary arch wire was placed. The mandibular stainless steel arch wire remained. Triangle elastics (3/16"; 4.5 oz.) were instructed to be worn for settling of the occlusion (Figures 8.38–8.42).

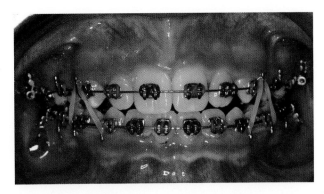

Figure 8.38 Anterior view of the dentition 16 weeks later. The Forsus springs have been removed and the maxillary arch wire was changed to .018 nickel-titanium. Triangle elastics were used to settle the buccal occlusion.

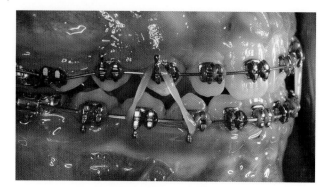

Figure 8.39 Right buccal view of the dentition 16 weeks later with triangle elastics used to settle the occlusion. Note the reduced overjet and improved overbite relationship.

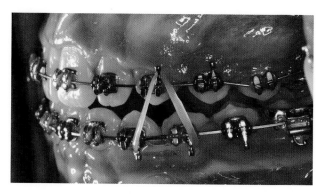

Figure 8.40 Left buccal view of the dentition 16 weeks later with a triangle elastic in place.

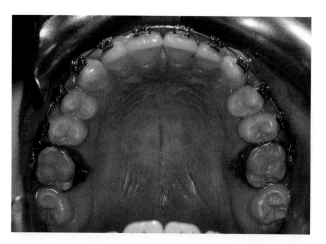

Figure 8.41 Occlusal view of the maxillary arch 16 weeks later.

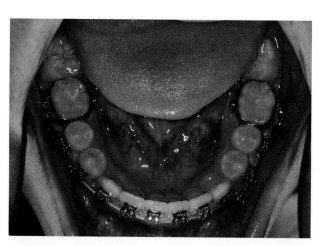

Figure 8.42 Occlusal view of the mandibular arch 16 weeks later.

Thirteenth Appointment

A progress panoramic radiograph was taken 6 weeks later (Figure 8.43). All root lengths appeared normal. An accentuated curve .017 × .025 nickel-titanium arch wire was placed on the maxillary arch. A reverse curve .017 × .025 nickel-titanium arch wire was placed on the mandible. Both arch wires were used to help open the bite after relapse of the Forsus springs. Elastomeric chain was placed from the maxillary first molar to first molar and

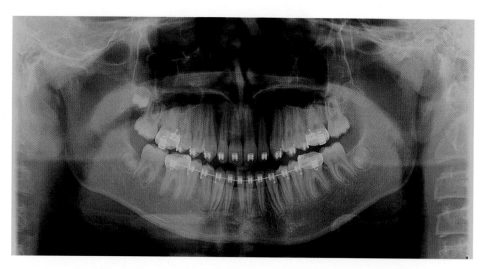

Figure 8.43 Progress panoramic radiograph indicating normal root lengths during therapy.

from the mandibular first molar to first molar. A triangle elastic was continued on the right side and a Class II elastic from the maxillary left canine to the mandibular left first molar (3/16"; 4.5 oz.) was placed on the left side. Note that the elastic was placed gingival to the mandibular first and second premolars to help settle the occlusion (Figures 8.44–8.48).

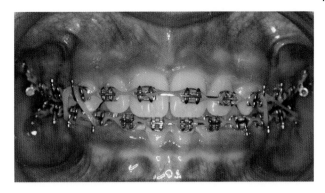

Figure 8.44 Anterior view of the dentition 6 weeks later. The maxillary arch wire was changed to .017×.025 nickel-titanium with an accentuated curve, and the mandibular arch wire was changed to .017×.025 nickel-titanium with a reverse curve to maintain bite opening. Elastomeric chain was placed in both arches from first molar to first molar.

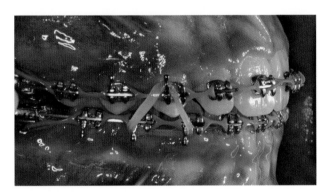

Figure 8.45 Right buccal view of the dentition 6 weeks later exhibiting the triangle elastic to aid in settling the occlusion.

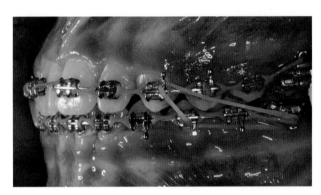

Figure 8.46 Left buccal view of the dentition 6 weeks later with a triangular Class II elastic to perfect the canine intercuspation.

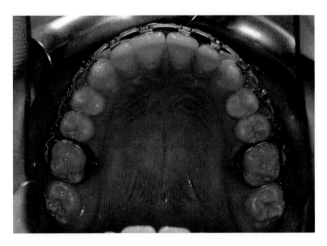

Figure 8.47 Occlusal view of the maxillary arch 6 weeks later displaying the improved arch form.

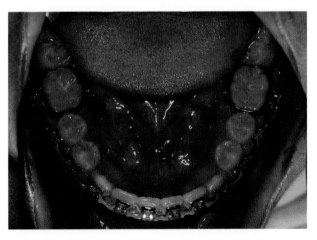

Figure 8.48 Occlusal view of the mandibular arch 6 weeks later with an improved arch form.

Fourteenth Active Appointment

Four weeks later, the maxillary arch wire was changed to .017 × .025 nickel-titanium and sectioned distal to the lateral incisors. The mandibular arch wire was changed to .016 × .022 nickel-titanium and sectioned distal to the canines. Elastomeric chain was placed between the maxillary lateral incisor to lateral incisor and a continuous stainless steel ligature was used from canine to canine. Settling elastics (3/8"; 4 oz.) were to be used daily (Figures 8.49–8.51). As the lack of cooperation was a serious factor in the treatment of this patient, it was once again stressed to wear these elastics as instructed to expedite the removal of the appliances.

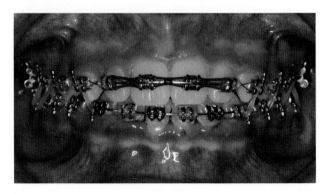

Figure 8.49 Anterior view of the dentition 4 weeks later with a sectioned .017 × .025 nickel-titanium maxillary arch wire and a sectioned .016 × .022 nickel-titanium mandibular arch wire.

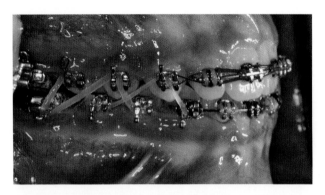

Figure 8.50 Right buccal view of the dentition 4 weeks later exhibiting settling elastics in place.

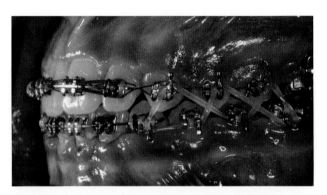

Figure 8.51 Left buccal view of the dentition 4 weeks later exhibiting settling elastics in place.

Fifteenth Appointment

Six weeks later, it was apparent that the patient was compliant with the settling elastics and the appliances were debonded. The patient's occlusion was Class I with a normal overbite and overjet. The arch forms are broad and U-shaped (Figures 8.52–8.59). The soft tissues were esthetic and balanced. Impressions were taken for immediate Essix retainers (DENTSPLY Raintree Essix, Sarasota, FL, USA). Photographs, a cephalogram, and an iTero scan (Align Technology, Inc, San Jose, CA, USA) were performed. The patient was instructed to wear the retainers at night and during sleep and was to be observed for compliance 1 month and every 3 months after appliance removal for the first year. Total treatment time was 16 months. The overall superimposition mainly indicated horizontal growth and forward positioning of the mandible due to the Forsus appliance (Figures 8.60 and 8.61; Table 8.3). The occlusal plane tipped downward. Regional superimpositions indicated that bite opening occurred via extrusion of the mandibular molar and retraction of both the maxillary and mandibular incisors, which was overshadowed by the horizontal growth vector.

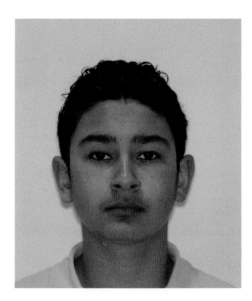

Figure 8.52 Full-face view on the day of appliance removal.

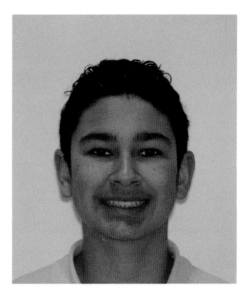

Figure 8.53 Full-face view with smile on the day of appliance removal.

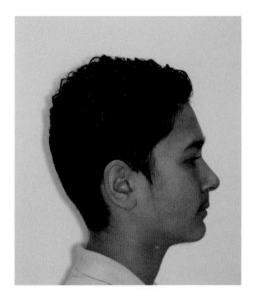

Figure 8.54 Right lateral view of the profile on the day of appliance removal.

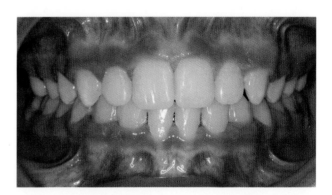

Figure 8.55 Anterior view of the dentition on the day of appliance removal.

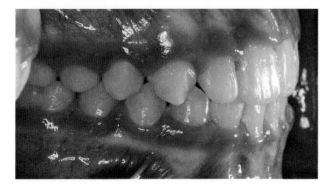

Figure 8.56 Right buccal view of the dentition on the day of appliance removal.

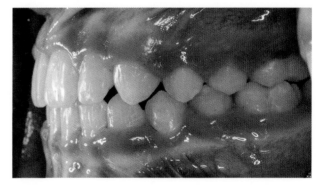

Figure 8.57 Left buccal view of the dentition on the day of appliance removal.

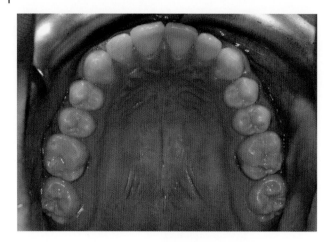

Figure 8.58 Occlusal view of the maxillary arch on the day of appliance removal.

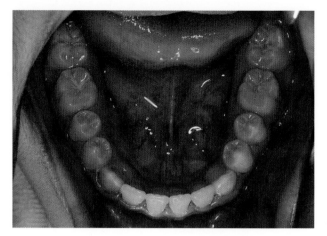

Figure 8.59 Occlusal view of the mandibular arch on the day of appliance removal.

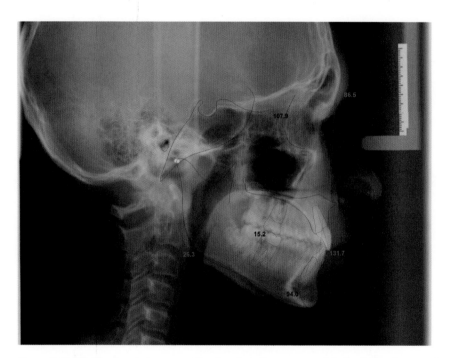

Figure 8.60 Digitized cephalogram on the day of appliance removal, indicating an improved maxillary and mandibular relationship.

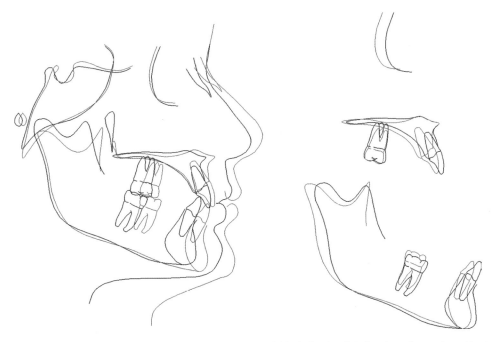

Figure 8.61 Overall and regional superimposition (initial, black; final, red) indicating a forward positioning of the mandible as a result of growth and appliance therapy and maintenance of the incisor angulations with minimal retraction.

Table 8.3 Significant pre-treatment and post-treatment cephalometric values

	Norm	Pre-treatment	Post-treatment
SNA	82°	86.4°	86.5°
SNB	80°	82.7°	83.6°
ANB	2°	+3.7°	+2.9°
WITS appraisal	−1 to +1 mm	+0.7 mm	−2.6 mm
FMA	21°	23°	22.7°
SN-GoGn	32°	27.8°	26.3°
Maxillary incisor to SN	105°	103.8°	107.9°
Mandibular incisor to GoGn	95°	96.3°	94°
Soft tissue			
Lower lip to E-plane	−2.0 mm	−3.1 mm	−3.5 mm
Upper lip to E-plane	−1.6 mm	−3.1 mm	−4.3 mm

SNA, sella-nasion-A point; SNB, sella-nasion-B point; ANB, A point-nasion-B point; WITS appraisal, Witwatersrand appraisal; FMA, Frankfort horizontal-mandibular plane; SN-GoGn, sella nasion-gonion gnathion.

Commentary

The issue of compliance and the following of instructions relates to all age ranges of patients, whether it is concerned with oral hygiene issues or the wearing of elastics or any other auxiliaries. There comes a time in the course of treatment when non-compliant modes of therapy may have to be introduced or the treatment terminated with the agreement that "this is the best we can do" based upon the patient's participation in their own care.

Review Questions

1 What procedure on the mandibular premolar was the elastomeric chain used for in this case?

2 Growth modification may be accomplished with an extraoral appliance such as a headgear. True or false?

3 What purpose was served by the closed coil springs placed in an edentulous site?

4 In a non-compliant patient, the used of a fixed auxiliary may correct the sagittal problem. True or false?

Suggested References

Albino J. Factors influencing adolescent cooperation in orthodontic treatment. Semin Orthod 6: 214–223, 2000.

Antonarakis GS, Kiliaridis S. Maxillary molar distalization with non-compliance intramaxillary appliances in Class II malocclusions. A systematic review. Angle Orthod 78: 1133–1140, 2008.

Patel MP, Janson G, Henriques JF et al. Comparative distaliization effects of Jones jig and pendulum appliances. Am J Orthod Dentofac Orthop 135: 336–342, 2009.

Sinha PK. Patient compliance in orthodontic practice. In: Nanda R, Kapila S, eds. Current Therapy in Orthodontics. St Louis, MO: Mosby Elsevier, 2010; pp. 9–14.

9

Skeletal Class II and Dental Class II Division 1 Subdivision: Four Premolar Extractions

---

LEARNING OBJECTIVES

- How to correct midline discrepancies
- How to create anchorage in the maxillary arch
- How to correct deep overbite relationships
- What appliances are available when compliance presents a problem

---

Interview Data

This is an 11 year old male with the chief complaint from both parents and himself of "needing braces".

- Development: pre-pubescent
- Motivation: good
- Medical history: non-contributory
- Dental history: previously seen by an oral and maxillofacial surgeon for temporomandibular (TMJ) joint sounds; possible diagnosis of condylar resorption and flattening of the condylar head
- Family history: non-contributory

- Habits: none
- Limitations: none
- Facial form: convex profile, ovoid, symmetric mesoprosopic form, retrognathic mandible with deficient chin
- Facial proportions: slightly increased lower third of face and symmetric

Clinical Examination

- Incisor-stomion (Figures 9.1 and 9.2):
  - At rest: 2 mm
  - Smiling: 6 mm

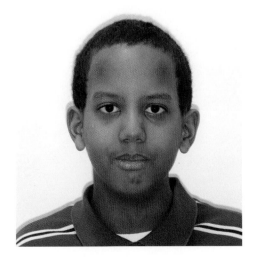

Figure 9.1 Full face at rest displaying an ovoid, symmetric face.

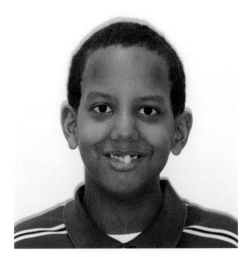

Figure 9.2 Full face with smile displaying 2 mm of gingival and incisor protrusion.

Atlas of Orthodontic Case Reviews, First Edition. Marjan Askari and Stanley A. Alexander.
© 2017 John Wiley & Sons, Inc. Published 2017 by John Wiley & Sons, Inc.

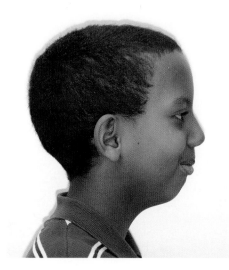

Figure 9.3 Lateral view of right profile indicating a convex form, retrognathic mandible, and deficient chin.

- Breathing: nasal
- Lips: incompetent at rest and strained
- Severe crowding with blocked out mandibular canines
- Mentalis strain
- Soft tissue profile: convex with recessive chin (Figure 9.3)
- Nasolabial angle: slightly obtuse
- High mandibular plane angle

Dentition (Figure 9.4)

- Teeth clinically present

7654321	123456
765421	124567

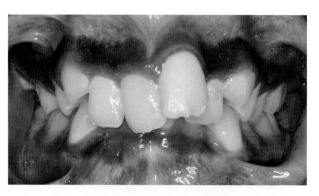

Figure 9.4 Anterior view of the dentition displaying deep overbite, severe overjet, and severe crowding.

- Early permanent dentition with blocked out mandibular canines
- Overjet: 12 mm for maxillary left central incisor; 8 mm for maxillary right central incisor
- Overbite: 10 mm with palatal impingement
- Midlines: maxillary midline 2 mm left of face; mandibular midline 1 mm right of face
- Anterior crossbite: none
- Posterior crossbite: none

Right Buccal View (Figure 9.5)

- Molar: Class II end-on
- Curve of Spee: deep
- Crossbite: none
- Caries: none

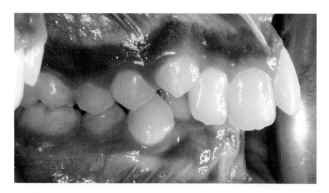

Figure 9.5 Right buccal view of the dentition displaying a Class II end-on molar and canine occlusion and a deep curve of Spee.

Left Buccal View (Figure 9.6)

- Molar: Class I
- Curve of Spee: deep
- Crossbite: none
- Caries: none

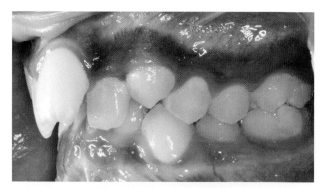

Figure 9.6 Left buccal view of the dentition displaying a Class I molar and canine occlusion and a deep curve of Spee.

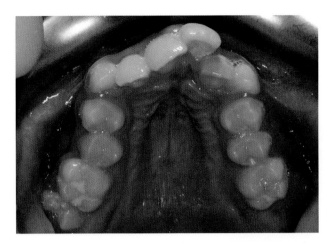

Figure 9.7 Occlusal view of the maxillary arch exhibiting an asymmetric form and severe crowding.

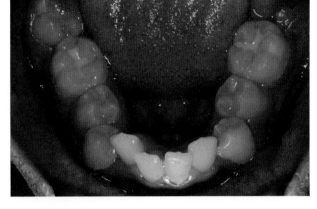

Figure 9.8 Occlusal view of the mandibular arch exhibiting a U-shaped arch form with severe crowding and blocked-out canines.

Maxillary Arch (Figure 9.7)

- Asymmetric catenary curve arch form with severe crowding
- Rotated first molars
- No caries

Mandibular Arch (Figure 9.8)

- U-shaped arch form with severe crowding and blocked out canines

Function

- Normal range of motion without discomfort: maximum opening = 40 mm; lateral excursion right = 8 mm; lateral excursion left = 10 mm; protrusive = 7 mm
- Centric relation-centric occlusion: coincident
- Slight crepitus of left TMJ
- Early permanent dentition with blocked out mandibular canines
- Root lengths and periodontium appear normal
- Left condyle appears to be flattened (Figure 9.9)

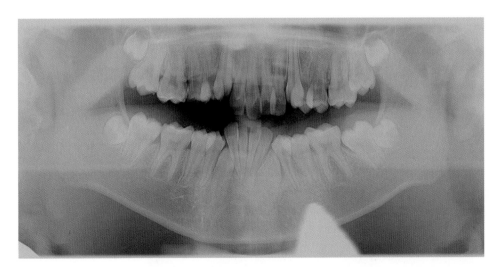

Figure 9.9 Panoramic radiograph demonstrating a severely crowded dentition with blocked-out mandibular canines and normal root structures.

Diagnosis and Treatment Plan

The patient presents with a Class II skeletal and Class II dental (subdivision right) pattern, possible TMJ pathology, completely blocked-out mandibular canines, severe crowding, deep impinging overbite, and excessive overjet (Figures 9.10 and 9.11; Tables 9.1 and 9.2). The treatment plan was discussed with the mother and a consult for evaluation of the TMJ was recommended prior to orthodontic treatment.

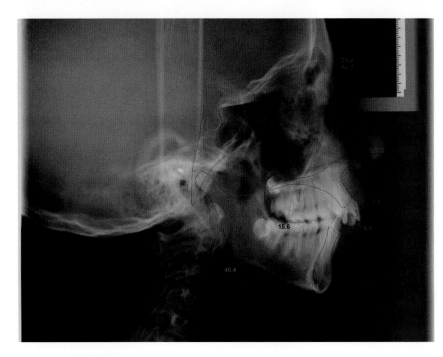

Figure 9.10 Digitized cephalogram exhibiting a Class II skeletal pattern, high mandibular plane angle and severely upright maxillary and mandibular incisors.

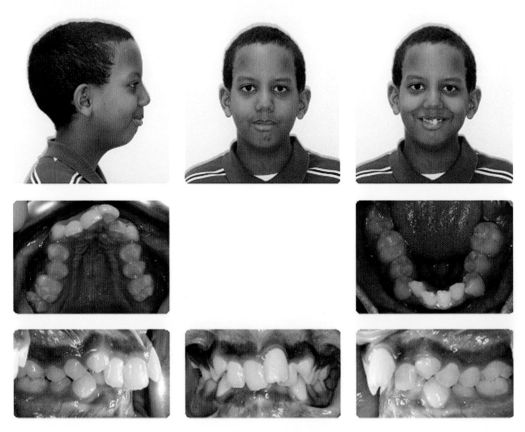

Figure 9.11 Pre-treatment extraoral and intraoral composite photograph.

Table 9.1 Significant cephalometric values

	Norm	Patient pre-treatment
SNA	80°	73.4°
SNB	78°	68.2°
ANB	2°	+5.2°
WITS appraisal	−1 to +1 mm	+10.0 mm
FMA	21°	35.4°
SN-GoGn	32°	40.4°
Maxillary incisor to SN	105°	97.5°
Mandibular incisor to GoGn	95°	87.1°
Soft tissue		
Lower lip to E-plane	−2 mm	+5.8 mm
Upper lip to E-plane	−1.6 mm	+2.9 mm

SNA, sella-nasion-A point; SNB, sella-nasion-B point; ANB, A point-nasion-B point; WITS appraisal, Witwatersrand appraisal; FMA, Frankfort horizontal-mandibular plane; SN-GoGn, sella nasion-gonion gnathion.

Table 9.2 The patient's problem list in three dimensions

	Transverse	Sagittal	Vertical
Soft tissue	Normal	Convex profile; obtuse nasolabial angle; retrognathic mandible; deficient chin prominence	Hyperdivergent
Dental	Severe space deficiency	Early adult dentition; Class II molar subdivision (right) with blocked-out mandibular canines and excessive overjet	10 mm overbite with palatal impingement
Skeletal	Normal	Severe Class II	Hyperdivergent

Treatment Objectives

To achieve the desired objectives, the extraction of four premolars was recommended to relieve the dental crowding. A referral to a specialist for the treatment of TMJ disorders was emphasized before orthodontic treatment would commence. The need for a genioplasty in the future was also discussed to help mask the mandibular retrognathia (Figure 9.12).

Treatment Options

1) No treatment – obviously not a choice due to the severe dental and skeletal issues the patient presents with at this time.
2) Non-extraction therapy with growth modification and expansion/reproximation of the dentition.

3) Extraction of four first premolars.
4) Orthognathic surgery to address the severe skeletal discrepancy.

The parents chose option 3, based upon the perceived level of cooperation. There was no desire for a major surgical intervention, which they felt was not necessary.

First Active Appointment

After clearance to begin treatment (the TMJ disorder will be reviewed periodically during the course of orthodontic treatment), separators were placed between all four first permanent molars. One week later, bands were cemented with glass ionomer to the mandibular first permanent molars. Brackets were bonded to the maxillary canines

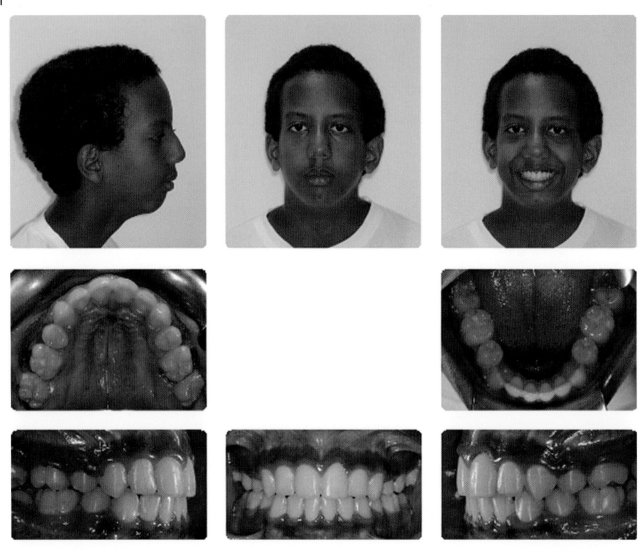

Figure 9.12 Post-treatment extraoral and intraoral composite photograph.

and second premolars and mandibular incisors and second premolars, but no arch wires were placed. Bands were fitted to the maxillary first permanent molars and an impression was taken for the construction of a Nance appliance to augment maxillary anchorage. The appliance was cemented to the molars during the following week. At this time, all four first premolars were extracted. Maxillary and mandibular .014 nickel-titanium wires were placed and cinched, but not engaging all of the teeth. A sectional .016 × .022 β-titanium wire was placed into the utility tube between the maxillary first permanent molars and canines for canine retraction with elastomeric chain. Closed coil springs were placed in the mandibular canine areas to maintain space on the right side of the arch and to allow for the mandibular dental shifting to the left side (Figures 9.13–9.17).

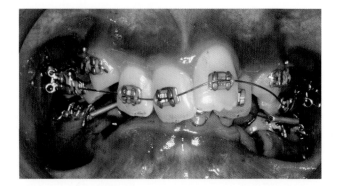

Figure 9.13 Anterior view of the dentition at the beginning of treatment – .014 nickel-titanium base arch wires have been placed in the maxillary and mandibular arches; sectional .016 × .022 β-titanium arch wires have been ligated from the maxillary canine to first molar to initiate canine retraction with elastomeric chain.

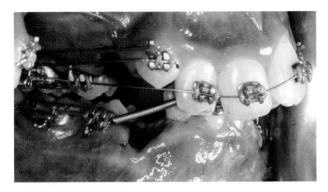

Figure 9.14 Right buccal view of the dentition displaying the sectional arch wire for maxillary canine retraction. The closed coil spring was placed on the mandibular arch to hold extraction space.

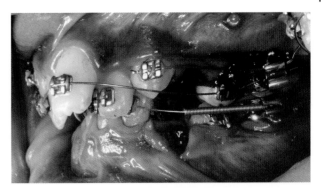

Figure 9.15 Left buccal view of the dentition displaying the sectional arch wire for maxillary canine retraction. The short, closed coil spring was placed on the mandibular arch to allow for the incisors to shift to the left into the extraction space.

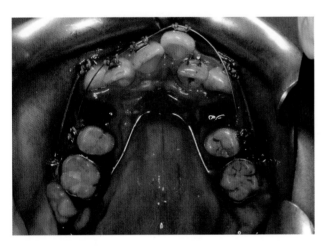

Figure 9.16 Occlusal view of the maxillary arch with Nance anchorage appliance in place on the day of extraction and placement of the bonded appliance.

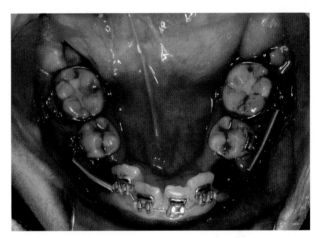

Figure 9.17 Occlusal view of the mandibular arch on the day of appliance placement.

Second Active Appointment

One month later, the sectional wire was removed. All teeth were engaged on the .016 nickel-titanium wire and retraction of the canines was performed with elastomeric chain. The mandibular arch wire was changed to .016 × .022 nickel-titanium with closed coil springs placed between the lateral incisors and second premolars (Figures 9.18–9.22).

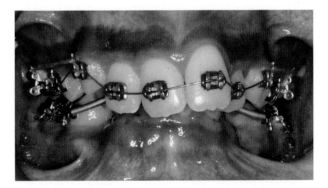

Figure 9.18 Anterior view of the dentition 4 weeks later. The sectional arch was removed and continuous .016 nickel-titanium wire was inserted for canine retraction with elastomeric chain on the maxillary arch.

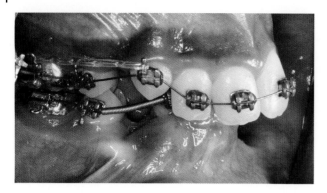

Figure 9.19 Right buccal view of the dentition 4 weeks later displaying the elastomeric retraction chain on the continuous maxillary arch wire.

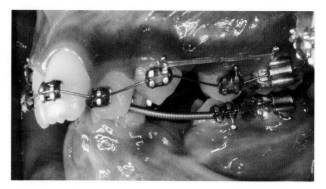

Figure 9.20 Left buccal view of the dentition 4 weeks later displaying the elastomeric retraction chain on the continuous maxillary arch wire.

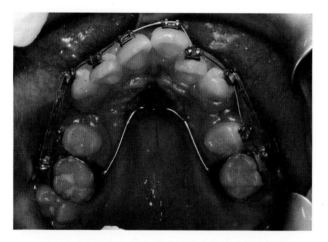

Figure 9.21 Occlusal view of the maxillary arch 4 weeks later.

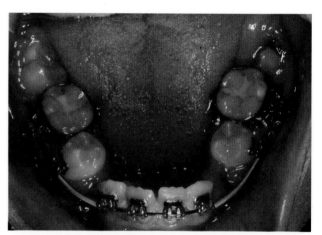

Figure 9.22 Occlusal view of the mandibular arch 4 weeks later.

Third Active Appointment

Five weeks later, the maxillary arch wire was changed to a .016 × .022 nickel-titanium wire with a .017 × .025 stainless steel "piggyback" overlay with an off-centered "V" bend placed in front of the molar tube and ligated between the central incisors for incisor intrusion and for correction of the axial inclination of the incisors (Figure 9.23). Elastomeric chain was placed from maxillary canine to maxillary canine for space consolidation and from maxillary canines to first molars for canine retraction. The mandibular arch wire was changed to .017 × .025 nickel-titanium with an open coil spring between the right lateral incisor and second premolar for a midline shift to the left, and a closed coil spring between the left lateral incisor and second premolar to maintain space for canine eruption (Figures 9.24–9.27).

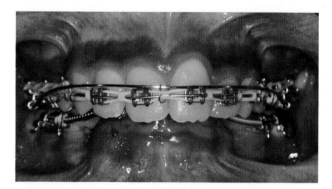

Figure 9.23 Anterior view of the dentition 5 weeks after the previous appointment. The base arch wire was changed in the maxilla to .016 × .022 nickel-titanium with an overlay .017 × .025 stainless steel wire for anterior intrusion and improvement of the incisor angulation. Elastomeric chain has been ligated to the maxillary arch from first molar to first molar for space consolidation.

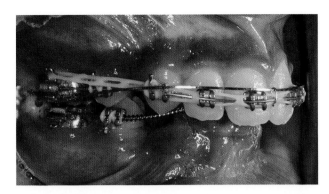

Figure 9.24 Right buccal view of the dentition 5 weeks after the previous appointment. The mandibular wire has been changed to .017 × .025 nickel-titanium and an open coil spring has been added to shift the mandibular midline to the left.

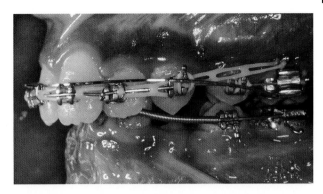

Figure 9.25 Left buccal view of the dentition 5 weeks after the previous appointment. The mandibular wire has been changed to .017 × .025 nickel-titanium and a closed coil spring has been added between the second premolar and lateral incisor to maintain space for the erupting canine.

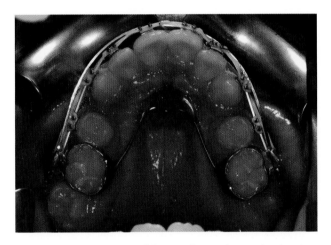

Figure 9.26 Occlusal view of the maxillary arch 5 weeks after the previous appointment displaying the improved arch form.

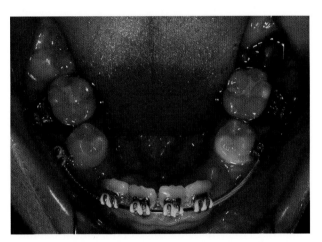

Figure 9.27 Occlusal view of the mandibular arch 5 weeks after the previous appointment, demonstrating the midline shift to the left with the open coil spring on the right quadrant and the maintenance of canine space with the closed coil spring on the left quadrant.

Fourth and Fifth Active Appointments

Five weeks later, the maxillary arch wire was changed to .017 × .025 nickel-titanium and the same intrusion mechanics and retraction mechanics were being performed. The mandibular arch wire was changed to .017 × .025 stainless steel with an activated open coil spring for the midline shift and a closed coil spring for space maintenance (Figures 9.28 and 9.29). The same mechanics were employed for the next 5 weeks.

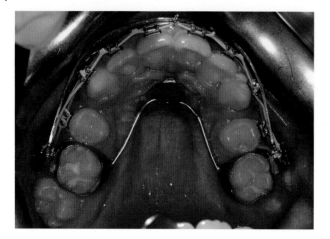

Figure 9.28 Occlusal view of the maxillary arch 5 weeks later demonstrating space closure.

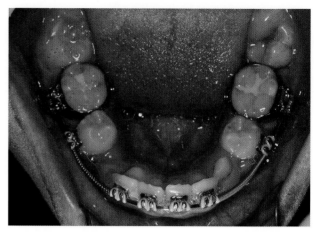

Figure 9.29 Occlusal view of the mandibular arch 5 weeks later. The arch wire has been changed to .017×.025 stainless steel.

Sixth Active Appointment

After an additional 4 weeks, the Nance appliance was removed and all maxillary first and second molars were banded due to a crossbite of the maxillary left second molar. A sectional .014 nickel-titanium wire was overlaid from the first molar to the second molar for alignment and leveling. The same intrusion mechanics were continued. An elastomeric chain extended from the first molar to first molar for space consolidation. An arch wire stop (arrow) was placed on the mandibular right canine area to increase the force of the coil for the midline shift to the left (Figures 9.30–9.34).

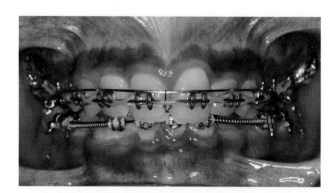

Figure 9.30 Anterior view of the dentition 14 weeks later. Note the improvement of the overbite relationship.

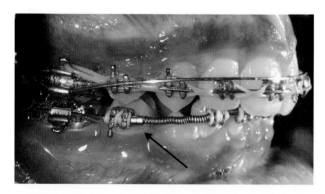

Figure 9.31 Right buccal view of the dentition 14 weeks later. The Nance appliance was removed and first and second molars were banded. The same arch wires were in place with the addition of a sectional .014 nickel-titanium wire to align the maxillary second molar. An arch wire stop was placed mesial to the second premolar to increase the activity of the open coil spring (arrow).

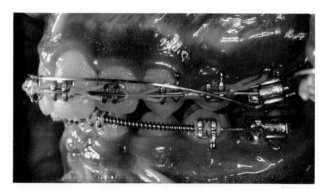

Figure 9.32 Left buccal view of the dentition 14 weeks later. The Nance appliance was removed and first and second molars were banded. The same arch wires were in place with the addition of a sectional .014 nickel-titanium wire to align the maxillary second molar.

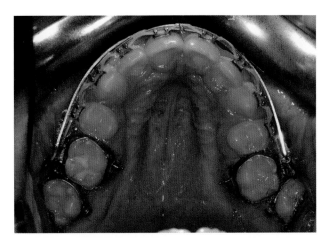

Figure 9.33 Occlusal view of the maxillary arch exhibiting the initial alignment of the second molars.

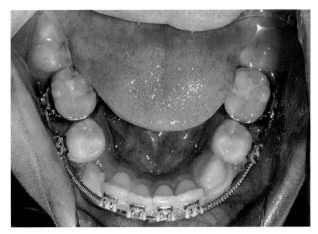

Figure 9.34 Occlusal view of the mandibular arch demonstrating further eruption of the canines.

Seventh Active Appointment

Four weeks later, the mandibular left canine was bonded and a "piggyback" .016 nickel-titanium wire was used for alignment while the midline shift was still being

perfected. Maxillary intrusion was still being performed, but the base arch wire was changed to .018 nickel-titanium as a result of debonding of the right canine bracket (Figures 9.35 and 9.36).

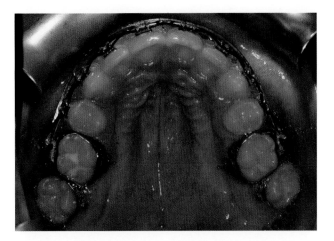

Figure 9.35 Occlusal view of the maxillary arch 4 weeks later. Note the improvement in the position of the second molar.

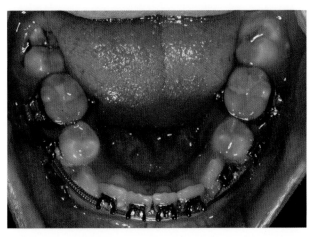

Figure 9.36 Occlusal view of the mandibular arch 4 weeks later. A "piggyback" .016 nickel-titanium wire was placed to align the newly bonded left canine.

Eighth Active Appointment

The mandibular second molars and the mandibular right canine were bonded. The maxillary base wire was changed to .016 × .022 nickel-titanium and the mandibular wire to .016 nickel-titanium. Elastometric chain was placed between the maxillary canines for space consolidation and between the maxillary canines and first molars for retraction. An occlusal build-up with glass ionomer of the palatal cusps of the maxillary first molars was placed to aid in the correction of the crossbite of the maxillary left second molars by temporarily separating them from occlusion (Figures 9.37–9.41).

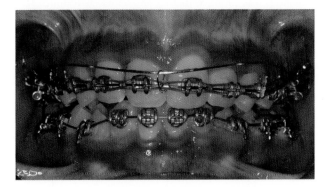

Figure 9.37 Anterior view of the dentition at the eighth appointment. The appearance of bite opening was achieved by the temporary placement of glass ionomer blocks on the maxillary first molars.

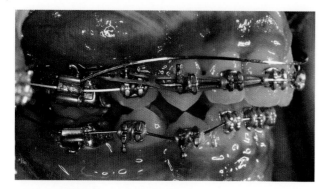

Figure 9.38 Right buccal view of the dentition at the eighth appointment. The mandibular arch wire was changed to .016 nickel-titanium to engage the newly bonded second molars and right canine.

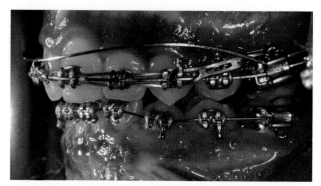

Figure 9.39 Left buccal view of the dentition at the eighth appointment.

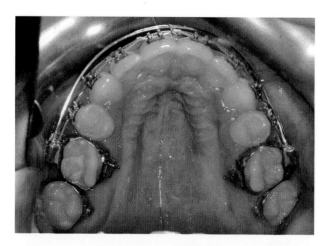

Figure 9.40 Occlusal view of the maxillary arch at the eighth appointment. Note the improvement in the position of the second molars and temporary placement of glass ionomer overlays on the palatal cusps of the molars.

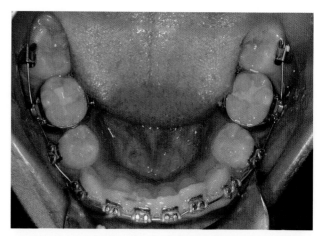

Figure 9.41 Occlusal view of the mandibular arch at the eighth appointment with the newly bonded second molars and right canine.

Ninth Active Appointment

Five weeks later, the occlusal build-up of the palatal cusps of the maxillary first molars was removed. The maxillary base arch was changed to .017 × .025 nickel-titanium and the same intrusion arch overlay was ligated between the maxillary central incisors. The mandibular arch wire was changed to a .016 × .022 nickel-titanium wire. Elastomeric chains were placed between the maxillary canines for space consolidation and from the maxillary canines and first molars to complete retraction. An additional elastomeric chain was attached lingually between the maxillary first and second molars for alignment of the second molars. The patient was required to wear Class II elastics (3/16″, 4.5 oz.) from the maxillary canines to the mandibular first molars for the overjet correction and attainment of a Class I relationship (Figures 9.42–9.46).

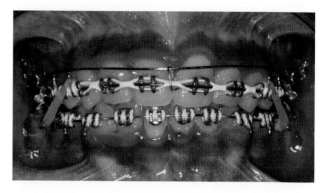

Figure 9.42 Anterior view of the dentition 5 weeks later. The maxillary arch wire was changed to .017 × .025 nickel-titanium with the same stainless steel overlay. The mandibular arch wire was changed to .016 × .022 nickel-titanium. The glass ionomer overlays on the maxillary molars have been removed. Note the improvement in the overbite relationship.

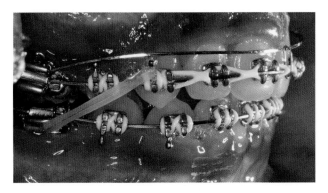

Figure 9.43 Right buccal view of the dentition 5 weeks later. Class II elastics were being worn to improve the overjet and Class I relationship.

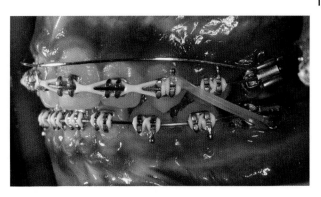

Figure 9.44 Left buccal view of the dentition 5 weeks later. Class II elastics were being worn to improve the overjet and Class I relationship.

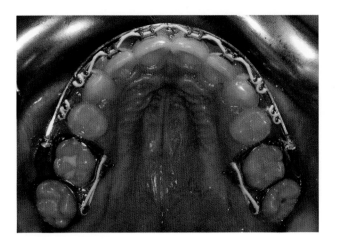

Figure 9.45 Occlusal view of the maxillary arch 5 weeks later. Elastomeric chain was being used on the lingual of first and second molars to gain improved alignment.

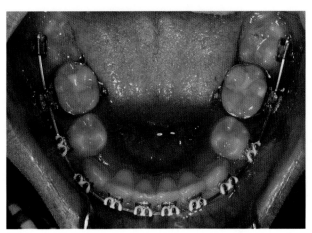

Figure 9.46 Occlusal view of the mandibular arch 5 weeks later. Note the improved arch form.

Tenth Active Appointment

Four weeks later, it was realized that compliance with the Class II elastics was poor. It was stressed that these elastics must be worn full-time or the overjet correction would not be achieved. The crossbite of the second molars was corrected. The maxillary intrusion arch was removed. Elastomeric chain was placed from maxillary first molar to maxillary first molar for final space consolidation (Figures 9.47–9.51).

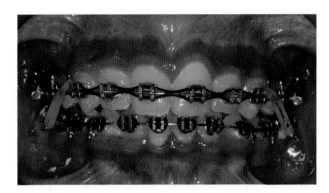

Figure 9.47 Anterior view of the dentition 4 weeks after the previous appointment. The intrusive overlay arch wire has been removed.

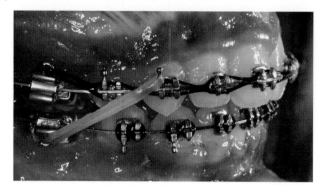

Figure 9.48 Right buccal view of the dentition 4 weeks after the previous appointment.

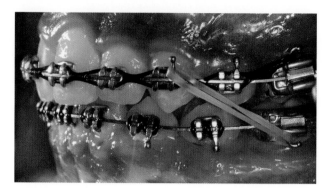

Figure 9.49 Left buccal view of the dentition 4 weeks after the previous appointment.

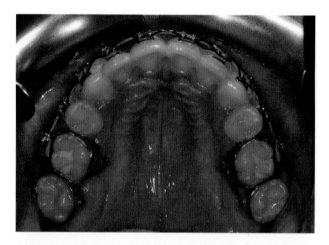

Figure 9.50 Occlusal view of the maxillary arch 4 weeks after the previous appointment.Note the improved positions of the first and second molars.

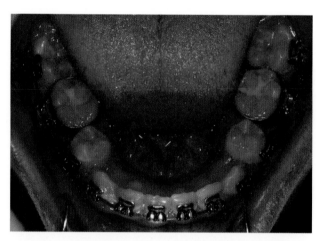

Figure 9.51 Occlusal view of the mandibular arch 4 weeks after the previous appointment.

Eleventh Active Appointment

Six weeks later, it was decided to place Forsus (3 M Unitek, Monrovia, CA, USA) springs to aid in the Class II correction as the patient's compliance with elastic wear was poor. Both maxillary and mandibular arch wires were changed to .017 × .025 stainless steel to maintain rigidity and prevent the Forsus springs from distorting the arch forms. Elastomeric chains were placed from the maxillary first molar to the maxillary first molar and from the mandibular first molar to the mandibular first molar. A 25 mm Forsus spring was placed bilaterally (Figures 9.52–9.54).

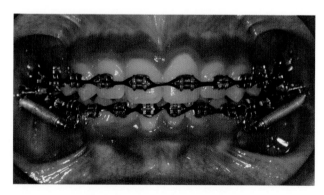

Figure 9.52 Anterior view of the dentition 6 weeks later. Both the maxillary and mandibular arch wires have been changed to .017 × .025 stainless steel. Elastomeric chain was placed from first molar to first molar to consolidate space.

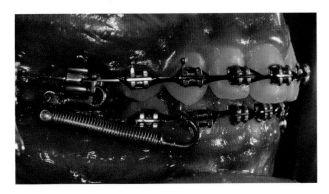

Figure 9.53 Right buccal view of the dentition 6 weeks later. The Forsus spring has been placed to improve the overjet and Class I relationship.

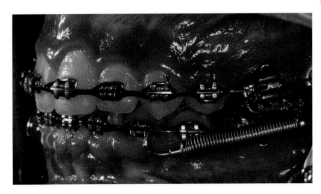

Figure 9.54 Left buccal view of the dentition 6 weeks later. The Forsus spring has been placed to improve the overjet and Class I relationship.

Twelfth Active Appointment

Four weeks later the same appliance and attachments were kept in place, but a 1 mm shim was added to the right spring rod to aid in the midline and Class II correction in the right quadrants (Figures 9.55–9.57).

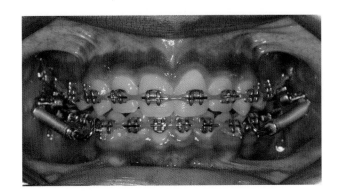

Figure 9.55 Anterior view of the dentition 4 weeks later.

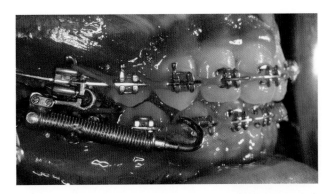

Figure 9.56 Right buccal view of the dentition 4 weeks later. A 1 mm shim has been added to the Forsus rod to increase spring length and to move the mandibular midline to the left.

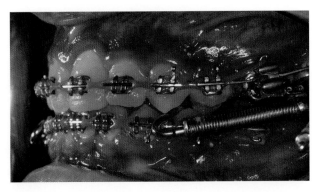

Figure 9.57 Left buccal view of the dentition 4 weeks later with Forsus spring in place.

Thirteenth Active Appointment

Six weeks later, the occlusion was over-corrected to an edge-to-edge position and the Forsus springs were removed. The maxillary arch wire was reformed with an accentuated curve of Spee for bite opening. The mandibular arch wire was changed to .017×.025 nickel-titanium. Elastomeric chain was continued from first molar to first molar in both arches. The patient was instructed to wear triangle elastics from the maxillary canines to the mandibular canines and second premolars (3/15", 4.5 oz.) for settling of the occlusion (Figures 9.58–9.60).

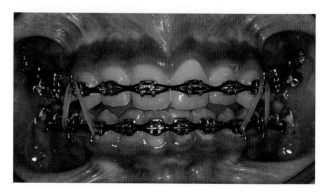

Figure 9.58 Anterior view of the dentition 6 weeks later with an over-corrected overjet relationship. The Forsus springs have been removed. Triangle elastics were being used to settle the occlusion.

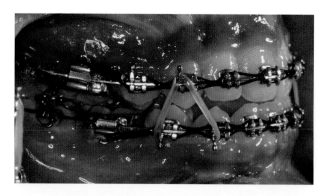

Figure 9.59 Right buccal view of the dentition 6 weeks later exhibiting an overcorrected overjet and edge to edge overbite relationship. The triangle elastic was being used to improve intercuspation.

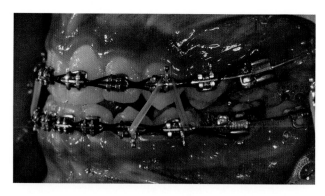

Figure 9.60 Left buccal view of the dentition 6 weeks later exhibiting an over-corrected overjet and edge-to-edge overbite relationship. The triangle elastic was being used to improve intercuspation.

Fourteenth Active Appointment

Six weeks later a progress panoramic radiograph was taken (Figure 9.61). As a result of the radiographic interpretation of root positions, it was decided to reposition the mandibular right lateral incisor, mandibular left central incisor, and both mandibular canines for better root alignment. The maxillary arch wire was sectioned distal to the lateral incisors and a .016 nickel-titanium wire was ligated to the mandibular teeth. An elastomeric chain

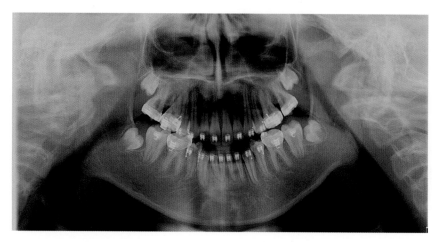

Figure 9.61 Progress panoramic radiograph 6 weeks after the previous appointment. All root lengths appear normal. The mandibular right lateral incisor root position is still in need of improvement.

was placed from maxillary lateral incisor to lateral incisor. The patient was instructed to wear settling elastics (3/8", 4.5 oz.) to finalize the occlusion. The wearing of these elastics was stressed because compliance with the Class II elastics was poor (Figures 9.62–9.64).

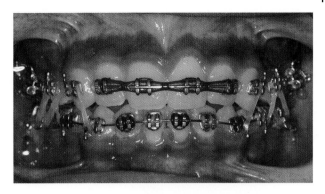

Figure 9.62 Anterior view of the dentition 6 weeks after the previous appointment. The maxillary arch wire was sectioned distal to the lateral incisors, and elastomeric chain was placed to maintain space closure.

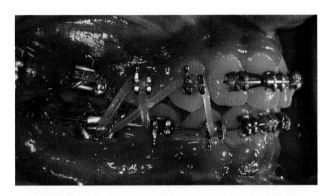

Figure 9.63 Right buccal view of the dentition 6 weeks after the previous appointment. Settling elastics were used to improve intercuspation.

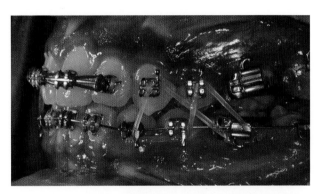

Figure 9.64 Left buccal view of the dentition 6 weeks after the previous appointment. Settling elastics were used to improve intercuspation.

Fifteenth to 17th Active Appointments

The patient was unable to wear the settling elastics for the previous 4 weeks. For the following 8 weeks the patient was given triangle elastics (3/16", 6 oz.) from the maxillary canines to the mandibular canines and second premolars which he found to be more tolerant to insert. The maxillary arch wire was changed to .016 × .022 nickel-titanium and the mandibular arch wire was changed to .016 × .022 reverse curve nickel-titanium to maintain bite opening.

Eighteenth Appointment

The patient was debonded and impressions were taken for delivery of immediate Essix retainers (DENTSPLY Raintree Essix, Sarasota, FL, USA). Instructions were given for the retainers to be worn in the evenings and while sleeping. Photographs and a final cephalometric radiograph were taken (Figures 9.65–9.73). An iTero scan (Align Technology, Inc, San Jose, CA, USA) of the occlusion was to be taken 1 month after the gingiva had time to improve and retainer compliance was evaluated. Treatment time required was 74 weeks.

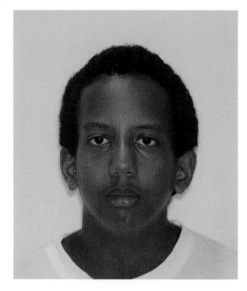

Figure 9.65 Full-face view 12 weeks after the previous appointment and with the appliances removed.

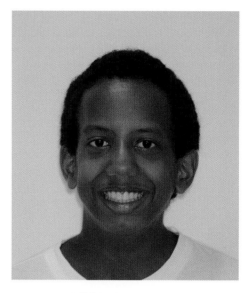

Figure 9.66 Full-face view with smile twelve weeks after the previous appointment.

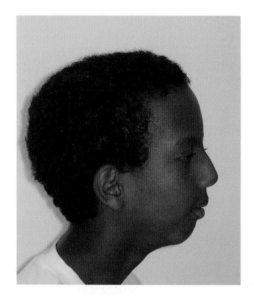

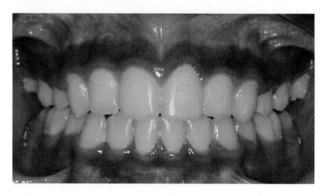

Figure 9.68 Anterior view of the dentition at the completion of treatment with an improved alignment, overbite, and overjet relationship.

Figure 9.67 Lateral view of the right profile 12 weeks after the previous appointment and at the completion of treatment. The deficient chin projection is still apparent.

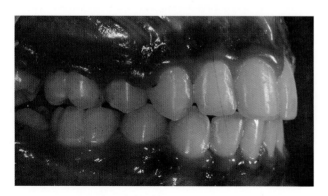

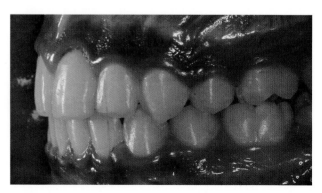

Figure 9.69 Right buccal view of the dentition at the completion of treatment, demonstrating a Class I molar and canine relationship and improved overbite and overjet.

Figure 9.70 Left buccal view of the dentition at the completion of treatment demonstrating a Class I molar and canine relationship and improved overbite and overjet.

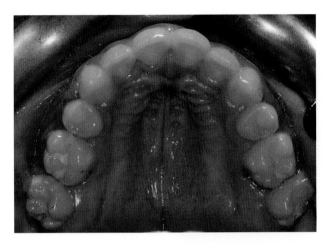

Figure 9.71 Occlusal view of the maxillary arch at the completion of treatment demonstrating an improved arch form.

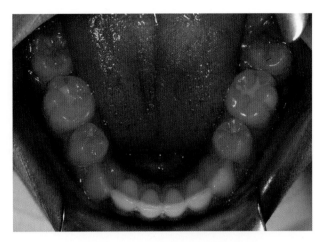

Figure 9.72 Occlusal view of the mandibular arch at the completion of treatment demonstrating an improved arch form.

Upon measurement, growth over the treatment time was predominantly in a vertical direction. As a result of treatment, the occlusal plane tipped down anteriorly, which improved the WITS appraisal, while the mandibular incisor was flared. The majority of space closure was the result of posterior protraction. Soft tissue analysis remained the same, as the patient would still benefit from a genioplasty because the chin projection was deficient (Table 9.3; Figures 9.73 and 9.74).

Commentary

During the course of treatment, there were no side-effects to the TMJ and the patient did not require supportive therapy as the result of the extractions and dental movements. The left joint continued to make sounds upon movement and slight crepitus was observed, but no pain was involved. The overall esthetic result may be improved with a genioplasty due to an insufficient chin projection once the patient completes growth.

Table 9.3 Significant pre-treatment and post-treatment cephalometric values

	Norm	Pre-treatment	Post-treatment
SNA	82°	73.4°	74.0°
SNB	80°	68.2°	68.9°
ANB	2°	+5.2°	+5.1°
WITS appraisal	−1 to +1 mm	+10.0 mm	+4.4 mm
FMA	21°	35.4°	33.8°
SN-GoGn	32°	40.4°	40.0°
Maxillary incisor to SN	105°	97.5°	94.6°
Mandibular incisor to GoGn	95°	87.1°	100.6°
Soft tissue			
Lower lip to E-plane	−2.0 mm	+5.8 mm	+5.6 mm
Upper lip to E-plane	−1.6 mm	+2.9 mm	+4.1 mm

SNA, sella-nasion-A point; SNB, sella-nasion-B point; ANB, A point-nasion-B point; WITS appraisal, Witwatersrand appraisal; FMA, Frankfort horizontal-mandibular plane; SN-GoGn, sella nasion-gonion gnathion.

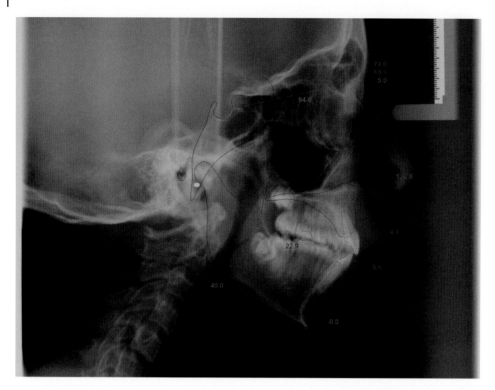

Figure 9.73 Digitized cephalogram at the completion of treatment with an improved skeletal and incisal relationship.

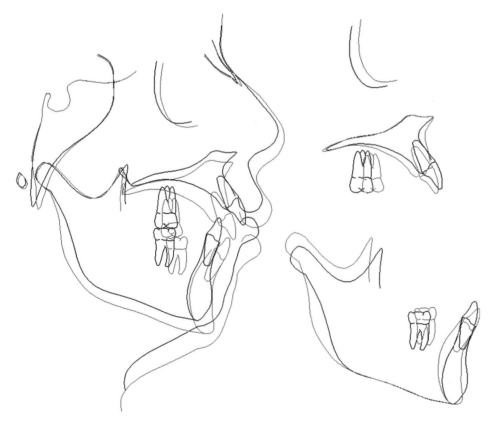

Figure 9.74 The overall skeletal changes were vertical (initial, black; final, red) with the mandible predominantly moving downward due to the vertical growth pattern. Regional changes indicated flaring of the mandibular incisor and overall maintenance of the maxillary incisor angulation.

Review Questions

1 How was the midline shift to the mandibular dentition accomplished?

2 What was the purpose of adding glass ionomer to the maxillary molar palatal cusps?

3 What method of therapy was used to help in the correction of the deep overbite relationship?

4 The lack of compliance with Class II elastics resulted in what type of appliance placement?

Suggested References

Gianelly AA. Treatment of crowding in the mixed dentition. Am J Orthod Dentofac Orthop 121(6): 569–571, 2002.

Proffit WR, Fields HW Jr, Sarver DM. Orthodontic treatment planning: From problem list to specific plan. In: Proffit WR, Fields HW Jr, Sarver DM eds. Contemporary Orthodontics, 5th edn. St Louis, MO: Mosby, 2012; pp. 220–275.

10

Class III Skeletal Tendency and Class I Dental: Four Premolar Extractions

---

LEARNING OBJECTIVES

- Precautionary measures to be taken with Class III tendencies
- Anchorage requirements with high angle cases
- Prevention of round tripping or guarding against root resorption

---

Interview Data

The parent's chief complaint was that they believe their 10-year-old daughter needed braces; the patient "does not like the way my teeth look."

- Development: pre-pubescent
- Motivation: good, but non-talkative
- Medical history: non-contributory
- Dental history: seen in a pediatric dentistry clinic for care
- Family history: no malocclusion seen in family
- Habits: none
- Facial form: ovoid, symmetric leptoprosopic facial form
- Facial proportions: long lower face

Clinical Examination

- Incisor-stomion (Figures 10.1 and 10.2):
  - At rest: 2 mm
  - Smiling: 5 mm
- Breathing: nasal
- Lips: together at rest
- Severe crowding with space maintainers in place
- Soft tissue profile: convex (Figure 10.3)
- Nasolabial angle: obtuse
- High mandibular plane angle

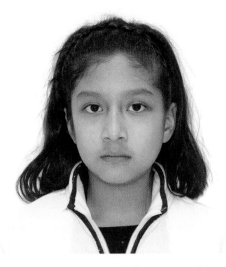

Figure 10.1 Full face at rest displaying an ovoid, long symmetric form.

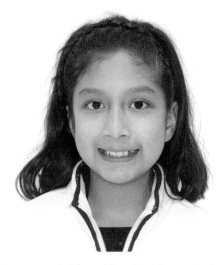

Figure 10.2 Full face with smile without a gingival display.

Atlas of Orthodontic Case Reviews, First Edition. Marjan Askari and Stanley A. Alexander.
© 2017 John Wiley & Sons, Inc. Published 2017 by John Wiley & Sons, Inc.

- Anterior crossbite: none
- Posterior crossbite: none

Right Buccal View (Figure 10.5)

- Molar: Class I
- Curve of Spee: flat
- Crossbite: none
- Caries: none

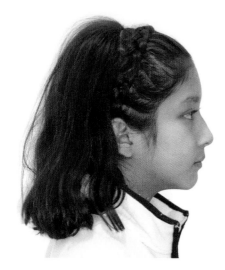

Figure 10.3 Right lateral view of profile exhibiting a mild convex profile and obtuse nasolabial angle.

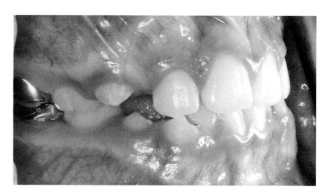

Figure 10.5 Right buccal view of the dentition displaying a Class I molar relationship and flat curve of Spee in the mixed dentition.

Dentition (Figure 10.4)

- Teeth clinically present

6e421	124e6
6e4321	1234e6

- Late mixed dentition
- Overjet: 2 mm
- Overbite: 5 mm
- Midlines: maxillary midline coincident with face; mandibular midline 1 mm shifted to left

Left Buccal View (Figure 10.6)

- Molar: Class I
- Curve of Spee: flat
- Crossbite: none
- Caries: none

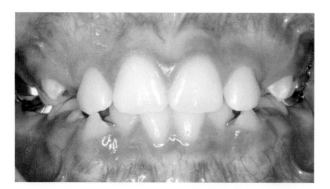

Figure 10.4 Anterior view of the dentition with the maxillary midline coincident with the face and the mandibular midline 1 mm to the left. The overbite is 5 mm and the overjet is 2 mm.

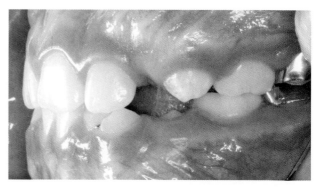

Figure 10.6 Left buccal view of the dentition displaying a Class I molar relationship and flat curve of Spee in the mixed dentition.

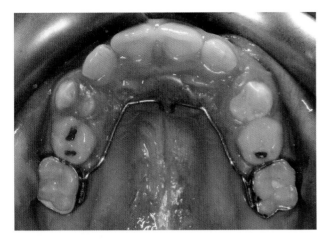

Figure 10.7 Occlusal view of the maxillary arch with a U-shaped arch form and Nance appliance in place.

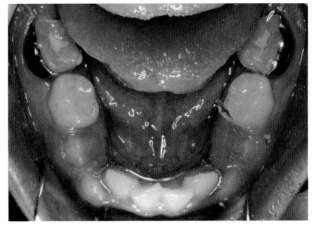

Figure 10.8 Occlusal view of the mandibular arch with a tapered U-shaped arch form and lingual holding arch in place.

Maxillary Arch (Figure 10.7)
- U-shaped arch form
- No caries
- Nance appliance in place

Mandibular Arch (Figure 10.8)
- Tapered U-shaped arch form
- Crowded incisors
- Lingual arch in place

Function

- Normal range of motion without pain
- Centric relation-centric occlusion: coincident
- Maximum opening: 45 mm
- Right excursive: 7 mm
- Left excursive: 9 mm
- Protrusive: 6 mm
- Late mixed dentition with development of second molars
- Root lengths and periodontium appear normal for the patient's age
- Condyles appear normal
- Maxillary and mandibular space maintainers are in place (Figure 10.9)

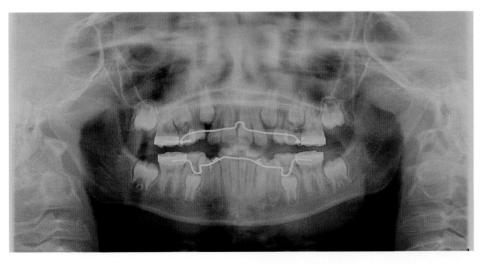

Figure 10.9 Panoramic radiograph displaying a late mixed dentition with normal root formation, tooth development, and space maintainers in place.

Diagnosis and Treatment Plan

The patient displays a Class I late mixed dentition with severe crowding and a Class III hyperdivergent skeletal pattern (Tables 10.1 and 10.2; Figure 10.10). The correction of the orthodontic problem will be comprehensive, incorporating a four first premolar extraction protocol, while also monitoring the Class III skeletal growth.

Table 10.1 Significant cephalometric values

	Norm	Patient pre-treatment
SNA	80°	77.6°
SNB	78°	75.4°
ANB	2°	+2.2°
WITS appraisal	−1 to +1 mm	−5.0 mm
FMA	21°	28.3°
SN-GoGn	32°	45.9°
Maxillary incisor to SN	105°	95.3°
Mandibular incisor to GoGn	95°	83.4°
Soft tissue		
Lower lip to E-plane	−2 mm	−1.2 mm
Upper lip to E-plane	−1.6 mm	−1.4 mm

SNA, sella-nasion-A point; SNB, sella-nasion-B point; ANB, A point-nasion-B point; WITS appraisal, Witwatersrand appraisal; FMA, Frankfort horizontal-mandibular plane; SN-GoGn, sella nasion-gonion gnathion.

Table 10.2 The patient's problem list in three dimensions

	Transverse	Sagittal	Vertical
Soft tissue	Normal	Convex profile; obtuse nasolabial angle	Hyperdivergent
Dental	Severe crowding	Normal late mixed dentition relationship of molars with crowding	5 mm overbite
Skeletal	Normal	Class III	Hyperdivergent

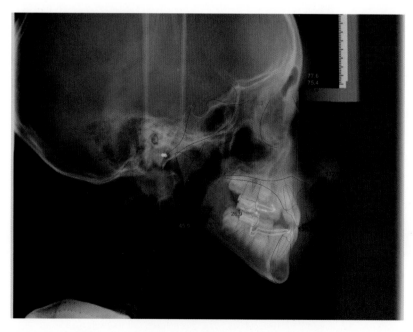

Figure 10.10 Digitized cephalogram exhibiting a Class III skeletal pattern, high mandibular plane angle, and upright maxillary and mandibular incisors.

Treatment Objectives

The parent's and patient's chief complaint will be addressed by the correction of the severely crowded dentition through the implementation of symmetric extractions of the four first premolars. As the patient is also hyperdivergent, the extraction of premolars will reduce the facial convexity and lead to a more stable incisor and soft tissue relationship without the flaring of teeth. The Class III skeletal growth pattern will also be monitored and treated if necessary (Figures 10.11 and 10.12).

Treatment Options

1) No treatment at this time – treatment to begin once the full permanent dentition is erupted.
2) Treatment as indicated with the extraction of the four first premolars.
3) Non-extraction treatment with air-rotor stripping of the dentition to alleviate the crowding.

The patient and parent both chose option 2. The possibility that the Class III growth pattern would interfere with this course of treatment was discussed. A surgical course of treatment would be implemented if conventional orthodontic treatment was unable to correct this additional problem.

Passive Appointments

One week prior to band fitting and impressions, elastic separators were placed mesial to the maxillary and mandibular molars. Bands were fitted and impressions were taken for fabrication of a lower lingual holding arch and a passive Hyrax appliance with soldered hooks to support a reverse pull face mask if needed during treatment due to the Class III tendency.

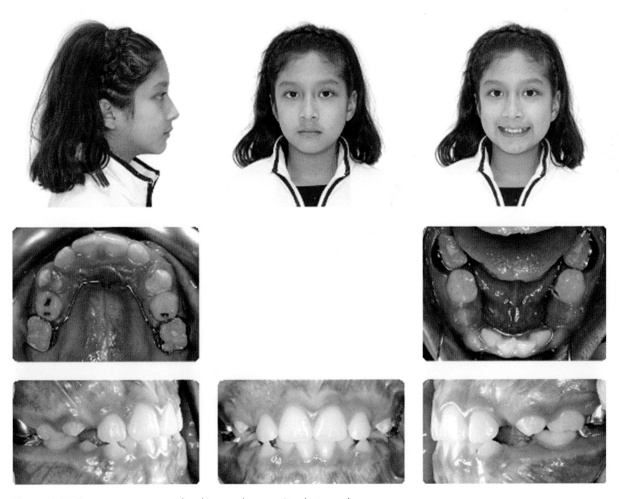

Figure 10.11 Pre-treatment extraoral and intraoral composite photograph.

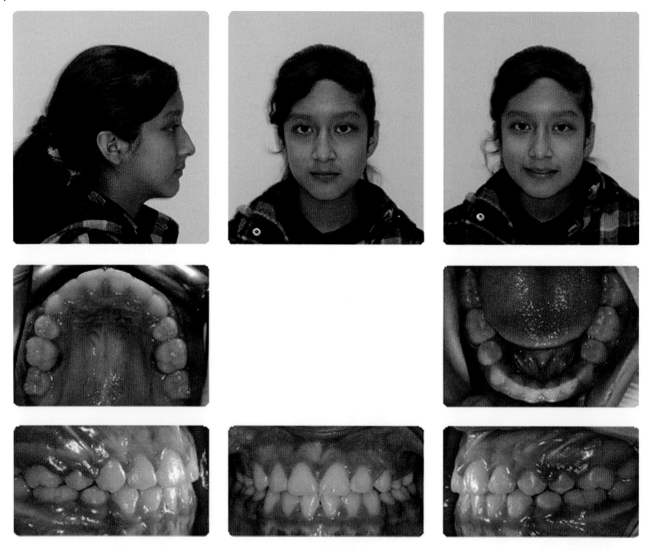

Figure 10.12 Post-treatment extraoral and intraoral composite photograph.

First Active Appointment

The Hyrax appliance and lower lingual holding arch were cemented. The maxillary incisors and the mandibular canines and incisors were bonded with bi-dimensional brackets. At the same visit, all four first premolars were extracted. A maxillary .016 nickel-titanium arch wire and mandibular .017 × .025 nickel-titanium were ligated with figure 8 elastomeric ties. The maxillary arch wire was offset in the midline to prevent wire slippage through the buccal tubes (arrow in Figure 10.13). An elastomeric chain was attached to the mandibular molars and canines for canine retraction. A bumper sleeve was inserted over the mandibular arch wire between the right and left canines for comfort and to avoid flaring of the lower incisors which were not ligated to the arch wire

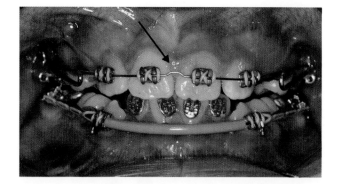

Figure 10.13 Anterior view of the dentition with initial bonding with bi-dimensional brackets and cementation of a Hyrax appliance and lingual holding arch. The maxillary arch wire (arrow) has been offset to prevent the wire slipping through the molar buccal tubes and the mandibular incisors have been bypassed to prevent "round tripping" of the roots during treatment.

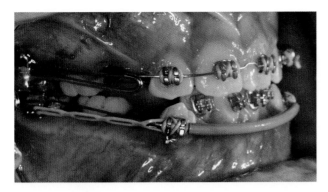

Figure 10.14 Right buccal view of the dentition on the day of appliance placement. The maxillary arch wire was .016 nickel-titanium and the mandibular arch wire was .017×.025 nickel-titanium. The mandibular canine was being retracted with elastomeric chain.

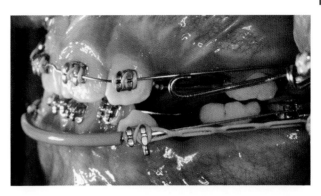

Figure 10.15 Left buccal view of the dentition on the day of appliance placement. The maxillary arch wire was .016 nickel-titanium and the mandibular arch wire was .017×.025 nickel-titanium. The mandibular canine was being retracted with elastomeric chain.

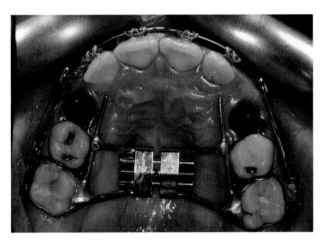

Figure 10.16 Occlusal view of the maxillary arch on the day of appliance placement. The Hyrax appliance with buccal hooks is in place in case a reverse pull face mask is required later in treatment. Note the extraction sites of the first premolars which were performed at this appointment.

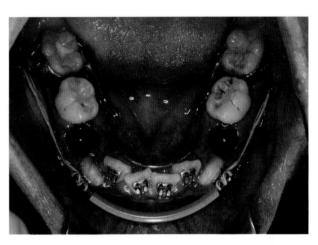

Figure 10.17 Occlusal view of the mandibular arch on the day of appliance placement. Note the extraction sites of the first premolars and the bypass of the incisors as the canines are being retracted.

(Figures 10.13–10.17). The non-ligation of the mandibular incisors at this early stage in treatment had three purposes: it would prevent the labialization of the incisors if the Class III tendency further expressed itself; it would prevent round tripping and possible root resorption as a result, if the lower incisors were in need of retraction; and it would allow the natural unraveling of the incisors as the canines were being retracted.

Second Active Appointment

One month later, the patient returned and the arch wires were re-tied with figure 8 elastomeric ties and elastomeric chain was re-attached to the mandibular canines and molars (Figures 10.18 and 10.19). Note the soft tissue healing of the extraction sites when compared with Figures 10.16 and 10.17.

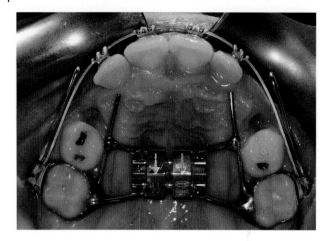

Figure 10.18 Occlusal view of the maxillary arch 1 month later. Note the healed extraction sites.

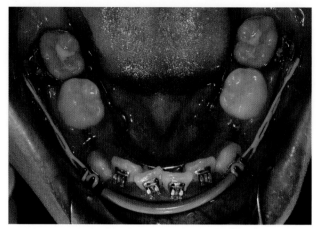

Figure 10.19 Occlusal view of the mandibular arch 1 month later. Note the healed extraction sites and initial retraction of the left canine.

Third Active Appointment

Six weeks later, the mandibular canines were retracted sufficiently to unravel the four incisors, which were now ligated to the arch wire. Closed coil springs were placed between the mandibular molars and canines to maintain the space. The maxillary incisors were consolidated with elastomeric chain (Figures 10.20–10.24).

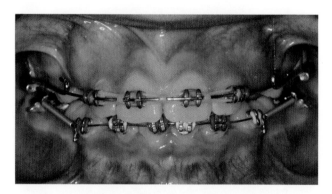

Figure 10.20 Anterior view of the dentition 6 weeks later. The mandibular incisors have now been engaged. Elastomeric chain was placed on the maxillary incisors for space consolidation.

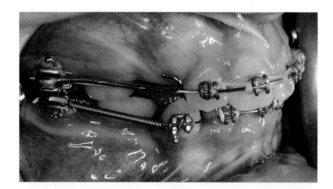

Figure 10.21 Right buccal view of the dentition 6 weeks later. The mandibular canine has been retracted sufficiently to allow alignment of the incisors. A closed coil spring has been placed to maintain the space.

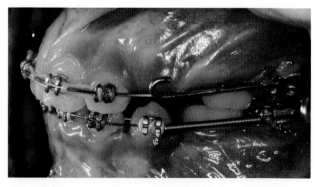

Figure 10.22 Left buccal view of the dentition 6 weeks later. The mandibular canine has been retracted sufficiently to allow alignment of the incisors. A closed coil spring has been placed to maintain the space.

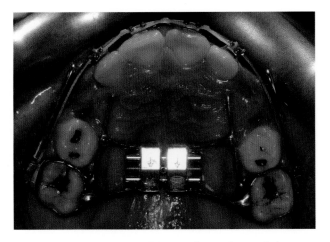

Figure 10.23 Occlusal view of the maxillary arch 6 weeks later.

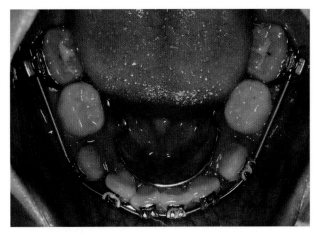

Figure 10.24 Occlusal view of the mandibular arch 6 weeks later. Note the incisal engagement and the prior retraction of the canines.

Fourth Active Appointment

Six weeks later, the maxillary arch wire was changed to a .017 × .025 nickel-titanium wire. The face mask hooks were removed as they were unnecessary at this stage of treatment. An elastomeric chain was placed on the maxillary left molar and four incisors to consolidate space and to shift the midline to the patient's left. A closed coil spring was also placed in the maxillary left quadrant to allow for a precise shift to the left once the midline was established. The mandibular arch wire remained the same with the closed coil springs still in place and the incisors and canines ligated. Note the alignment of the anterior segment (Figures 10.25–10.29).

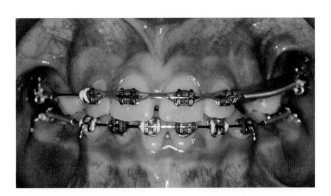

Figure 10.25 Anterior view of the dentition at the fourth active appointment. The maxillary arch wire was changed to .017×.025 nickel-titanium. An elastomeric chain was placed from the maxillary right lateral incisor to the left first molar to shift the midline. A closed coil spring was placed in the maxillary left quadrant to allow precision space closure.

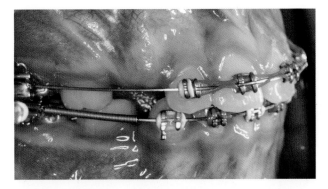

Figure 10.26 Right buccal view of the dentition at the fourth active appointment.

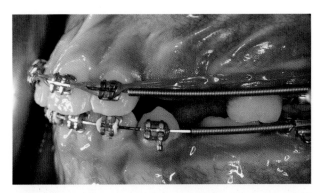

Figure 10.27 Left buccal view of the dentition at the fourth active appointment.

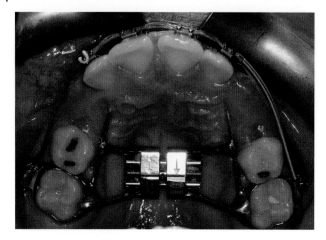

Figure 10.28 Occlusal view of the maxillary arch at the fourth active appointment. The buccal hooks have been removed from the Hyrax appliance.

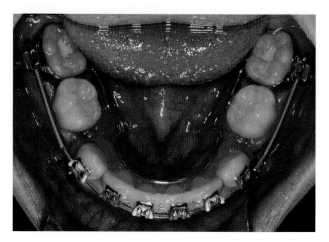

Figure 10.29 Occlusal view of the mandibular arch at the fourth active appointment. Note the improved arch form.

Fifth Active Appointment

For the next 4 months the same mechanics were employed to shift the maxillary midline. During this time, the second primary molars were exfoliated and the erupting second premolars were bonded. The Hyrax appliance and lower lingual holding arch were removed and new molar bands were cemented. A .016 nickel-titanium arch wire was placed in the maxillary arch and ligated with elastomeric chain to consolidate the incisors. A .018 nickel-titanium arch wire was ligated to the mandibular teeth (Figures 10.30–10.34).

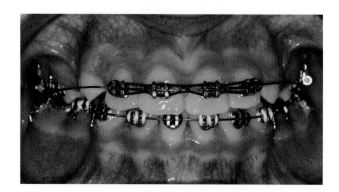

Figure 10.30 Anterior view of the dentition 4 months later. Elastomeric chain was being used to consolidate space while waiting for the exfoliation of the remaining primary teeth.

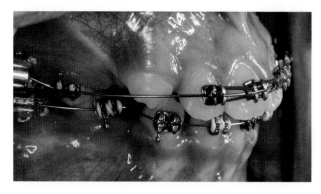

Figure 10.31 Right buccal view of the dentition 4 months later.

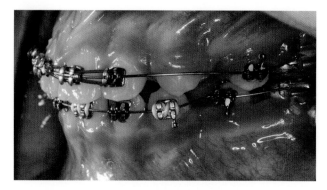

Figure 10.32 Left buccal view of the dentition 4 months later.

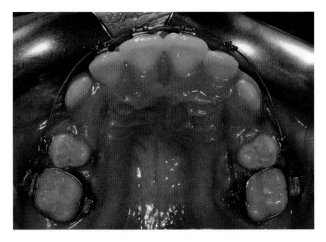

Figure 10.33 Occlusal view of the maxillary arch 4 months later. The Hyrax appliance was removed, new molar bands were cemented and a .016 nickel-titanium arch wire was placed.

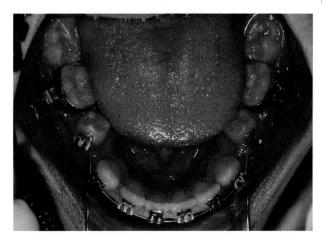

Figure 10.34 Occlusal view of the mandibular arch 4 months later. The lingual arch has been removed and new molar bands have been cemented. The second premolars were bonded and were being rotated to correct position with a .018 nickel-titanium arch wire.

Sixth to Eighth Active Appointments

One month later, both the upper and lower arch wires were changed to .016 × .022 nickel-titanium arch wires. The maxillary canines were bonded during the eight appointment. Triangle elastics (3/16", 4 oz.) were placed from the maxillary canines to the mandibular canines and second premolars and the patient was instructed to change the elastics daily. These were used to settle the occlusion during active alignment (Figures 10.35–10.39).

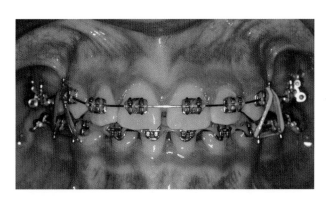

Figure 10.35 Anterior view of the dentition 4 weeks later. Both maxillary and mandibular arch wires were changed to .016 × .022 nickel-titanium.

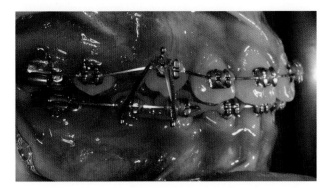

Figure 10.36 Right buccal view of the dentition 4 weeks later. The triangle elastic was being used to settle the occlusion.

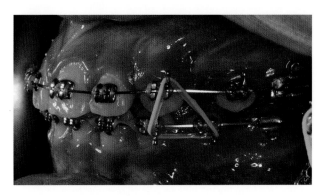

Figure 10.37 Left buccal view of the dentition 4 weeks later. The triangle elastic was being used to settle the occlusion.

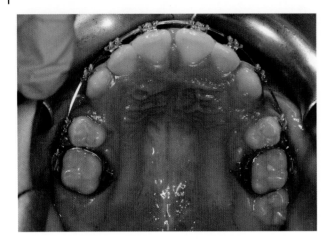

Figure 10.38 Occlusal view of the maxillary arch 4 weeks later.

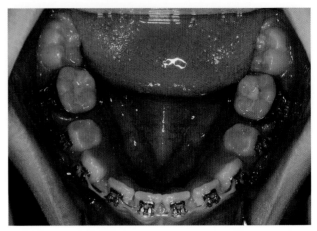

Figure 10.39 Occlusal view of the mandibular arch 4 weeks later. Elastomeric chain was used to consolidate space from canine to canine.

Ninth Active Appointment

One month later, both arch wires were changed to .017 × .025 nickel-titanium. Elastomeric chain was placed on the maxillary left canine to molar, maxillary left lateral incisor to the maxillary right central incisor, and the maxillary right canine and second premolar for space consolidation. Space closure and anterior anchorage of the mandibular arch were accomplished with elastomeric chain from the mandibular right canine to the mandibular left second premolar, and elastomeric chain from the right second premolar to the right canine. Triangle elastics were continued as previously instructed (Figures 10.40–10.44).

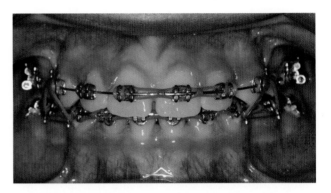

Figure 10.40 Anterior view of the dentition 4 weeks later. The maxillary and mandibular arch wires were changed to .017 × .025 nickel-titanium. Elastomeric chain was placed from maxillary right central incisor to left lateral incisor for space closure and midline correction.

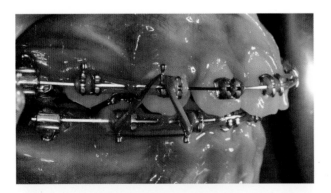

Figure 10.41 Right buccal view of the dentition 4 weeks later. Elastomeric chain was placed between the maxillary canine and second premolar for improved Class I canine position and space closure, and from the mandibular second premolar to second premolar for space closure. The triangle elastics have been continued.

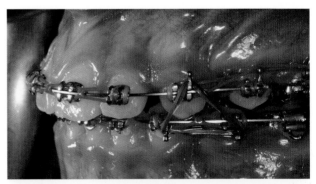

Figure 10.42 Left buccal view of the dentition 4 weeks later. Elastomeric chain was placed from the maxillary canine to the molar for space closure and improvement to the Class I canine position. Triangle elastics were continued.

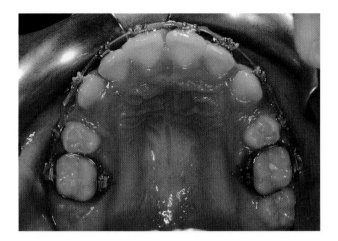

Figure 10.43 Occlusal view of the maxillary arch 4 weeks later.

Figure 10.44 Occlusal view of the mandibular arch 4 weeks later with space closure in progress.

Tenth to 11th Active Appointments

For the next 17 weeks, the patient was seen for two appointments. Elastomeric chain was continued for space closure, while the mandibular incisor brackets were repositioned upside down to reverse the torque expression of the brackets and to further labialize the crowns. A .017 × .025 β-titanium closing loop arch wire was ligated to the maxillary arch for anterior space closure. B-titanium wires are, on average, 40% less stiff than stainless steel wires of the same dimensions and have a greater range of activation. This wire was formed with an accentuated curve of Spee for improvement of the deep bite and to prevent further bite closure during retraction. Triangle elastics (3/16", 6 oz.) were continued from the mandibular first molars and second premolars to the maxillary canines in a Class II vector and for maintenance of the posterior bite closure (Figures 10.45–10.49).

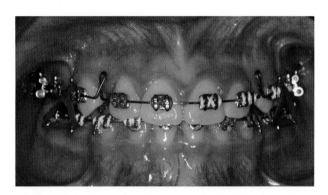

Figure 10.45 Anterior view of the dentition. For the next 17 weeks, space closure in the maxillary arch was accomplished with a .017 × .025 β-titanium closed loop arch wire.

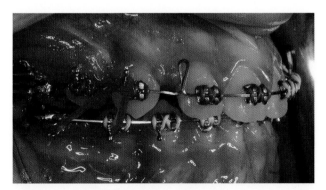

Figure 10.46 Right buccal view of the dentition over the 17-week period. Note the activity remaining in the looped arch wire with its legs criss-crossed. The triangle elastics were continued to help settle the occlusion.

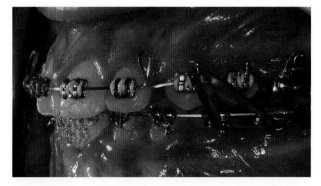

Figure 10.47 Left buccal view of the dentition over the 17-week period. Note the activity remaining in the looped arch wire with its legs criss-crossed. The triangle elastics were continued to help settle the occlusion.

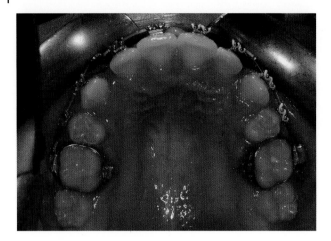

Figure 10.48 Occlusal view of the maxillary arch over the 17-week period exhibiting space closure.

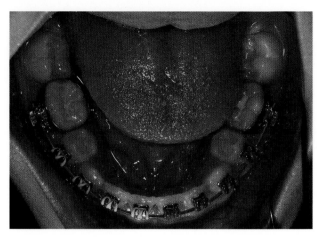

Figure 10.49 Occlusal view of the mandibular arch over the 17-week period exhibiting space closure.

Twelfth to 13th Active Appointments

For the next 12 weeks, anterior space closure was accomplished and the deep overbite improved. The maxillary closing loop arch wire was replaced with a .017 × .025 nickel-titanium wire and elastomeric chain was used to close the remaining posterior spaces. Triangle elastics were placed on the right mandibular canine and second premolar and maxillary canine and Class II elastics on the left mandibular first molar and left maxillary canine (3/16", 6 oz.) (Figures 10.50–10.54).

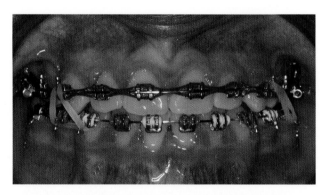

Figure 10.50 Anterior view of the dentition over the next 12 weeks. The maxillary arch wire was changed to .017 × .025 nickel-titanium. The remainder of maxillary space was closed with elastomeric chain from first molar to first molar. Note the improvement in the overbite relationship.

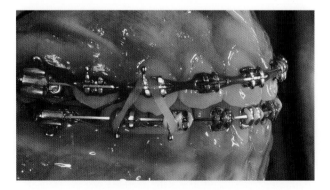

Figure 10.51 Right buccal view of the dentition over the next 12 weeks. The molar and canine are Class I. The triangle elastic was still used for improvement in the intercuspation.

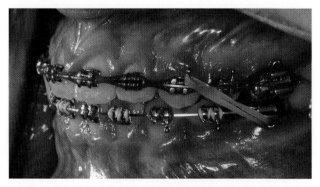

Figure 10.52 Left buccal view of the dentition over the next 12 weeks. The Class II elastic was being used to perfect the Class I relationship.

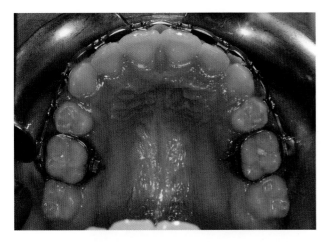

Figure 10.53 Occlusal view of the maxillary arch over the next 12 weeks. Space consolidation was continued with elastomeric chain.

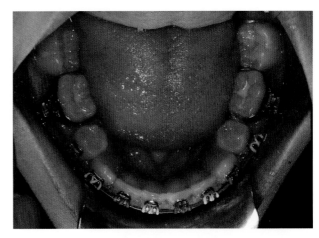

Figure 10.54 Occlusal view of the mandibular arch over the next 12 weeks.

Fourteenth Active Appointment

A progress panoramic radiograph was taken to evaluate root positioning and to identify any side-effects of space closure such as root resorption (Figure 10.55). Roots appeared upright and minimal resorption was noted on the maxillary incisors and the maxillary and mandibular second premolars. Elastomeric chains were placed in both the maxillary and mandibular arches from first molar to first molar to complete space closure. Triangle and Class II elastics were continued as previously instructed.

Fifteenth Active Appointment

One month later the patient was debonded, impressions taken for immediate Essix retainers (DENTSPLY Raintree Essix, Sarasota, FL, USA), and final records (photographs, cephalometric radiograph, and i-model records) were taken (Figures 10.56–10.63). The first molars and canines were corrected to a Class I relationship with a normal overjet and 2 mm overbite. Arch forms were broad and U-shaped. The patient was instructed to wear the retainers only at night and while

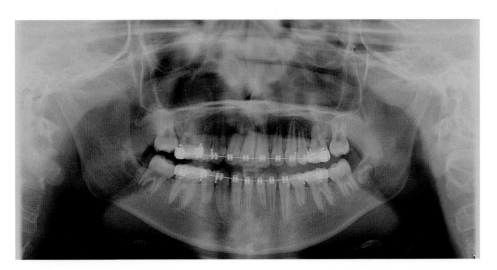

Figure 10.55 Panoramic radiograph at the 14th active appointment. There appears to be minimal root blunting of the incisors and mandibular second molars as a result of space closure.

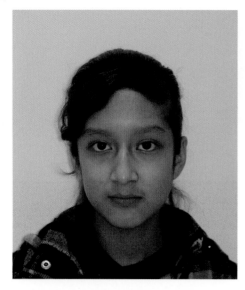

Figure 10.56 Full-face view at the time of appliance removal.

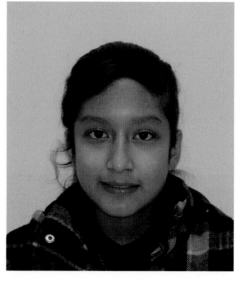

Figure 10.57 Full-face view with smile at the time of appliance removal.

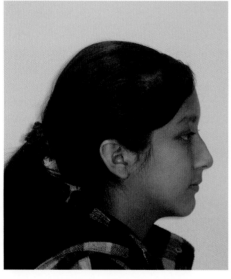

Figure 10.58 Right lateral view of profile displaying an esthetic result and mild facial convexity.

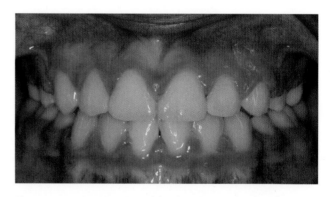

Figure 10.59 Anterior view of the dentition on the day of appliance removal. Note the improvement in the overbite and midline relationship.

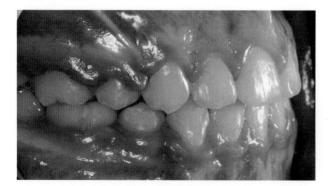

Figure 10.60 Right buccal view of the dentition on the day of appliance removal. Note the Class I molar and canine relationship.

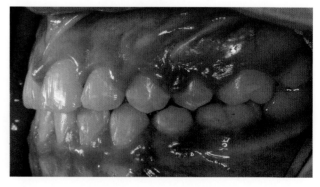

Figure 10.61 Left buccal view of the dentition on the day of appliance removal. Note the Class I molar and canine relationship.

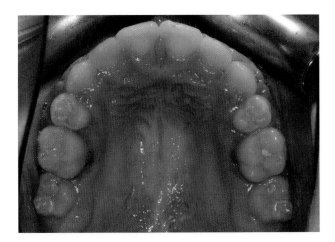

Figure 10.62 Occlusal view of the maxillary arch on the day of appliance removal.

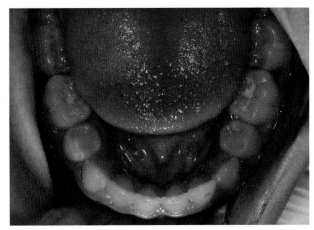

Figure 10.63 Occlusal view of the mandibular arch on the day of appliance removal.

sleeping. The occlusion was allowed to settle and function throughout the day. The patient was scheduled for a 1 month retainer check, followed by checks every 3 months for the first year post-treatment. The total treatment time was 23 months.

Upon measurement, there was an improvement in the WITS appraisal which decreased from −5.7 to −2.2 mm. Both the maxillary incisor angulation and mandibular incisor angulation improved from 91.5° to 103.6° and from 77.9° to 88.9°, respectively. Soft tissue measurements indicated an improvement of the lower lip position to the E-plane from −1.6 to −3.5 mm. All other measurements remained the same clinically (Figure 10.64; Table 10.3).

Overall superimposition of pre-treatment (black) and post-treatment (red) indicated that growth displacement of the skeleton and dentition occurred equally in a downward and forward direction (Figure 10.65). Regional superimposition of the maxilla indicated that the maxillary incisor was retracted and torqued to a proper position. The mandibular superimposition revealed that extraction space closure occurred by both anterior retraction and posterior protraction. The mandibular incisor angulation also improved.

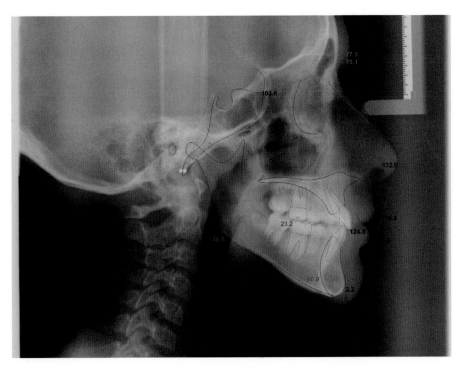

Figure 10.64 Digitized cephalogram on the day of appliance removal showing the improved skeletal, incisor, and soft tissue relationships.

Table 10.3 Significant pre-treatment and post-treatment cephalometric values

	Norm	Pre-treatment	Post-treatment
SNA	82°	78.6°	77.3°
SNB	80°	76.1°	75.1°
ANB	2°	+2.1°	+2.2°
WITS appraisal	−1 to +1 mm	−5.7 mm	−2.2 mm
FMA	21°	31.5°	32.4°
SN-GoGn	32°	45.7°	43.5°
Maxillary incisor to SN	105°	91.5°	103.6°
Mandibular incisor to GoGn	95°	77.9°	88.9°
Soft tissue			
Lower lip to E-plane	−2.0 mm	−1.6 mm	−3.5 mm
Upper lip to E-plane	−1.6 mm	−2.2 mm	−4.4 mm

SNA, sella-nasion-A point; SNB, sella-nasion-B point; ANB, A point-nasion-B point; WITS appraisal, Witwatersrand appraisal; FMA, Frankfort horizontal-mandibular plane; SN-GoGn, sella nasion-gonion gnathion.

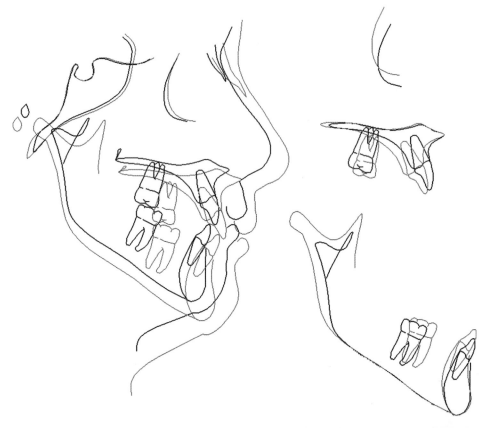

Figure 10.65 Overall superimposition (initial, black; final, red) indicated that growth occurred equally in the horizontal and vertical vectors. Regional superimposition indicated improved torque of the maxillary incisors and reciprocal space closure in the mandibular arch.

Commentary

This case represents a typical and straightforward approach to the extraction of four premolar teeth to resolve a malocclusion. Anecdotally, as well as evidence-based, in order to gain stability to the final result, the mandibular incisors were positioned upright in relation to the mandibular plane. This objective was due to the extreme vertical growth tendency of the patient rather than locating the incisors to a more angulated position as would be the case in patients with more average growth vector tendencies.

Review Questions

1 What qualities do β-titanium wires possess to make them ideal for use in space closure?

2 What type of movement to the dentition may be achieved with an accentuated curve of Spee to an arch wire placed in the maxilla?

3 What type of changes in the patient can be displayed with overall superimpositions of cephalometric tracings?

Suggested References

Krull JT, Krull GE, Dean JA. Cephalometrics and facial aesthetics: the key to complete treatment planning. In: McDonald and Avery's Dentistry for the Child and Adolescent, 10th edn. Elsevier, 2016; pp. 390–414.

Proffit WR. Mechanical principles in orthodontic force control. In: Proffit WR, Fields H, Sarver D, eds. Contemporary Orthodontics, 5th edn. CV Mosby Co., 2013; pp. 314–318.

Proffit WR. The second stage of comprehensive treatment. In: Proffit WR, Fields H, Sarver D, eds. Contemporary Orthodontics, 5th edn. CV Mosby Co., 2013; pp. 556–581.

11

Class III Skeletal and Class III Dental: Non-Extraction and Non-Surgical

LEARNING OBJECTIVES

- The problem list for Class III malocclusions
- The clinical and radiographic examination prior to treatment
- The development of treatment objectives and formation of a treatment plan
- The biomechanical plan
- The rationale and development of a retention plan for the correction of Class III malocclusions

Interview Data

- Development: post-pubescent
- Motivation: good
- Medical history: non-contributory
- Dental history: seen regularly for examinations
- Family history: no history of malocclusion
- Limitations: none
- Habits: none
- Facial form: mesoprosopic and ovoid
- Facial proportions: slightly decreased lower third

This 15-year-old Hispanic male wanted his teeth aligned, required orthognathic surgery that was recommended by a previous consult, but only wanted "braces." His past medical history was non-contributory and he had routine dental care.

Clinical Examination

- Incision-stomion (Figures 11.1 and 11.2):
  - At rest: 0 mm
  - Smiling: 9 mm

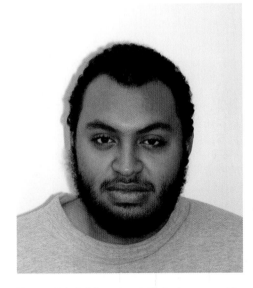

Figure 11.1 Full face at rest displaying an ovoid, symmetric face with full lips.

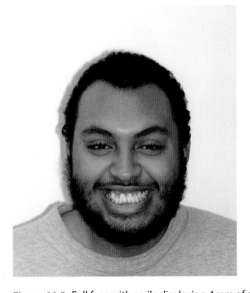

Figure 11.2 Full face with smile displaying 4 mm of gingiva.

Atlas of Orthodontic Case Reviews, First Edition. Marjan Askari and Stanley A. Alexander.
© 2017 John Wiley & Sons, Inc. Published 2017 by John Wiley & Sons, Inc.

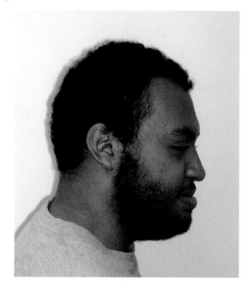

Figure 11.3 Right lateral view of profile exhibiting a concave form, acute nasolabial angle, and full lower lip.

- Smile line: 3 mm of gingival display
- Breathing: nasal
- Lips: together at rest
- Soft tissue profile: concave (Figure 11.3)
- Broad nose
- Acute nasolabial angle
- Prominent lower lip and chin
- Normal mandibular plane angle

Dentition (Figure 11.4)

- Teeth present clinically:

7654321	1234567
7654321	1234567

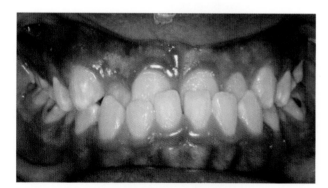

Figure 11.4 Anterior view of the dentition displaying an anterior crossbite, coincident midlines, and a 4 mm overbite.

- Overjet: −3 mm
- Overbite: 4 mm
- Midlines: coincident
- Rotated maxillary premolars

Right Buccal View (Figure 11.5)
- Molar: Class III
- Canine: Class III
- Curve of Spee: deep
- Crossbite: none
- Caries: none

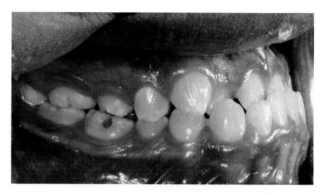

Figure 11.5 Right buccal view of the dentition displaying a Class III molar and canine relationship and deep curve of Spee.

Left Buccal View (Figure 11.6)
- Molar: Class III
- Canine: Class I
- Curve of Spee: deep
- Crossbite: none
- Caries: none

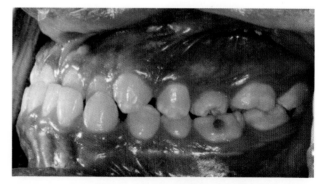

Figure 11.6 Left buccal view of the dentition displaying a Class III molar relationship, Class I canine relationship, and deep curve of Spee.

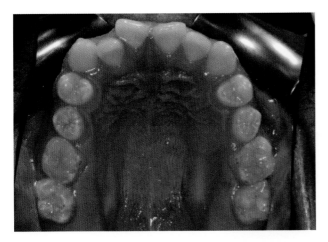

Figure 11.7 Occlusal view of the maxillary arch displaying an ovoid, symmetric arch form with crowding.

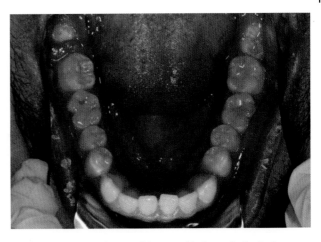

Figure 11.8 Occlusal view of the mandibular arch displaying a tapered, symmetric arch form.

Maxillary Arch (Figure 11.7)
- Symmetric, ovoid arch form with crowding
- No caries

Mandibular Arch (Figure 11.8)
- Tapered arch form and not coordinated with maxillary form
- Incisor rotations with spacing distal to canines
- No caries

Function

- Maximum opening = 45 mm
- Centric relation-centric occlusion = 2 mm
- Maximum excursive movements: right = 7 mm; left = 10 mm; protrusive = 4 mm
- Temporomandibular joint palpation: normal
- Right and left masseter: negative to palpation
- Habits: none
- Speech: normal
- All 32 teeth are present (Figure 11.9)
- Root length, periodontium, and bony architecture are normal
- Condyles appear normal

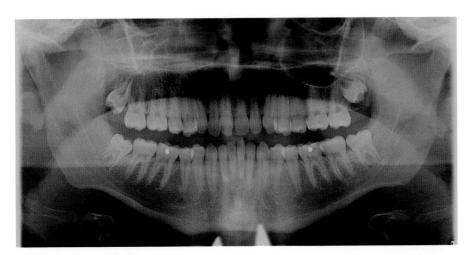

Figure 11.9 Panoramic radiograph exhibiting an adult dentition with all third molars erupting or developing. The condyles, periodontium and root lengths appear normal.

Diagnosis and Treatment Plan

As the molar relationship was Class III and the canine relationship closer to a Class I occlusion with a centric relation-centric occlusion discrepancy of 2 mm, the overall dental malocclusion in reality was closer to a Class I malocclusion. However, the severe skeletal Class III occlusion as represented by the −10.2 mm WITS appraisal compounds the problem of this case if further growth becomes a factor (Figure 11.10; Tables 11.1 and 11.2).

Maxilla – the maxillary molars were banded and all remaining teeth bonded with brackets or tubes

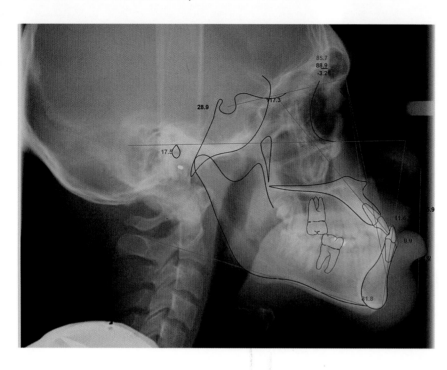

Figure 11.10 Digitized cephalogram indicating a severe Class III skeletal relationship, flat mandibular plane angle, and dentally compensated maxillary and mandibular incisors.

Table 11.1 Significant cephalometric values

	Norm	Patient pre-treatment
SNA	82°	85.7°
SNB	80°	88.9°
ANB	2°	−3.2°
WITS appraisal	−1 to +1 mm	−10.2 mm
FMA	21°	18.6°
SN-GoGn	32°	27.6°
Maxillary incisor to SN	105°	113°
Mandibular incisor to GoGn	95°	80.1°
Soft tissue		
Lower lip to E-plane	−2.0 mm	+4.2 mm
Upper lip to E-plane	−1.6 mm	−5.9 mm

SNA, sella-nasion-A point; SNB, sella-nasion-B point; ANB, A point-nasion-B point; WITS appraisal, Witwatersrand appraisal; FMA, Frankfort horizontal-mandibular plane; SN-GoGn, sella nasion-gonion gnathion.

Table 11.2 The patient's problem list in three dimensions

	Transverse	Sagittal	Vertical
Soft tissue	Normal	Concave profile; full lower lip; acute nasolabial angle	Hypodivergent
Dental	Normal	Class III molar; Class I canine; anterior crossbite; anterior dental compensation	4 mm overbite
Skeletal	Normal	Class III	Hypodivergent

(bi-dimensional, slot size .018 central and lateral incisors and .022 canines, premolars, and molars). The arch was leveled and aligned with specific arch wires during the treatment and Class III elastics and selective interproximal reduction (IPR) were performed during the sequence of treatment. Finally, the arch would be coordinated with the mandibular arch throughout treatment.

Mandibular – the mandibular first molars were banded and the remaining teeth bonded with brackets or tubes as indicated for the maxillary arch. The arch was leveled and aligned as above.

Once the maxilla and mandible were coordinated and in proper alignment, the arches would be detailed and finished. It was predicted that the treatment duration would be 30 months, and that retention would be provided with the use of Essix retainers (DENTSPLY Raintree Essix, Sarasota, FL, USA) followed by Hawley retainers after 6 months of retention with the clear retainers.

Treatment Objectives

The patient's chief complaint was to be immediately addressed by aligning the dental arches. The creation of a positive overjet would be attempted. Esthetics and function would be enhanced. Although the patient and parent indicated that surgery was not desired, it was made evident that if the patient continued to grow in a Class III direction, the treatment results could be outgrown, which would require a surgical procedure.

Treatment Options

The options presented to the patient were five-fold:

1) No treatment.
2) Dental decompensation and setup for one- or two-jaw surgery.
3) Extraction of one mandibular incisor.
4) Extraction of mandibular first premolars.
5) Non-extraction with leveling and alignment followed by IPR, and Class III elastic traction.

The patient wanted option 5. As a compromised treatment plan was desired by the patient, it was understood that the skeletal component of the malocclusion was not to be addressed (Figures 11.11 and 11.12). With regard to acceptable esthetics as a result of this compromise, the maxillary dental arch was to be proclined and the mandibular dental arch retroclined through the process of reproximation of the anterior dentition and the use of Class III elastics to augment the leveling and slight distalization of the mandibular dentition.

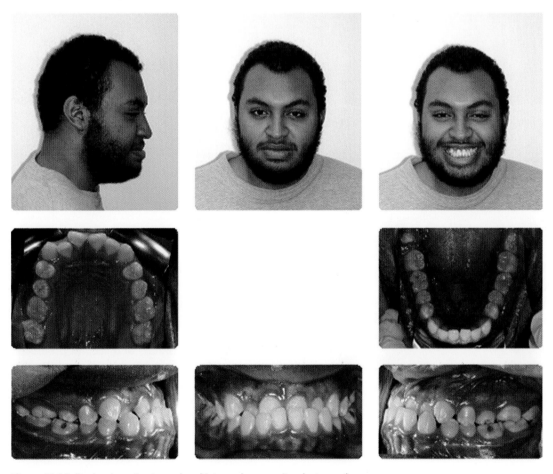

Figure 11.11 Pre-treatment extraoral and intraoral composite photograph.

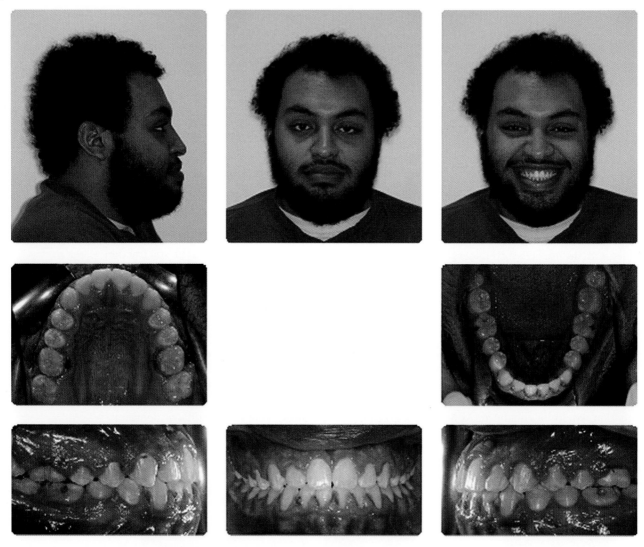

Figure 11.12 Post-treatment extraoral and intraoral composite photograph.

First Active Appointment with Full Appliances Placed

The banding and bonding of all teeth was performed (Figures 11.13–11.17). A 0.014 nickel-titanium wire was placed in the maxillary arch. The bracket on the maxillary right lateral incisor was placed upside down to aid in the crossbite correction by adjusting the torque delivery (Figure 11.13) once a rectangular wire was inserted. Figure 11.16 shows an elastomeric chain placed on the maxillary molars and second premolars to aid in the rotation of the premolars. Topical fluoride treatment, oral hygiene, diet, and emergency protocol were discussed and reinforced with the Aquarium software (Dolphin Imaging and Management Solutions, Chatsworth, CA, USA).

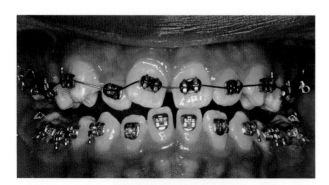

Figure 11.13 Anterior view of the dentition at the first active appointment. A .014 nickel-titanium arch wire was placed on the maxillary arch and the right lateral incisor bracket was bonded upside down to aid in the crossbite correction.

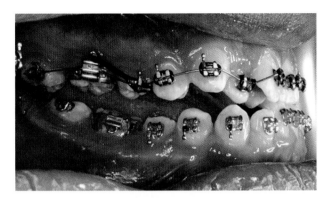

Figure 11.14 Right buccal view of the dentition at the first active appointment. Elastomeric chain was used for premolar rotation.

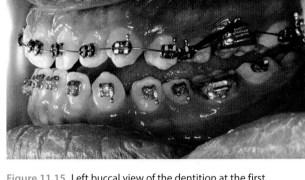

Figure 11.15 Left buccal view of the dentition at the first appointment. Elastomeric chain was used for premolar rotation.

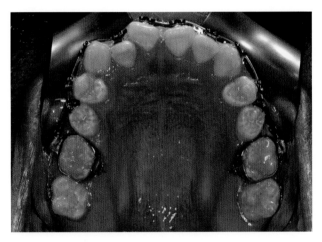

Figure 11.16 Occlusal view of the maxillary arch displaying elastomeric chain from first molars to second premolars to correct the premolar rotations.

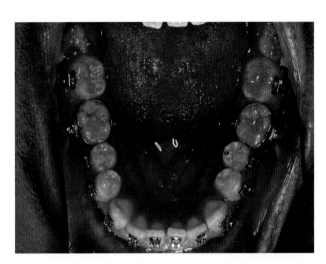

Figure 11.17 Occlusal view of the mandibular arch with brackets in place at the first active visit.

Second Active Appointment

Six weeks later, a 0.016 nickel-titanium arch wire was placed in the maxilla for premolar rotation (Figures 11.18 and 11.19). Note the improved alignment since the first visit 1 month prior to this. No arch wire was placed in the mandible. At this appointment, oral hygiene instruction and flossing were emphasized.

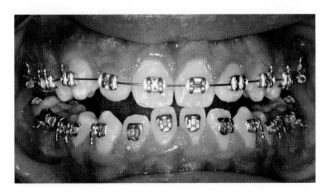

Figure 11.18 Anterior view of the dentition 6 weeks later. The maxillary arch wire was changed to .016 nickel-titanium. Note the improvement in alignment.

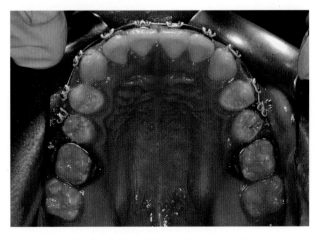

Figure 11.19 Occlusal view of the maxillary arch with improved rotation of the second premolars.

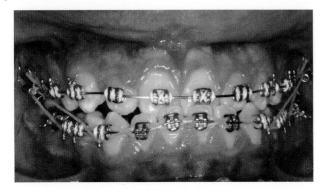

Figure 11.20 Anterior view of the dentition 5 weeks later at the third active appointment. The maxillary arch wire was changed to .017 × .025 nickel-titanium, and a .016 nickel-titanium mandibular arch wire was inserted.

Third Active Appointment

The maxillary arch wire was changed to a .017 × .025 nickel-titanium wire (Figures 11.20–11.24). The wire was passed gingival to the bracket wings of the maxillary second premolars for extrusion (arrows in Figures 11.21 and 11.22) and an elastomeric chain connected the first molars to the second premolars for rotation. A maxillary 0.016 nickel-titanium wire was placed in the mandible and an elastomeric chain was attached to the mandibular six anterior teeth for space consolidation. Class III triangular elastics (1/4", 4.5 oz) were connected from the mandibular canines and premolars to the maxillary second molars and instructed to be worn full-time to aid in the anterior crossbite correction.

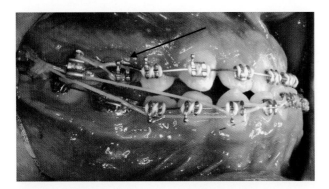

Figure 11.21 Right buccal view of the dentition at the third appointment. Class III elastics were being worn to improve the overjet. Note that the maxillary arch wire was placed gingival to the second premolar to gain extrusion (arrow).

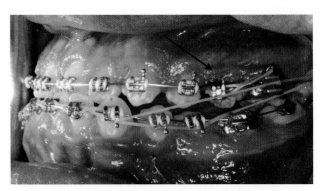

Figure 11.22 Left buccal view of the dentition at the third appointment. Class III elastics were being worn to improve the overjet. Note that the maxillary arch wire was placed gingival to the second premolar to gain extrusion (arrow).

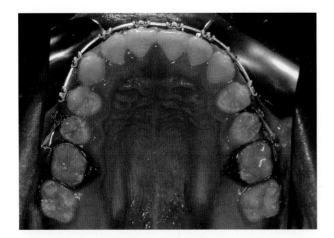

Figure 11.23 Occlusal view of the maxillary arch at the third appointment. Note the improved arch form and rotation of the second premolars.

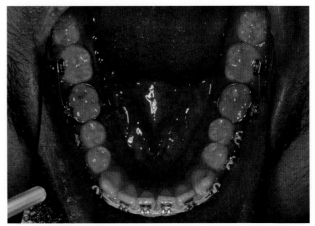

Figure 11.24 Occlusal view of the mandibular arch at the third appointment.

Fourth Active Appointment

The patient presented with a positive overjet (Figures 11.25–11.29) over the following 4 weeks. A maxillary .017 × .025 stainless steel wire was placed and an expanded .018 stainless steel wire was placed in the mandible with a continuous elastomeric module from the mandibular right canine to the mandibular left canine for space closure. Elastomeric modules were still placed between the maxillary molars and second premolars for de-rotation of the premolars. Class III triangular elastics (3/16″, 4.5 oz.) were placed from the mandibular canines and first premolars to the maxillary first molars for the Class III correction. Oral hygiene was reinforced.

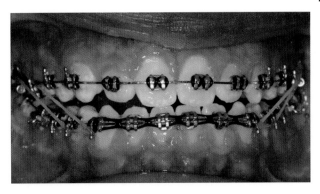

Figure 11.25 Anterior view of the dentition at the fourth appointment 4 weeks later. The maxillary arch wire was changed to .017 × .025 stainless steel and the mandibular arch wire was changed to expanded .018 stainless steel. Elastomeric chain was attached from mandibular canine to canine for space closure. A positive overjet has been obtained.

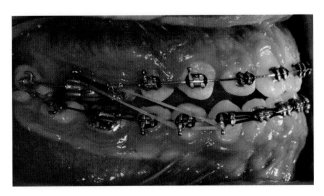

Figure 11.26 Right buccal view of the dentition at the fourth appointment.

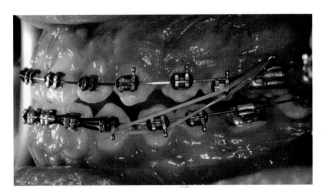

Figure 11.27 Left buccal view of the dentition at the fourth appointment.

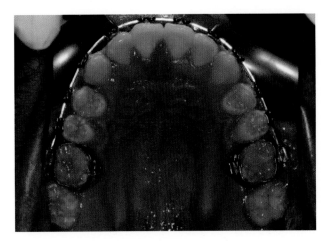

Figure 11.28 Occlusal view of the maxillary arch at the fourth appointment. Note the improved rotations of the second premolars.

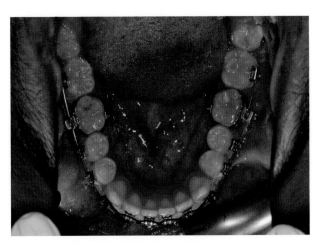

Figure 11.29 Occlusal view of the mandibular arch at the fourth appointment.

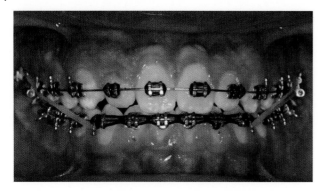

Figure 11.30 Anterior view of the dentition at the fifth appointment. The maxillary arch wire was changed to .016×.022 due to the repositioning of the second premolar brackets. The positive overjet has been maintained.

Fifth Active Appointment

The positive overjet had been maintained (Figures 11.30–11.34) and the patient reported that he was more comfortable and masticated food with ease. The maxillary second premolar brackets were repositioned to improve the rotational and eruptive corrections. The maxillary wire was replaced with a .016 × .022 nickel-titanium wire due to the re-bracketing of the premolars, while the triangular elastics were replaced (1/4", 4.5 oz). The elastomeric modules were continued from the mandibular canine to canine.

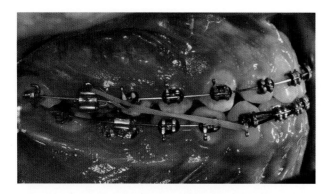

Figure 11.31 Right buccal view of the dentition at the fifth appointment.

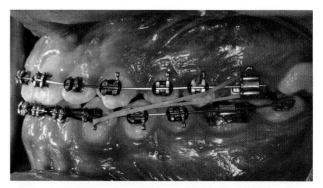

Figure 11.32 Left buccal view of the dentition at the fifth appointment.

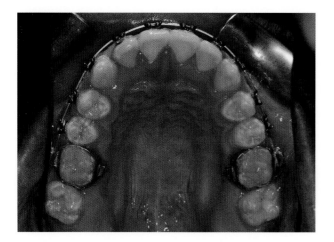

Figure 11.33 Occlusal view of the maxillary arch at the fifth appointment.

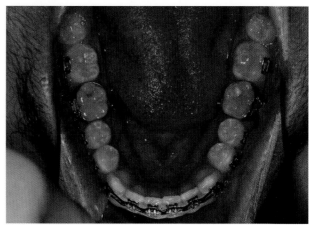

Figure 11.34 Occlusal view of the mandibular arch at the fifth appointment.

Sixth Active Appointment

The maxillary arch wire was replaced with a .017 × .025 nickel-titanium wire. Class III elastics (3/16", 4.0 oz.) were to be worn on the patient's right side to maintain the midline correction, and triangular elastics on the left side from the maxillary canine to the mandibular canine and first premolar for settling of the buccal occlusion. Elastomeric modules were to be continued on the mandibular canine to canine and from the maxillary canine to canine for space closure (Figures 11.35–11.37).

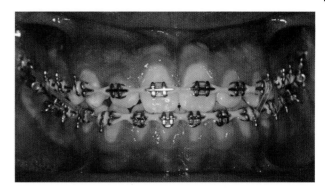

Figure 11.35 Anterior view of the dentition at the sixth appointment. The maxillary arch wire was changed to .017 × .025 nickel-titanium. Elastomeric chain was placed from maxillary canine to canine for space closure and continued on the mandibular arch for space closure.

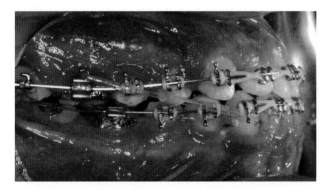

Figure 11.36 Right buccal view of the dentition at the sixth appointment. Class III elastics were used to maintain the positive overjet and midline improvement.

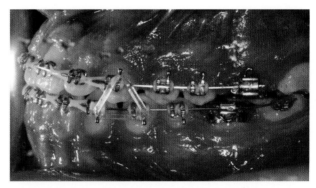

Figure 11.37 Left buccal view of the dentition at the sixth appointment. A triangle elastic was used to improve canine intercuspation.

Seventh Active Appointment

The maxillary lateral incisor brackets and the maxillary right canine bracket were repositioned. The maxillary arch wire was changed to .016 × .022 nickel-titanium because of the repositioning and for flexibility. Elastomeric chain was placed from maxillary first molar to first molar and from mandibular canine to mandibular canine for space consolidation. Settling elastics were placed from canines to molars in both arches for maximizing intercuspation of the buccal occlusion (Figures 11.38–11.42).

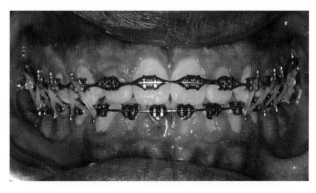

Figure 11.38 Anterior view of the dentition at the seventh appointment. Elastomeric chain was placed on the maxillary arch from first molar to first molar for space consolidation.

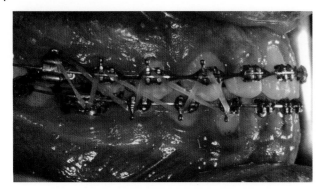

Figure 11.39 Right buccal view of the dentition at the seventh appointment. Settling elastics were being used to gain improved intercuspation of the occlusion.

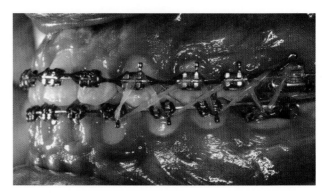

Figure 11.40 Left buccal view of the dentition at the seventh appointment; settling elastics were being used to gain improved intercuspation of the occlusion.

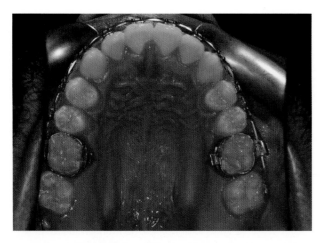

Figure 11.41 Occlusal view of the maxillary arch at the seventh appointment.

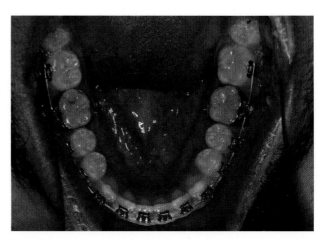

Figure 11.42 Occlusal view of the mandibular arch at the seventh appointment.

Eighth and Ninth Active Appointments

Elastomeric chains were continued to consolidate space, and settling elastics were continued for ideal intercuspation.

The patient was debonded. Final records were taken (Panoramic and cephalometric radiographs, photos, and digital model records; Figures 11.43–11.52). Impressions were taken for Essix retainers to be delivered immediately, and care and instructions for retainer wear were given. The patient was scheduled for a 1-month retainer check followed by observation every 3 months for the first year. Total treatment time was 15 months.The post-treatment panoramic radiograph indicates normal bony architecture, periodontium and no root resorption (Figure 11.51).

Upon measurement, the post-treatment cephalometric radiograph indicates a sella-nasion-A point (SNA) angle of 86.4°, a sella-nasion-B point (SNB) angle of 87.7°, an A point-nasion-B point (ANB) angle of −1.3°, and a WITS relationship of −7.2 mm. The mandibular plane angles are 16.2° (Frankfort horizontal-mandibular plane, FMA), 28.7° (sella nasion-gonion gnathion, SN-GoGn), the mandibular incisor to the mandibular plane (1:GoGn) at 77.3°, and the maxillary incisor to the SN plane at 118.7°. The soft tissue values improved for the lower lip, going from 4.2 to 3.6 mm, and for the upper lip they decreased from −5.9 to −1.0 mm (Figure 11.52; Table 11.3).

Overall and regional superimposition of this case was not possible due to changes in office software during the course of treatment. However, the post-treatment measurements indicate an improvement in the dental and bony architecture, albeit through dental compensations.

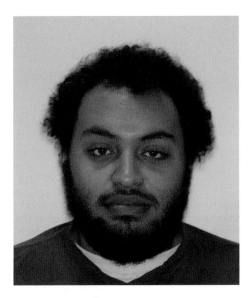

Figure 11.43 Full-face view on the day of appliance removal.

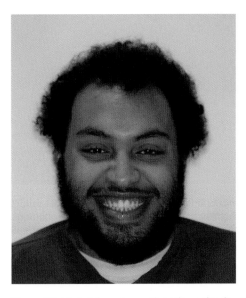

Figure 11.44 Full-face view with smile on the day of appliance removal.

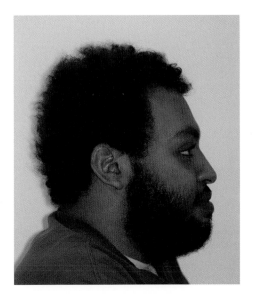

Figure 11.45 Right lateral view of profile on the day of appliance removal.

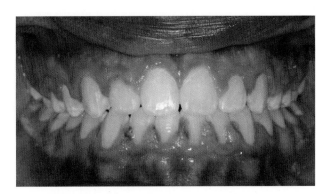

Figure 11.46 Anterior view of the dentition on the day of appliance removal. Note the improved overjet relationship.

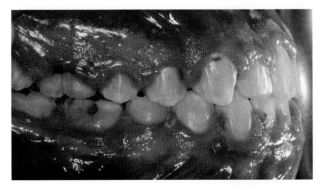

Figure 11.47 Right buccal view of the dentition on the day of appliance removal. Note the improved molar and canine relationship.

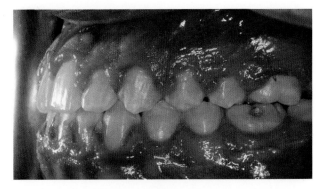

Figure 11.48 Left buccal view of the dentition on the day of appliance removal. Note the improved molar and canine relationship.

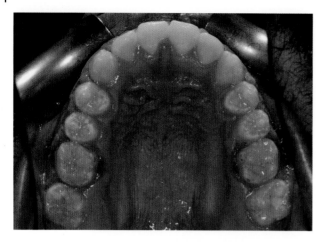

Figure 11.49 Occlusal view of the maxillary arch on the day of appliance removal.

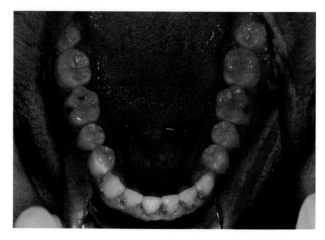

Figure 11.50 Occlusal view of the mandibular arch on the day of appliance removal.

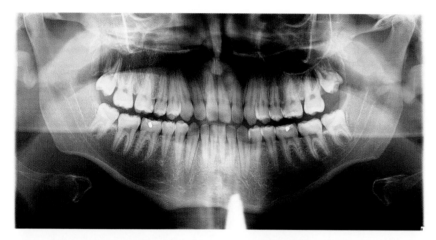

Figure 11.51 Panoramic radiograph on the day of appliance removal. Root lengths and periodontium are normal.

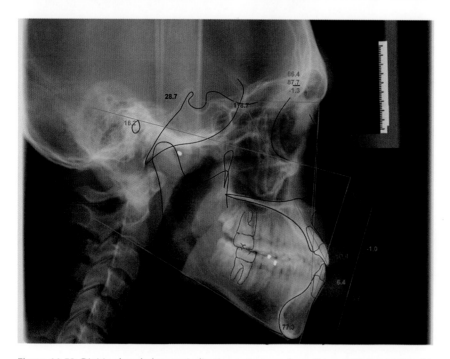

Figure 11.52 Digitized cephalogram indicating an improved maxillomandibular relationship and soft tissue balance.

Table 11.3 Significant pre-treatment and post-treatment cephalometric values

	Norm	Pre-treatment	Post-treatment
SNA	82°	85.7°	86.4°
SNB	80°	88.9°	87.7°
ANB	2°	−3.2°	−1.3°
WITS appraisal	−1 to +1 mm	−10.2 mm	−7.2 mm
FMA	21°	18.6°	16.2°
SN-GoGn	32°	27.6°	28.7°
Maxillary incisor to SN	105°	113°	118.7°
Mandibular incisor to GoGn	95°	80.1°	77.3°
Soft tissue			
Lower lip to E-plane	−2.0 mm	+4.2 mm	+3.6 mm
Upper lip to E-plane	−1.6 mm	−5.9 mm	−1.0 mm

SNA, sella-nasion-A point; SNB, sella-nasion-B point; ANB, A point-nasion-B point; WITS appraisal, Witwatersrand appraisal; FMA, Frankfort horizontal-mandibular plane; SN-GoGn, sella nasion-gonion gnathion.

Commentary

With growth completed, what would have been a straightforward orthognathic surgical case manifested into conventional orthodontic treatment with camouflage and acceptable dental compensations in place. Facial esthetics was not compromised and the patient avoided the extra risks and costs of a combined surgical procedure.

Review Questions

1 What are the required orthodontic records needed to produce a diagnosis and treatment plan?

2 What components of the orthodontic record are used in developing a problem list?

3 What properties are associated with the initial arch wires inserted into a fully bonded and banded arch?

4 What type of material is used for arch wire ligation?

5 In a Class III malocclusion treated without extractions or surgery, why is the maxillary arch treated prior to the mandibular arch?

6 What type of movement do intraoral elastics provide to the maxillary and mandibular arches in a Class III malocclusion?

Suggested References

Musich DR, Chemello PD. Orthodontic aspects of orthognathic surgery. In: Graber LW, Vanarsdall RL, Vig KWL, eds. Orthodontics Current Principles and Techniques, 5th edn. Philadelphia, PA: Elsevier Mosby, 2012; pp. 897–963.

Proffit WR, Sarver DM, Ackerman JL. Orthodontic diagnosis: the problem oriented approach. In: Proffit WR, Fields HW Jr, Sarver DM, eds. Contemporary Orthodontics, 5th edn. St Louis, MO: CV Mosby Co., 2013; pp. 151–219.

Proffit WR, Sarver DM. Combined surgical and orthodontic treatment. In: Proffit WR, Fields HW Jr, Sarver DM, eds. Contemporary Orthodontics, 5th edn. St Louis, MO: Mosby, 2013; pp. 685–714.

Sinha PK. Patient compliance in orthodontic practice. In Nanda R, Kapila S, eds. Current Therapy in Orthodontics. St Louis, MO: Mosby Elsevier, 2010; pp. 9–14.

12

Class III Skeletal and Class III Dental: Non-Extraction

LEARNING OBJECTIVES

- Treatment with camouflaging of a post-pubescent female (non-growth) with a skeletal Class III malocclusion
- A method to avoid occlusal interference during crossbite correction

---

Interview Data

The patient was previously in treatment with another orthodontist who retired due to health concerns. The patient's and parents' chief complaint was the continuation and completion of treatment. It was decided to take new photographic and radiographic records in order to generate a new treatment plan. The current appliances, however, were not removed for the clinical photographs and radiographs. New appliances would be placed once a new treatment plan was generated.

- Development: 13-year-old post-pubescent female, 2 years after menses initiation
- Motivation: good
- Medical history: non-contributory

- Dental history: seen for routine care by a local dentist in the community
- Family history: older brother was treated for a Class III malocclusion
- Habits: none
- Facial form: ovoid, asymmetric leptoprosopic facial form with chin deviating to the left
- Facial proportions: slightly long lower face

Clinical Examination

- Incisor-stomion (Figures 12.1 and 12.2):
  - At rest: 3 mm
  - Smiling: 8 mm

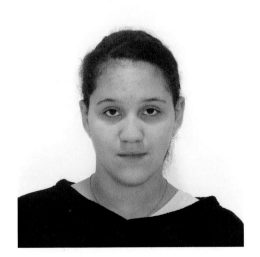

Figure 12.1 Full face at rest displaying a long, ovoid form with chin deviating to the left.

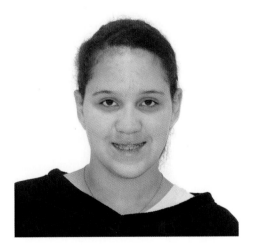

Figure 12.2 Full face with smile showing no gingival display.

Atlas of Orthodontic Case Reviews, First Edition. Marjan Askari and Stanley A. Alexander.
© 2017 John Wiley & Sons, Inc. Published 2017 by John Wiley & Sons, Inc.

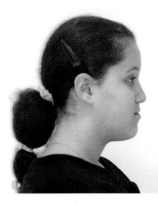

Figure 12.3 Right lateral view of profile exhibiting a concave form with an acute nasolabial angle.

- Smile line: 0 mm gingival display
- Breathing: nasal
- Lips together at rest
- Soft tissue profile: slightly concave (Figure 12.3)
- Nasolabial angle: slightly acute
- Normal mandibular plane angle

Dentition (Figure 12.4)

7654321	12c4567
7654321	1234567

- Overjet: −2 mm with anterior crossbite from canine to canine
- Overbite: 1 mm

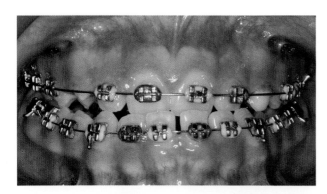

Figure 12.4 Anterior view of the dentition with previous appliances in place and an anterior crossbite with the mandibular midline shifted to the left.

- Midlines: maxillary midline is coincident with the face; mandibular midline is 2 mm to the left of the maxillary midline; diastema is present between mandibular central incisors

Right Buccal View (Figure 12.5)

- Molar: Class III
- Canine: Class III
- Curve of Spee: deep
- Crossbite: anterior crossbite
- Caries: none

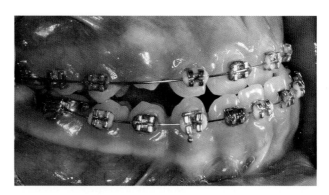

Figure 12.5 Right buccal view of the dentition prior to treatment, displaying a Class III molar and canine occlusion and a deep curve of Spee.

Left Buccal View (Figure 12.6)

- Molar: Class III
- Canine: Class III
- Curve of Spee: deep
- Crossbite: anterior crossbite
- Caries: none

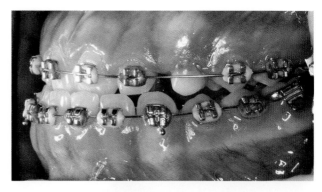

Figure 12.6 Left buccal view of the dentition prior to treatment, displaying a Class III molar and canine occlusion and a deep curve of Spee.

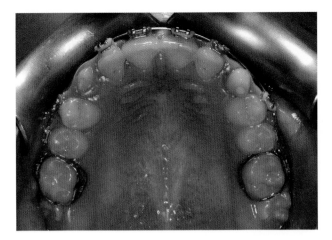

Figure 12.7 Occlusal view of the maxillary arch displaying a symmetric broad, U-shaped form in the late mixed dentition.

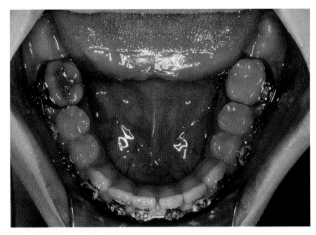

Figure 12.8 Occlusal view of the mandubular arch exhibiting a U-shaped form.

Maxillary Arch (Figure 12.7)
- Symmetric, broad, U-shaped arch form in late mixed dentition with appliance in place
- No caries

Mandibular Arch (Figure 12.8)
- U-shaped arch form with appliance in place
- No caries

Function

- Normal range of motion with slight deviation to the patient's left while opening; 40 mm maximum opening; bilateral right and left excursions = 8 mm; protrusive = 4 mm.
- Temporomandibular joint palpation: normal without pain
- Late mixed dentition with all 32 teeth present or developing
- Root lengths and periodontium appear normal
- Condyles appear normal (Figure 12.9)

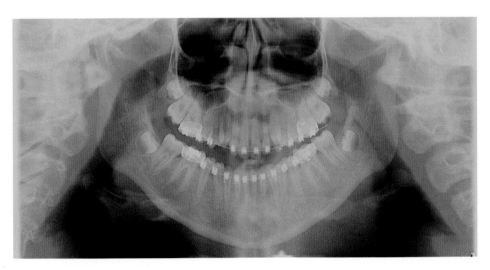

Figure 12.9 Panoramic radiograph with the previous appliances in place in the late mixed dentition. All permanent teeth are present or developing.

Diagnosis and Treatment Plan

The patient was a 13-year-old post-pubescent female with a skeletal and dental Class III malocclusion with maxillary and mandibular dental compensations

(Figure 12.10; Tables 12.1 and 12.2). Both the patient and parents wanted to avoid a surgical correction. A non-extraction, non-surgical treatment plan was presented to camouflage the existing skeletal and dental malocclusion through further dental compensation

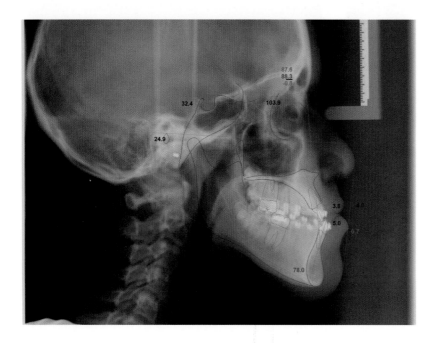

Figure 12.10 Digitized cephalogram indicating a skeletal Class III malocclusion, normal mandibular plane angle, and upright mandibulat incisors.

Table 12.1 Significant cephalometric values

	Norm	Patient pre-treatment
SNA	80°	87.6°
SNB	78°	88.3°
ANB	2°	−0.7°
WITS appraisal	−1 to +1 mm	−9.0 mm
FMA	21°	24.4°
SN-GoGn	32°	32.0°
Maxillary incisor to SN	105°	103.9°
Mandibular incisor to GoGn	95°	81°
Soft tissue		
Lower lip to E-plane	−2 mm	+0.70 mm
Upper lip to E-plane	−1.6 mm	−4.0 mm

SNA, sella-nasion-A point; SNB, sella-nasion-B point; ANB, A point-nasion-B point; WITS appraisal, Witwatersrand appraisal; FMA, Frankfort horizontal-mandibular plane; SN-GoGn, sella nasion-gonion gnathion.

Table 12.2 The patient's problem list in three dimensions

	Transverse	Sagittal	Vertical
Soft tissue	Normal	Concave profile; acute nasolabial angle; prognathic mandible	Normodivergent
Dental	Anterior crossbite	Late mixed dentition; Class III molar and canines and reverse overjet	1 mm overbite
Skeletal	Normal	Class III	Normodivergent

without affecting the facial esthetics. Both the patient and parents were informed that if latent growth expressed itself, an orthognathic surgical approach would be recommended during treatment or after the completion of treatment if relapse due to growth occurred.

Treatment Objectives

The anterior crossbite due to the skeletal and dental Class III malocclusion was to be addressed through dental compensation, while the facial esthetics would be maintained. A non-extraction mode of therapy would be delivered so as not to compromise orthognathic surgery if skeletal growth continued and this mode of correction became necessary.

Treatment Options

1) Orthognathic surgery to correct the skeletal and dental problems – this option was rejected initially as neither patient nor parents wanted a surgical approach.
2) Non-extraction correction with dental compensations and maintenance of the facial esthetics – this mode of therapy was desired by the patient. However, it was stressed that if growth continued, a surgical approach would be required to establish a functional occlusion and improve the facial esthetics.
3) Extraction of maxillary second premolars and mandibular first premolars to correct the anterior crossbite and create a Class I molar and canine occlusion.

Option 2 was chosen (Figures 12.11 and 12.12).

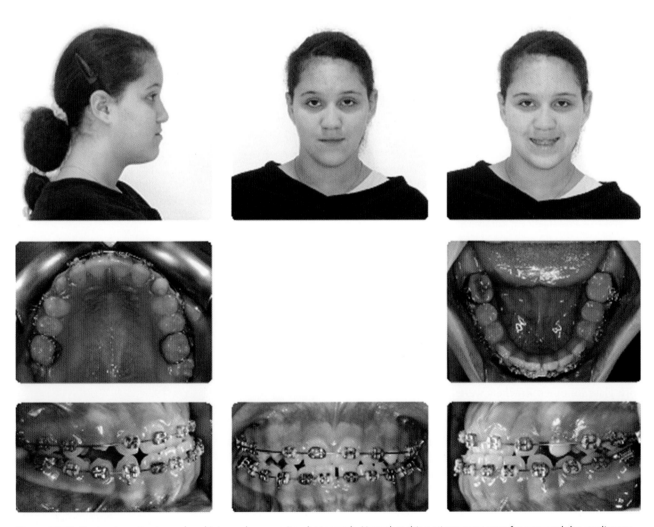

Figure 12.11 Pre-treatment extraoral and intraoral composite photograph. Note that this patient was a transfer case and the appliances were already in place.

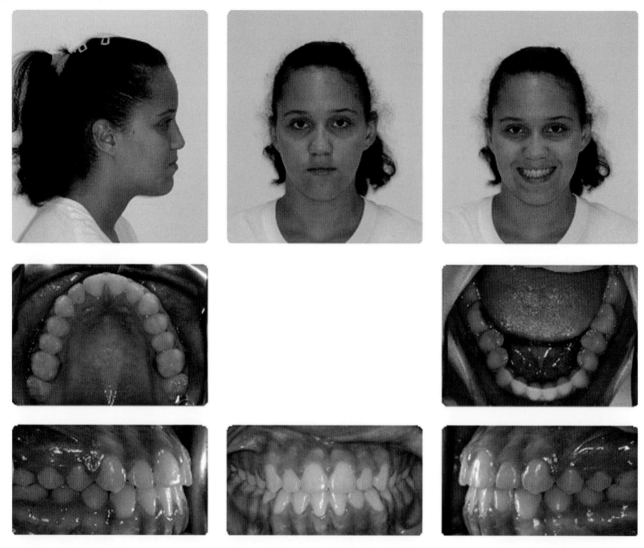

Figure 12.12 Post treatment extraoral and intraoral composite photograph.

First Active Appointment

This appointment included the removal of the previous appliance and placement of a bi-dimensional system. Band space was available and new molar bands were cemented to the maxillary and mandibular first molars with glass ionomer. Brackets were bonded from second premolar to second premolar. A .018 nickel-titanium wire was placed on the maxilla and a .016 nickel-titanium wire was ligated to the mandible with an elastomeric chain from first molar to first molar to consolidate space. An occlusal build-up with glass ionomer was placed on the maxillary first molar palatal cusps to prevent inter-cuspation of the teeth and to allow for easier crossbite correction (Figures 12.13–12.17).

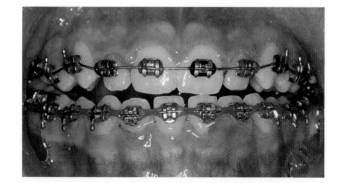

Figure 12.13 Anterior view of the dentition on the first day when new appliances were bonded. A .018 nickel-titanium arch wire was placed on the maxillary arch and a .016 nickel-titanium arch wire was placed on the mandibular arch. Elastomeric chain was placed from mandibular first molar to first molar.

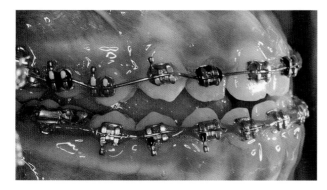

Figure 12.14 Right buccal view of the dentition on the first day when new appliances were bonded to the patient.

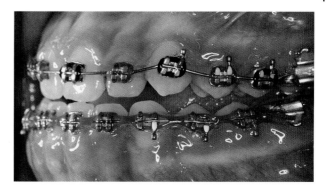

Figure 12.15 Left buccal view of the dentition on the first day when new appliances were bonded to the patient.

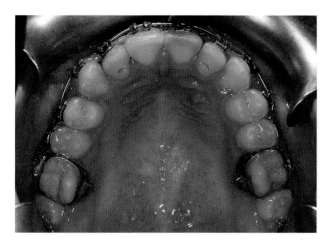

Figure 12.16 Occlusal view of the maxillary arch displaying glass ionomer occlusal build-up on the palatal cusps to disocclude the dentition.

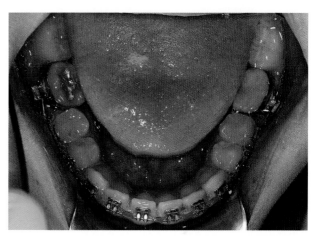

Figure 12.17 Occlusal view of the mandibular arch exhibiting the elastomeric chain extending from first molar to first molar.

Second Active Appointment

The patient returned 5 weeks later. Maxillary and mandibular arch wires were changed to .016 × .022 nickel-titanium, and elastomeric chain was placed from the right mandibular first premolar to the left mandibular first premolar. The patient was instructed to wear Class III elastics (1/4″, 4 oz.) and to change them daily. The occlusal build-up of glass ionomer was no longer present and the decision was made to not replace them at this time (Figures 12.18–12.22).

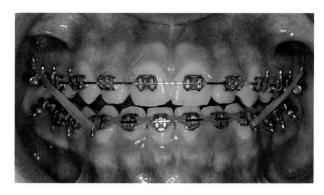

Figure 12.18 Anterior view of the dentition 5 weeks after the first appointment. The arch wires were changed to .016 × .022 nickel-titanium. Class III elastics were now being used to correct the anterior crossbite.

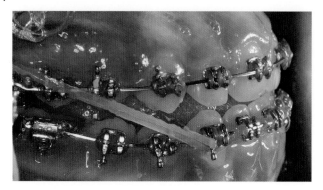

Figure 12.19 Right buccal view of the dentition 5 weeks later with a Class III elastic in place.

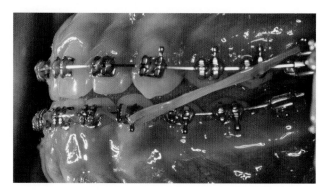

Figure 12.20 Left buccal view of the dentition 5 weeks later with a Class III elastic in place.

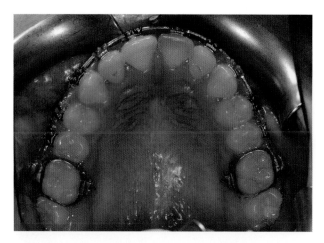

Figure 12.21 Occlusal view of the maxillary arch 5 weeks later. The glass ionomer build-up on the first molars was no longer present.

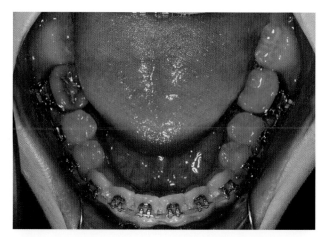

Figure 12.22 Occlusal view of the mandibular arch with elastomeric chain ligated from first premolar to first premolar.

Third Active Appointment

Four weeks later the patient returned for an appliance adjustment. The mandibular incisor brackets were removed and rebonded upside down to reverse the torque prescription in order to allow for the crowns to lingualize and to increase the dental compensation effect. The mandibular arch wire remained the same, but the maxillary arch wire was changed to .017 × .025 stainless steel to increase the arch rigidity and to express the full torque of the maxillary incisor brackets. Elastomeric chain was placed from the mandibular first premolar to first premolar for space consolidation. A Class III elastic was used on the right quadrant to shift the mandibular midline to the right, and a triangle elastic was used from the maxillary left canine to the mandibular canine and first premolar (3/16", 4.5 oz.). The elastics were to be changed daily (Figures 12.23–12.25). Note that the anterior crossbite had been corrected.

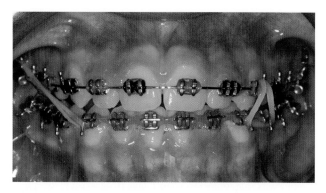

Figure 12.23 Anterior view of the dentition 4 weeks later. The maxillary arch wire was changed to .017 × .025 stainless steel. The mandibular incisor brackets were rebonded upside down to reverse the torque prescription and lingualize the crowns.

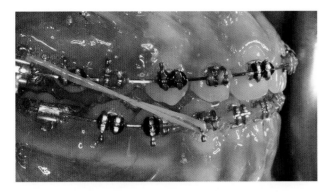

Figure 12.24 Right buccal view of the dentition 4 weeks later with a Class III elastic in place to shift the mandibular midline to the right.

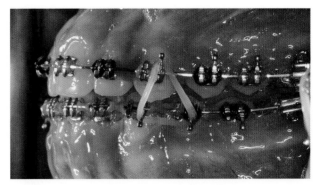

Figure 12.25 Left buccal view of the dentition 4 weeks later with a triangle elastic in place to improve intercuspation.

Fourth Active Appointment

Eight weeks later the mandibular right second molar was bonded with a tube due to its position. The mandibular arch wire was changed to .016 nickel-titanium in order to negotiate wire placement into the second molar tube. Glass ionomer build-up was placed on the maxillary second molar palatal cusps to allow for clearance of cusps and alignment of the mandibular second molar (Figures 12.26–12.30).

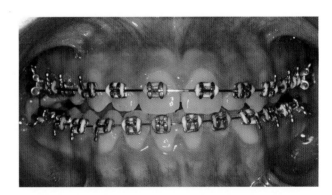

Figure 12.26 Anterior view of the dentition 8 weeks later. The mandibular second molars were bonded and a .016 nickel-titanium arch wire was placed on the mandibular arch.

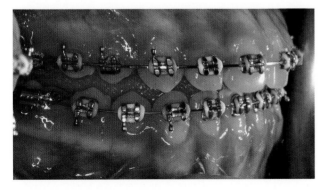

Figure 12.27 Right buccal view of the dentition 8 weeks later.

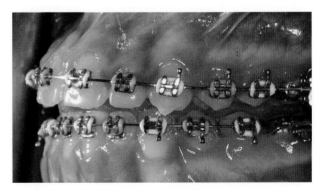

Figure 12.28 Left buccal view of the dentition 8 weeks later.

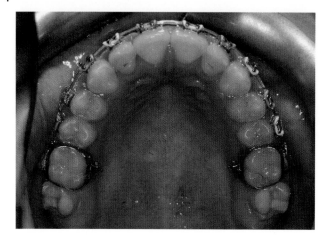

Figure 12.29 Occlusal view of the maxillary arch 8 weeks later with glass ionomer build-up on the second molars to allow for buccal tube placement on the mandibular second molar.

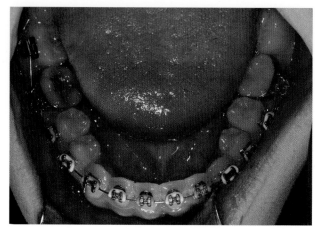

Figure 12.30 Occlusal view of the mandibular arch 8 weeks later.

Fifth Active Appointment

Six weeks later, the palatal build-up on the maxillary second molars was removed. The mandibular arch wire was changed to .016 × .022 nickel-titanium. An elastomeric chain was placed from the mandibular first molar to first molar. Class III elastics were placed (3/16", 4.5 oz.) and were to be changed daily (Figures 12.31–12.35).

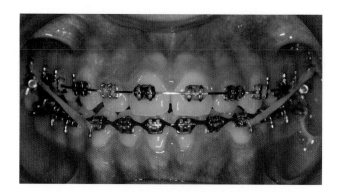

Figure 12.31 Anterior view of the dentition 6 weeks later. The mandibular arch wire was changed to .016 × .022 nickel-titanium and Class III elastics were replaced bilaterally.

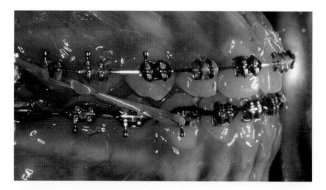

Figure 12.32 Right buccal view of the dentition 6 weeks later with a Class III elastic in place.

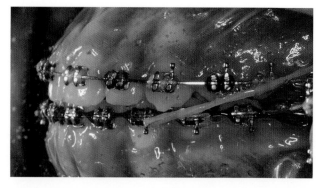

Figure 12.33 Left buccal view of the dentition 6 weeks later with a Class III elastic in place.

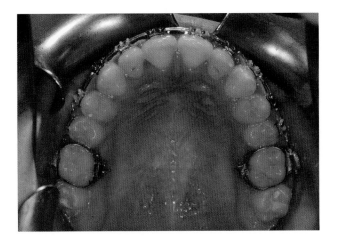

Figure 12.34 Occlusal view of the maxillary arch 6 weeks later. The glass ionomer build-up was removed.

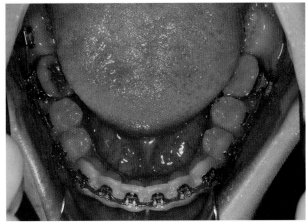

Figure 12.35 Occlusal view of the mandibular arch 6 weeks later with elastomeric chain extending from the first molar to the first molar.

Sixth Active Appointment

After 6 weeks, the mandibular arch wire was changed to .017 × .025 nickel-titanium, while the maxillary arch wire was kept as .017 × .025 stainless steel. Triangle elastics were instructed to be worn bilaterally from the maxillary canines to the mandibular canines and first premolars (3/16", 4.5 oz.). The overjet was corrected to 2 mm and the midlines were coincident (Figures 12.36–12.38).

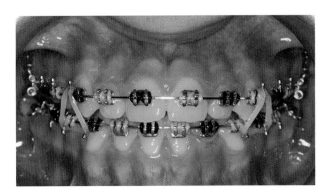

Figure 12.36 Anterior view of the dentition at the sixth active appointment 6 weeks later. The mandibular arch wire was changed to .017 × .025 nickel-titanium.

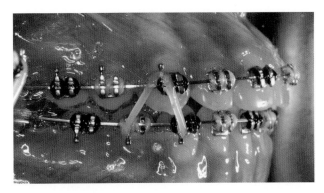

Figure 12.37 Right buccal view of the dentition at the sixth active appointment. Triangle elastics were used to settle the occlusion.

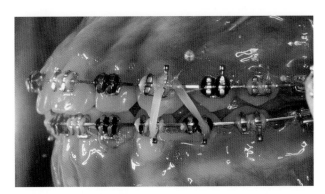

Figure 12.38 Left buccal view of the dentition at the sixth active appointment. Triangle elastics were used to settle the occlusion.

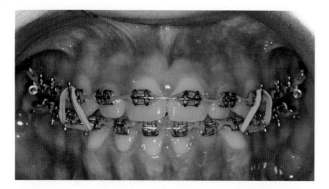

Figure 12.39 Anterior view of the dentition 5 weeks later. The maxillary arch wire was changed to .017×.025 nickel-titanium. Elastomeric chain was placed from first molar to first molar on both the maxillary and mandibular arches.

Seventh to Eighth Active Appointments

Five weeks later, the maxillary arch wire was changed to .017×.025 nickel-titanium. Elastomeric chain was ligated to both maxillary and mandibular arches from first molar to first molar. Triangle elastics (3/16″, 6 oz.) were to be changed daily. The use of nickel-titanium wire in both arches would allow for the settling of the buccal occlusion with elastic wear (Figures 12.39–12.41). The same mechanical plan continued for an additional 5 weeks.

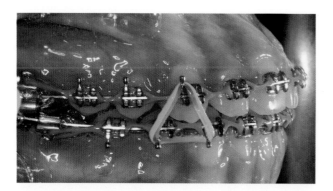

Figure 12.40 Right buccal view of the dentition 5 weeks later. Triangle elastics were still worn to settle the occlusion.

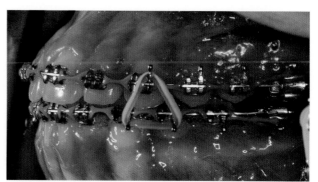

Figure 12.41 Left buccal view of the dentition 5 weeks later. Triangle elastics were still worn to settle the occlusion.

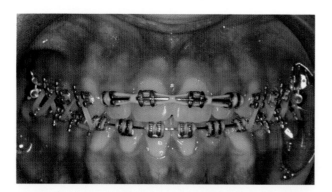

Figure 12.42 Anterior view of the dentition at the ninth active appointment. The maxillary arch wire was sectioned distal to the lateral incisors and the mandibular arch wire was sectioned distal to the canines. Elastomeric chain was placed from maxillary lateral incisor to lateral incisor.

Ninth Active Appointment

Four weeks later, the maxillary arch wire was sectioned distal to the lateral incisors and elastomeric chain was stretched from lateral incisor to lateral incisor. The mandibular arch was sectioned distal to the canines with individual ligation. Settling elastics (3/8″, 4.5 oz.) extended bilaterally from the mandibular first molar to the mandibular canine (Figures 12.42–12.44). A panoramic film was taken to observe root positions and morphology (Figure 12.45). The roots appeared normal and parallel without any indication of root resorption.

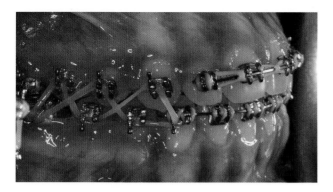

Figure 12.43 Right buccal view of the dentition at the ninth active appointment. Settling elastics were worn to improve intercuspation.

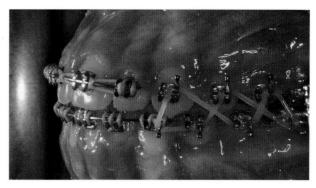

Figure 12.44 Left buccal view of the dentition at the ninth active appointment. Settling elastics were worn to improve intercuspation.

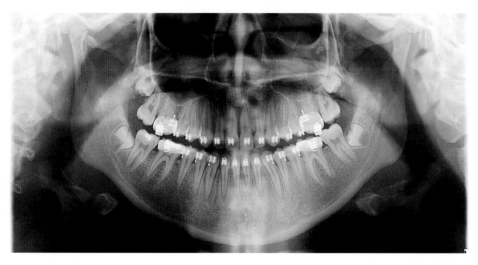

Figure 12.45 Panoramic radiograph on the ninth active appointment. All root lengths are normal and the periodontium appears healthy.

Tenth Active Appointment

Four weeks later, the patient returned and it was decided that greater anterior coupling was needed. A .016 × .022 reverse curve nickel-titanium wire was ligated to the mandibular arch. A .016 × .022 nickel-titanium sectional arch was tied to the maxillary arch from canine to canine. An elastomeric chain was placed between the maxillary canines. Settling elastics were continued as previously placed (Figures 12.46–12.48).

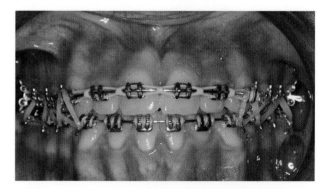

Figure 12.46 Anterior view of the dentition at the 10th active appointment 4 weeks later. A reverse curve .016×.022 nickel-titanium arch wire was placed on the mandibular arch and a sectional .016×.022 nickel-titanium arch wire was placed on the maxillary arch. Elastomeric chain was placed from the maxillary canine to canine.

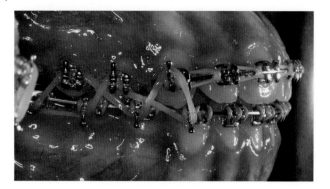

Figure 12.47 Right buccal view of the dentition at the 10th active appointment. Settling elastics were still being worn.

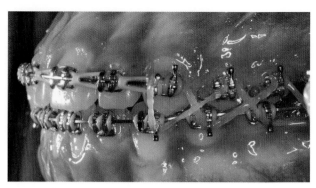

Figure 12.48 Left buccal view of the dentition at the 10th active appointment. Settling elastics were still being worn.

Tenth Appointment

The patient was debonded 3 weeks after the previous appointment. An iTero scan (Align Technology, Inc, San Jose, CA, USA), photographs, a cephalometric film, and impressions were taken for immediate Essix retainers (DENTSPLY Raintree Essix, Sarasota, FL, USA). These retainers were to be worn at night and during sleep. The patient was to return in 4 weeks for evaluation and compliance, and then every 3 months during the first year for observation, retention, and growth evaluation. The molar and canine relationships were Class I with a 2 mm overjet and 2 mm overbite. The patient's facial esthetics improved (Figures 12.49–12.56). Total treatment time was 13 months.

Minimal growth changes had taken place. However, Class III elastics resulted in a clockwise rotation of the mandible which aided in the correction. The WITS appraisal improved as a result of tipping of the occlusal plane. Regional superimposition indicated that the increased angulation of the maxillary incisor and retraction of the mandibular incisor helped to create a positive overjet through dental compensation and camouflage. The soft tissue drape slightly improved (Figures 12.57 and 12.58; Table 12.3).

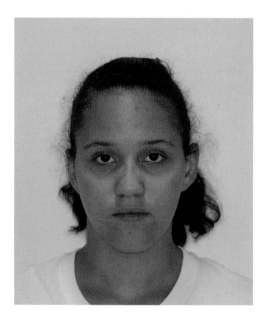

Figure 12.49 Full-face view on the day of appliance removal.

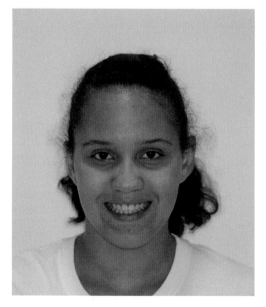

Figure 12.50 Full-face view with smile on the day of appliance removal.

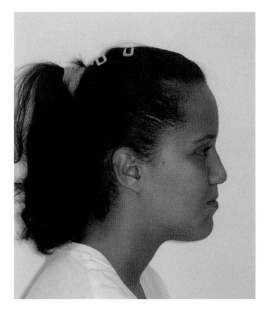

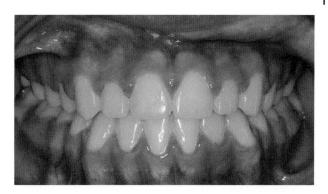

Figure 12.52 Anterior view of the dentition on the day of appliance removal. Note the improved overjet relationship.

Figure 12.51 Right lateral view of the profile on the day of appliance removal. Note the improved profile after treatment.

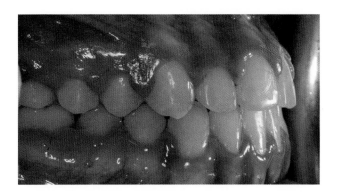

Figure 12.53 Right buccal view of the dentition on the day of appliance removal. Note the Class I molar and canine relationship.

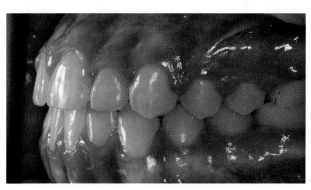

Figure 12.54 Left buccal view of the dentition on the day of appliance removal. Note the Class I molar and canine relationship.

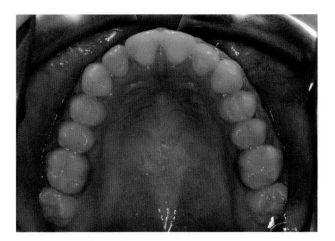

Figure 12.55 Occlusal view of the maxillary arch on the day of appliance removal.

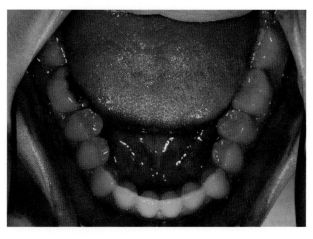

Figure 12.56 Occlusal view of the mandibular arch on the day of appliance removal.

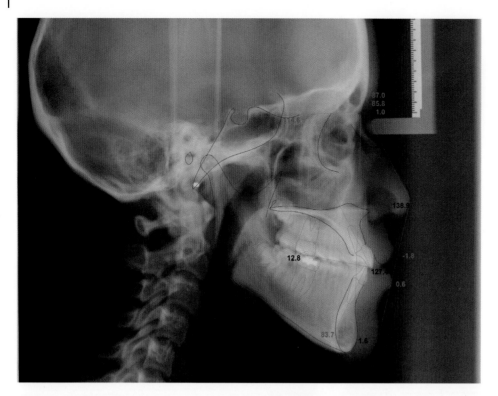

Figure 12.57 Digitized cephalogram exhibiting an improved skeletal relationship and ideal incisor relationships.

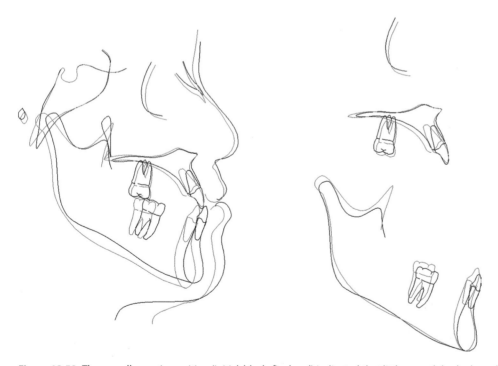

Figure 12.58 The overall superimposition (initial, black; final, red) indicated that little growth had taken place during treatment. The occlusal plane rotated clockwise as a result of Class III traction. Regional superimposition indicated an improved mandibular incisor position with slight mandibular retraction and torque of the maxillary incisor.

Table 12.3 Significant pre-treatment and post-treatment cephalometric values

	Norm	Pre-treatment	Post-treatment
SNA	82°	87.6°	87.0°
SNB	80°	88.3°	85.8°
ANB	2°	−0.7°	+1.2°
WITS appraisal	−1 to +1 mm	−9.0 mm	−4.3 mm
FMA	21°	24.4°	25.1°
SN-GoGn	32°	32.0°	32.2°
Maxillary incisor to SN	105°	103.9°	114.6°
Mandibular incisor to GoGn	95°	81.0°	83.7°
Soft tissue			
Lower lip to E-plane	−2.0 mm	+0.70 mm	+0.10 mm
Upper lip to E-plane	−1.6 mm	−4.0 mm	−2.0 mm

SNA, sella-nasion-A point; SNB, sella-nasion-B point; ANB, A point-nasion-B point; WITS appraisal, Witwatersrand appraisal; FMA, Frankfort horizontal-mandibular plane; SN-GoGn, sella nasion-gonion gnathion.

Commentary

Post-pubescent patients with anterior crossbites often present a debatable problem as to whether the minimal remaining growth will exacerbate the clinical problem or whether the Class III presentation may be camouflaged with selective extractions or with interproximal reduction, while still maintaining facial esthetics. This case demonstrated that the minimal growth remaining occurred in a clockwise direction, and therefore aided in camouflaging the anterior crossbite and the patient's facial esthetics.

Review Questions

1 With facial esthetics in mind, when can you consider camouflage treatment with a skeletal Class III malocclusion?

2 Tipping of the occlusal plane may aid in the non-surgical treatment of a Class III malocclusion. True or false?

3 Clockwise rotation of the mandible aids or hinders the non-surgical correction of a Class III malocclusion?

Suggested Reference

Proffit WR, Fields HW Jr, Sarver DM. Orthodontic treatment planning: From problem list to specific plan. In: Proffit WR, Fields HW Jr, Sarver DM eds. Contemporary Orthodontics, 5th edn. St. Louis, MO: Mosby, 2012; 220–275.

13

Class III Skeletal Pattern and Class II Dental: Non-Extraction

---

LEARNING OBJECTIVES

- Arch leveling with nickel-titanium wires
- Crossbite correction with nickel-titanium arch wires augmented with posterior bite blocks
- The use of reverse curve nickel-titanium arch wires for bite opening

---

Interview Data

This 15-year-old post-pubescent female with appliances in place voiced the chief complaint with her mother that she wanted to have her orthodontic care completed. She has not been under the care of an orthodontist for the past 2 years because of lack of finances.

- Development: post-pubescent
- Motivation: good
- Medical history: non-contributory
- Dental history: periodic care with a single restoration placed

- Family history: the mother of the child received orthodontic care as a growing child
- Habits: none
- Facial form: ovoid, leptoprosopic with mandible asymmetric to the patient's left
- Facial proportions: long lower face

Clinical Examination

- Incisor-stomion (Figures 13.1 and 13.2):
  - At rest: 2 mm
  - Smiling: 7 mm

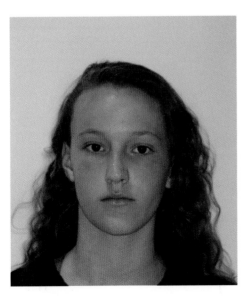

Figure 13.1 Full face at rest displaying a long, ovoid form with slight asymmetry of the mandible to the left.

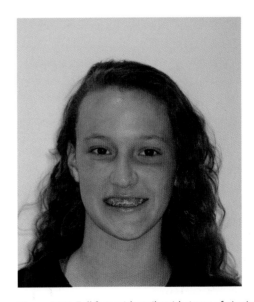

Figure 13.2 Full face with smile with 4 mm of gingival display.

Atlas of Orthodontic Case Reviews, First Edition. Marjan Askari and Stanley A. Alexander.
© 2017 John Wiley & Sons, Inc. Published 2017 by John Wiley & Sons, Inc.

- Lips: competent at rest
- Soft tissue profile: convex with a prominent chin deviating to the left (Figure 13.3)
- Nasolabial angle: normal
- Normal mandibular plane angle

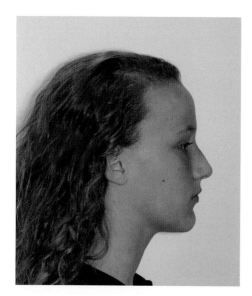

Figure 13.3 Right lateral view of profile exhibiting a slight facial convexity, normal nasolabial angle, and prominent chin.

Dentition (Figure 13.4)

- Teeth clinically present

7654321	1234567
7654321	1234567

- Overjet: 8 mm
- Overbite: 1 mm

- Midlines: the maxillary midline is 2 mm to the left of facial midline; the mandibular midline is 3 mm to the left of the maxillary midline

Right Buccal View (Figure 13.5)

- Molar: end-on
- Canine: Class II
- Curve of Spee: severe
- Caries: none

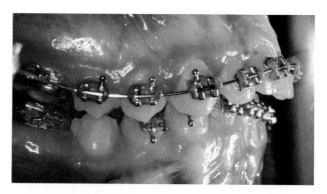

Figure 13.5 Right buccal view of the dentition displaying an end-on molar relationship, Class II canine relationship, and severe curve of Spee with original appliance in place.

Left Buccal View (Figure 13.6)

- Molar: Class II
- Canine: Class II
- Curve of Spee: severe
- Crossbite: maxillary left canine
- Caries: none

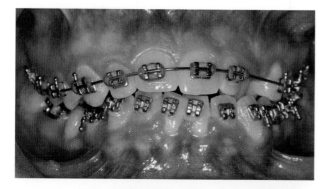

Figure 13.4 Anterior view of the dentition with original appliance in place displaying the maxillary midline 2 mm to the left of the patient's facial midline and the mandibular midline 3 mm to the left of the facial midline.

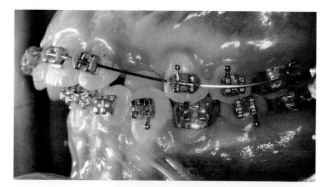

Figure 13.6 Left buccal view of the dentition displaying a Class II molar relationship, Class II canine relationship with the canine in crossbite, and severe curve of Spee with original appliance in place.

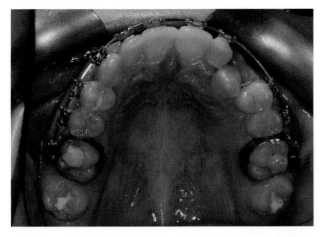

Figure 13.7 Occlusal view of the maxillary arch with the original appliance in place. The arch form is broad, U-shaped with the left canine out of the arch form.

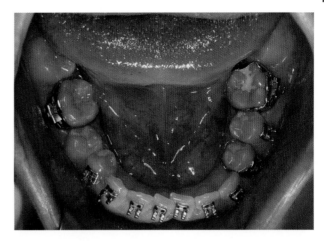

Figure 13.8 Occlusal view of the mandibular arch with original bands and brackets in place.

Maxillary Arch (Figure 13.7)
- Broad U-shaped arch form with left canine in lingual position
- No caries

Mandibular Arch (Figure 13.8)
- Broad U-shaped arch with "roller-coaster effect" due to bracket positions
- No caries

Function

- Centric relation-centric occlusion: coincident
- Normal range of motion: maximum opening = 40 mm; right lateral excursion = 8 mm; left lateral excursion = 7 mm; protrusive = 10 mm
- No pain upon palpation – there is a slight click without popping of the left joint
- Full permanent dentition with third molars developing
- All root lengths and periodontium appear normal
- "Roller-coaster effect" evident due to bracket positioning
- Condyles appear normal (Figure 13.9)

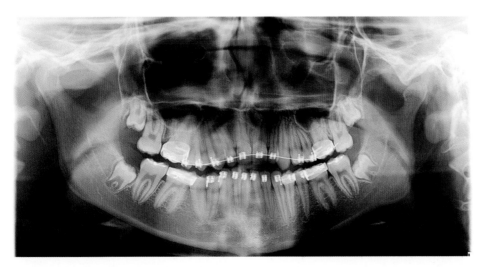

Figure 13.9 Panoramic radiograph displaying a "roller-coaster effect" due to original bracket positioning. The periodontium and condyles appear normal.

Diagnosis and Treatment Plan

The patient is a 15-year-old female with appliances in place, with poor oral hygiene and she has a mild Class III skeletal malocclusion, a Class II dental malocclusion, and severe overjet. The plan of treatment was to address the oral hygiene issue and continuation of orthodontic care if the home maintenance was improved. The manner of treatment would be non-extraction based upon the facial esthetics, skeletal pattern, and current position of the maxillary and mandibular incisors (Figure 13.10; Tables 13.1 and 13.2).

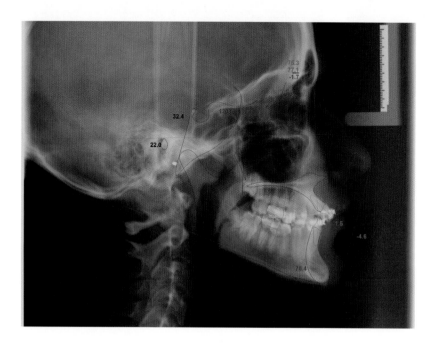

Figure 13.10 Digitized cephalogram exhibiting a normal skeletal relationship with a slight Class III skeletal tendency, normal mandibular plane angle, and severely flared maxillary incisors and upright mandibular incisors.

Table 13.1 Significant cephalometric values

	Norm	Patient pre-treatment
SNA	80°	77.3°
SNB	78°	78.4°
ANB	2°	−1.1°
WITS appraisal	−1 to +1 mm	−2.4 mm
FMA	21°	23.4°
SN-GoGn	32°	32.6°
Maxillary incisor to SN	105°	121.6°
Mandibular incisor to GoGn	95°	79.3°
Soft tissue		
Lower lip to E-plane	−2 mm	−5.4 mm
Upper lip to E-plane	−1.6 mm	−5.1 mm

SNA, sella-nasion-A point; SNB, sella-nasion-B point; ANB, A point-nasion-B point; WITS appraisal, Witwatersrand appraisal; FMA, Frankfort horizontal-mandibular plane; SN-GoGn, sella nasion-gonion gnathion.

Table 13.2 The patient's problem list in three dimensions

	Transverse	Sagittal	Vertical
Soft tissue	Asymmetric chin to the left	Convex profile; normal nasolabial angle; prominent chin	Normodivergent
Dental	Crossbite of maxillary left canine	Adult dentition; Class II molar and canines	1 mm overbite
Skeletal	Normal	Mild Class III	Normodivergent

Treatment Objectives

The objectives of treatment would entail the creation of a Class I molar and canine relationship, correction of the crossbite, and coordination of the arch forms, while maintaining facial esthetics. All would be predicated on the maintenance of good oral hygiene.

Treatment Options

1) Non-extraction treatment – this option was chosen by the patient and parent, based upon the criteria of facial esthetics and cessation of growth (Figures 13.11 and 13.12).
2) No treatment – this option was considered unacceptable due to the current positions of the dentition.
3) Extraction of the maxillary first molars only, the extraction of the maxillary first molars and mandibular first premolars, or extraction of the mandibular second premolars and maxillary first premolars – this option was discussed and would be implemented only if the non-extraction therapy was considered unsuccessful during the course of treatment.

First Active Appointment

The patient was completely debonded and elastic separators were placed between the maxillary and mandibular first molars. The patient was referred to a general dentist for an examination and caries restoration if necessary prior to re-treatment.

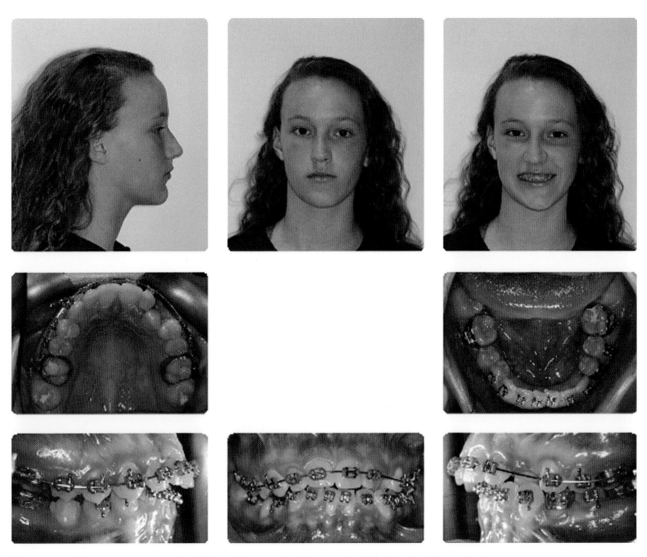

Figure 13.11 Pre-treatment extraoral and intraoral composite photograph with original appliances in place.

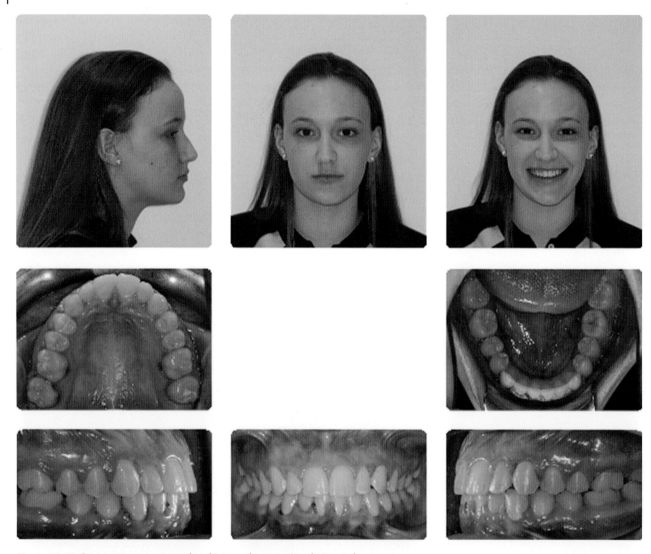

Figure 13.12 Post-treatment extraoral and intraoral composite photograph.

Second Active Appointment

Two weeks later, the maxillary first and second molars and mandibular first molars were banded and cemented with glass ionomer. Bi-dimensional brackets were placed on the remaining dentition. Maxillary and mandibular .014 nickel-titanium arch wires were placed. A glass ionomer build-up of the palatal cusps of the maxillary second molars was performed to disocclude the dentition and allow for the crossbite correction of the maxillary left canine. Oral hygiene and proper diet were stressed and home care instruction was reinforced (Figures 13.13–13.17).

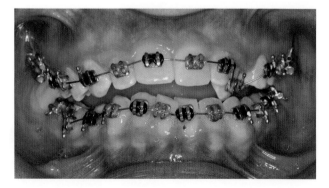

Figure 13.13 Anterior view of the dentition with new appliance in place –.014 nickel-titanium arch wires were ligated to both the maxillary and mandibular arches.

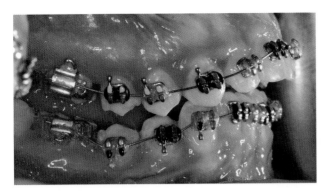

Figure 13.14 Right buccal view of the dentition on the day that new appliances were placed.

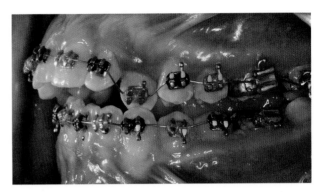

Figure 13.15 Left buccal view of the dentition on the day that new appliances were placed.

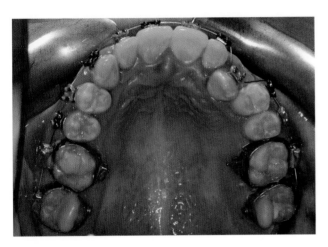

Figure 13.16 Occlusal view of the maxillary arch on the day new appliances were placed. Note the glass ionomer occlusal build-up on the palatal cusps of the second molars.

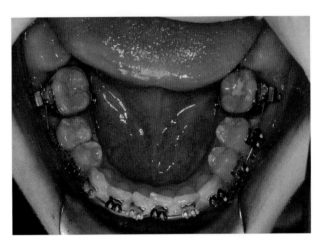

Figure 13.17 Occlusal view of the mandibular arch on the day that the new appliance was placed.

Third to Fourth Active Appointment

Four weeks later, the arch wires were changed to .016 nickel-titanium and the occlusal build-up on the second molars was removed and placed on the first molars (Figures 13.18–13.22). Eight weeks later, separators were placed for banding of the mandibular second molars.

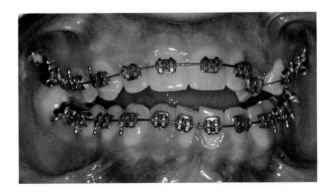

Figure 13.18 Anterior view of the dentition 4 weeks later. The arch wires have been changed to .016 nickel-titanium.

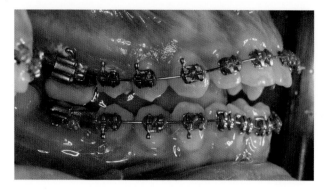

Figure 13.19 Right buccal view of the dentition 4 weeks later. Glass ionomer build-up has been placed on the first molar palatal cusps.

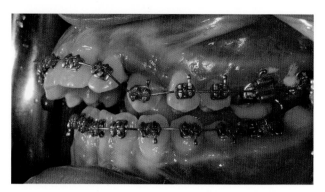

Figure 13.20 Left buccal view of the dentition 4 weeks later. Glass ionomer build-up has been placed on the first molar palatal cusps.

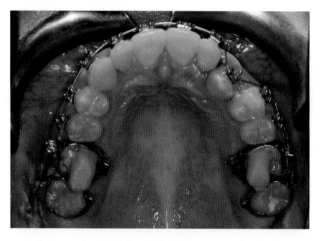

Figure 13.21 Occlusal view of the maxillary arch 4 weeks later. The glass ionomer has been removed from the second molars and replaced on the first molar palatal cusps.

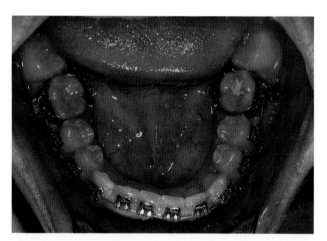

Figure 13.22 Occlusal view of the mandibular arch 4 weeks later.

Fifth Active Appointment

Five weeks later, the mandibular right second molar was banded, but the left second molar was left unbanded due to its appropriate position in the arch. A maxillary .016 × .022 nickel-titanium wire was ligated in place, while a .018 nickel-titanium wire was replaced on the mandibular arch to align the second molar. Note that the occlusal build-up was removed and the maxillary left canine crossbite has been corrected (Figures 13.23–13.27).

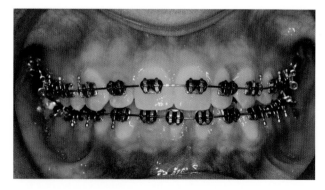

Figure 13.23 Anterior view of the dentition 4 weeks later. The maxillary arch wire was changed to .016 × .022 nickel-titanium and the mandibular arch wire was changed to .018 nickel-titanium.

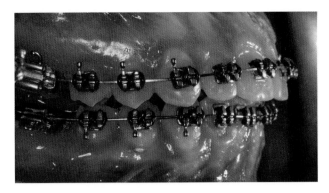

Figure 13.24 Right buccal view of the dentition 4 weeks later.

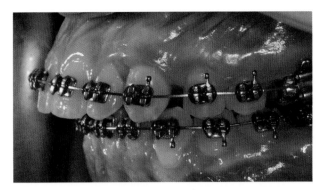

Figure 13.25 Left buccal view of the dentition 4 weeks later. Note the canine crossbite correction.

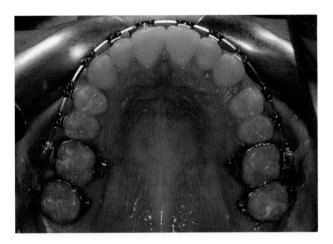

Figure 13.26 Occlusal view of the maxillary arch 4 weeks later. The glass ionomer build-up was removed.

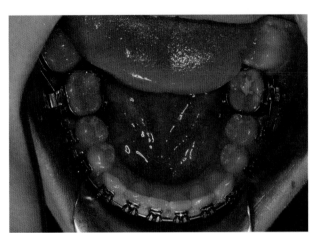

Figure 13.27 Occlusal view of the mandibular arch 4 weeks later. The right second molar was banded at this time.

Sixth Active Appointment

Four weeks later, the maxillary arch wire was changed to .017 × .025 nickel-titanium and the mandibular arch wire was changed to .016 × .022 nickel-titanium. A continuous elastomeric chain was attached to the maxillary first molar to maxillary first molar. The patient was instructed to wear a triangle elastic from the maxillary canine to the mandibular right canine and first premolar (3/16"; 4oz.) and a Class II elastic from the maxillary left canine to the mandibular left first molar (3/16"; 4oz.), the purpose of which was to settle the occlusion on the right side and shift the dental midline to the patient's right side (Figures 13.28–13.32).

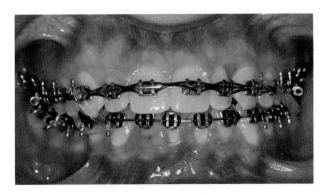

Figure 13.28 Anterior view of the dentition at the sixth appointment 4 weeks later. The maxillary arch wire was changed to .017 × .025 nickel-titanium and the mandibular arch wire was changed to .016 × .022 nickel-titanium. Elastomeric chain was placed from the maxillary first molar to first molar for space consolidation.

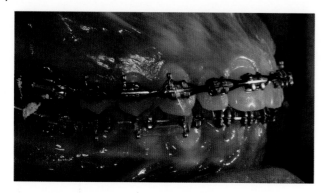

Figure 13.29 Right buccal view of the dentition on the sixth appointment. A triangle elastic was placed on the maxillary canine to the mandibular canine and first premolar to settle the occlusion.

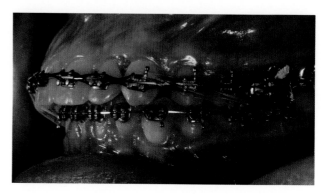

Figure 13.30 Left buccal view of the dentition on the sixth appointment. A Class II elastic was worn to shift the mandibular midline to the right and to correct the Class II canine position.

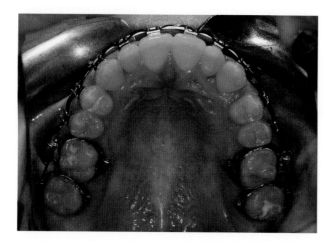

Figure 13.31 Occlusal view of the maxillary arch on the sixth appointment.

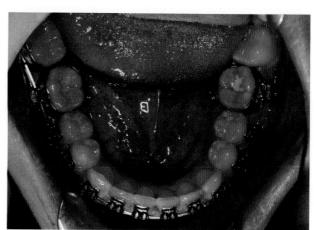

Figure 13.32 Occlusal view of the mandibular arch on the sixth appointment.

Seventh Active Appointment

Four weeks later the mandibular arch wire was changed to .017 × .025 nickel-titanium with a reverse curve for bite opening and flaring of the mandibular incisors. The elastomeric chain was continued on the maxillary arch. The patient was instructed to wear Class II elastics from the maxillary right canine to the mandibular right first molar and from the maxillary left canine to the mandibular left first molar (3/16"; 6 oz.). Note the midline improvement from the previous month (Figures 13.33–13.35).

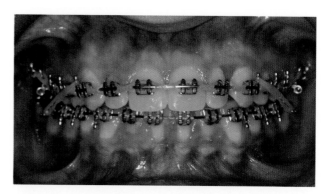

Figure 13.33 Anterior view of the dentition at the seventh appointment 4 weeks later. The mandibular arch wire was changed to .017 × .025 reverse-curved nickel-titanium. Elastomeric chain was continued on the maxillary arch. Class II elastics were now worn bilaterally to correct the Class II relationship. Note the improved midline correction since the sixth appointment.

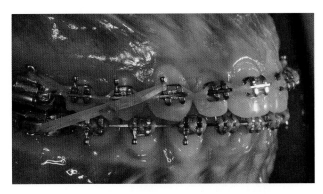

Figure 13.34 Right buccal view of the dentition at the seventh appointment. Class II elastics were worn to establish a Class I relationship.

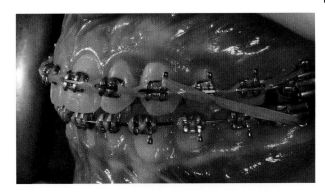

Figure 13.35 Left buccal view of the dentition at the seventh appointment. Class II elastics were worn to establish a Class I relationship.

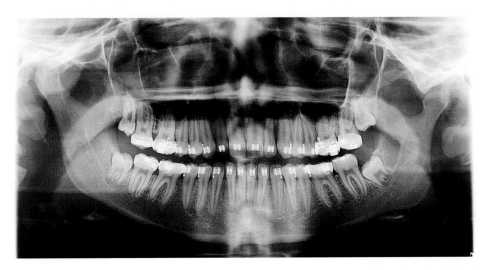

Figure 13.36 Panoramic radiograph at the eighth appointment 4 weeks later. All root lengths and periodontium appear normal.

Eighth Active Appointment

A progress panoramic radiograph was taken 4 weeks after the previous appointment. All root lengths appear normal and parallel. Extraction of the third molars was recommended after the completion of active orthodontic care (Figure 13.36).

Ninth Appointment

Eight weeks later, the patient was debonded. Alginate impressions were taken for immediate Essix retainers (DENTSPLY Raintree Essix, Sarasota, FL, USA). Photographs, an iTero scan (Align Technology, Inc, San Jose, CA, USA), and a cephalogram were taken. The patient was instructed to wear the retainers at night and while sleeping and was told to return in 1 month for observation for an iTero scan, followed by quarterly appointments during the first year after active orthodontic therapy was completed. The molar and canine relationships were in a Class I position and the overbite was improved. Maxillary and mandibular arch forms are broad and U-shaped. The facial esthetics appeared balanced and the patient and parents were pleased with the result. Active treatment time was 10 months (Figures 13.37–13.44).

The overall superimposition indicated little, if any, growth, contributing to the correction. Regional superimposition indicated that the maxillary incisor was tipped back to a more acceptable and stable position, while the mandibular incisor was inclined labially to a normal position. The soft tissue drape improved as a result of the improved incisor angulations (Figures 13.45 and 13.46; Table 13.3).

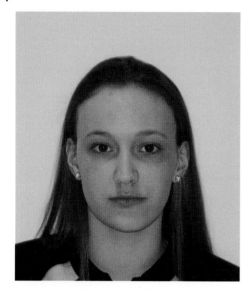

Figure 13.37 Full-face view 8 weeks later, on the day of appliance removal.

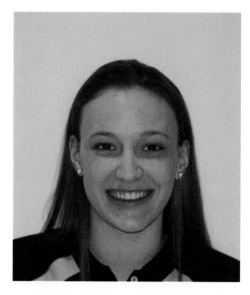

Figure 13.38 Full-face view with smile 8 weeks later, on the day of appliance removal.

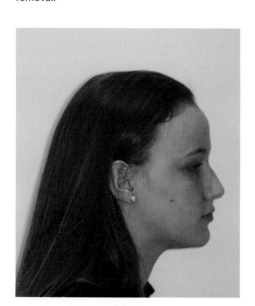

Figure 13.39 Right lateral view of profile 8 weeks later, on the day of appliance removal, displaying an esthetic relationship.

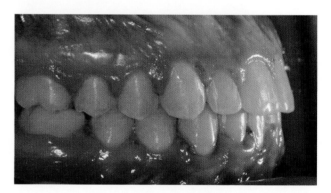

Figure 13.41 Right buccal view of the dentition on the day of appliance removal.

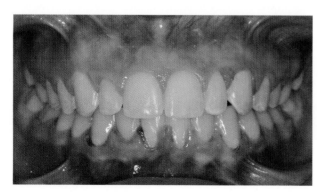

Figure 13.40 Anterior view of the dentition 8 weeks later, on the day of appliance removal.

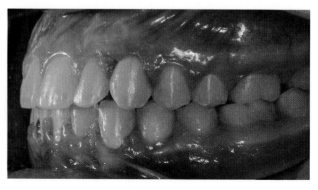

Figure 13.42 Left buccal view of the dentition on the day of appliance removal.

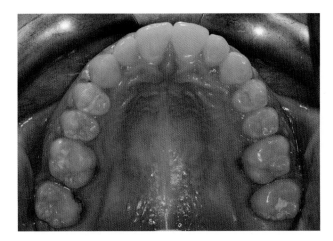

Figure 13.43 Occlusal view of the maxillary arch on the day of appliance removal.

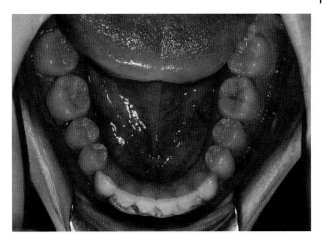

Figure 13.44 Occlusal view of the mandibular arch on the day of appliance removal.

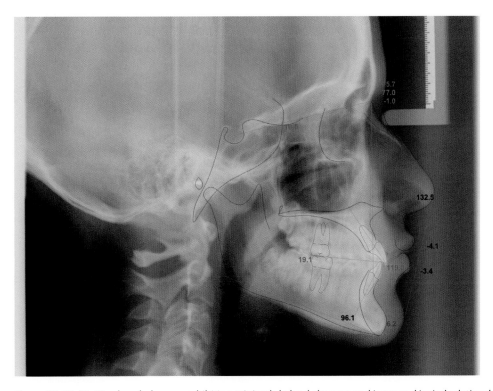

Figure 13.45 Digitized cephalogram exhibiting minimal skeletal changes and improved incisal relationships.

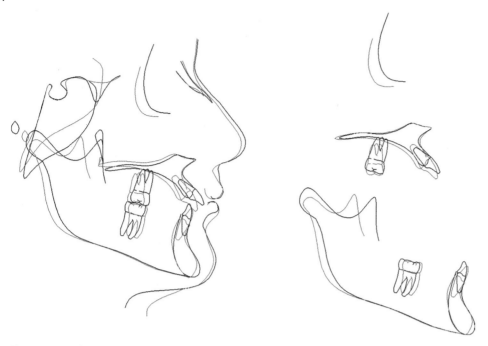

Figure 13.46 The overall superimposition (initial, black; final, red) indicated minimal skeletal change with little, if any, growth taking place during treatment. The regional superimposition indicated minimal change in the position of the molars, but improved incisor positions as the maxillary incisor was tipped lingually and the mandibular incisor was tipped labially.

Table 13.3 Significant pre-treatment and post-treatment cephalometric values

	Norm	Pre-treatment	Post-treatment
SNA	82°	77.3°	75.7°
SNB	80°	78.4°	77.0°
ANB	2°	−1.1°	−1.3°
WITS appraisal	−1 to +1 mm	−2.4 mm	−4.7 mm
FMA	21°	23.4°	26.6°
SN-GoGn	32°	32.6°	32.0°
Maxillary incisor to SN	105°	121.6°	110.5°
Mandibular incisor to GoGn	95°	79.3°	96.1°
Soft tissue			
Lower lip to E-plane	−2.0 mm	−5.4 mm	−3.4 mm
Upper lip to E-plane	−1.6 mm	−5.1 mm	−4.1 mm

SNA, sella-nasion-A point; SNB, sella-nasion-B point; ANB, A point-nasion-B point; WITS appraisal, Witwatersrand appraisal; FMA, Frankfort horizontal-mandibular plane; SN-GoGn, sella nasion-gonion gnathion.

Commentary

The evaluation of overall facial esthetics and the position of the mandibular incisor in its relation to the mandible on a classical and modern point of evaluation can often create a non-extraction mode of therapy. In this case, the extreme upright position of the mandibular incisor and relatively straight profile created a clinical situation in which the maintenance of the full complement of teeth became the treatment of choice.

Review Questions

1   What method was used to disocclude the dentition for correction of the maxillary left canine?

2   The correction of the patient's midline discrepancy was accomplished by what method?

3   Opening of the deep bite and flaring of the mandibular incisors was accomplished late in the treatment by what method?

Suggested References

Abdulaziz KA, Sadowsky S, BeGole EA. A comparison of the effects of rectangular and round arch wires in leveling the curve of Spee. Am J Orthod Dentofacial Orthop 116: 522–529, 1999.

Yitschaky O, Neuhof MS, Yitschaky M, Zini A. Relationship between dental crowding and mandibular incisor proclination during orthodontic treatment without extraction of permanent mandibular teeth. Angle Orthod 86(5): 727–733, 2016.

14

Class III Skeletal and Class I Dental: Four Premolar Extractions

Interview Data

An 11-year-old female transferred from another ortho-dontic office with appliances in place and four premolars already extracted. The parent wished for continued treatment.

- Development: pre-pubescent
- Motivation: good
- Medical history: controlled asthmatic
- Dental history: routine dental care; transferred from an orthodontic office with appliances in place and pre-molars already extracted
- Family history: non-contributory
- Habits: none

- Facial form: ovoid, symmetric leptoprosopic facial form
- Facial proportions: convex profile with long lower face and high mandibular plane angle

Clinical Examination

- Incisor-stomion (Figures 14.1 and 14.2):
  - At rest: 4 mm
  - Smiling: 9 mm
- Breathing: nasal
- Lips: together at rest
- Appliances in place
- Soft tissue profile: convex (Figure 14.3)
- Nasolabial angle: normal
- High mandibular plane angle

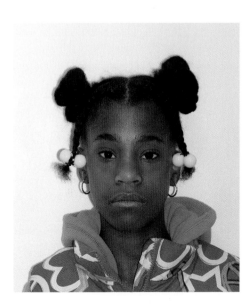

Figure 14.1 Full-face view with symmetric, ovoid form.

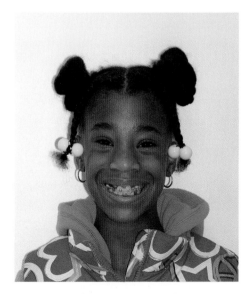

Figure 14.2 Full-face view with smile displaying 3 mm of gingiva.

Atlas of Orthodontic Case Reviews, First Edition. Marjan Askari and Stanley A. Alexander.
© 2017 John Wiley & Sons, Inc. Published 2017 by John Wiley & Sons, Inc.

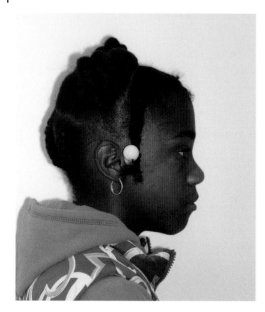

Figure 14.3 Right lateral view of profile displaying a convex form and high mandibular plane angle.

Dentition (Figure 14.4)

- Teeth clinically present:

6521	12356
65321	12356

- Overjet: 1.5 mm
- Overbite: 4 mm
- Crossbite: maxillary right and left lateral incisors
- Midlines: maxillary midline is 1 mm right of facial midline; mandibular midline is 2 mm to the right of maxillary dental midline and 3 mm to the right of facial midline

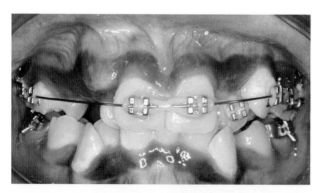

Figure 14.4 Anterior view of the dentition displaying previous appliances in place with severe crowding. The maxillary midline is 1 mm to the right of the facial midline and the mandibular midline is 2 mm to the right of the maxillary dental midline.

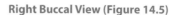

Right Buccal View (Figure 14.5)

- Molar: Class I
- Canine: not applicable
- Curve of Spee: deep
- Crossbite: maxillary lateral incisor
- Caries: none

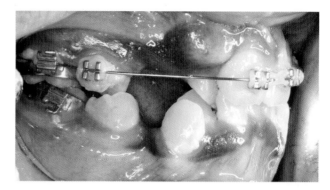

Figure 14.5 Right buccal view of the dentition with a Class I molar relationship, a deep curve of Spee and crossbite of the maxillary lateral incisor.

Left Buccal View (Figure 14.6)

- Molar: Class I
- Canine: not applicable
- Curve of Spee: deep
- Crossbite: maxillary lateral incisor
- Caries none

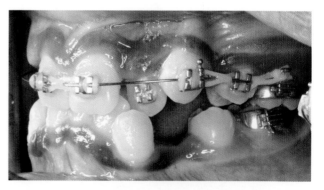

Figure 14.6 Left buccal view of the dentition displaying a Class I molar relationship, deep curve of Spee, and crossbite of the maxillary lateral incisor.

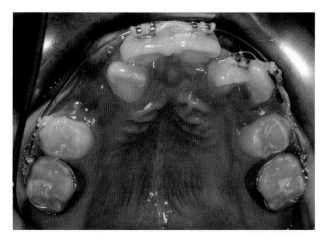

Figure 14.7 Occlusal view of the maxillary arch exhibiting a broad, U-shaped arch form with severe crowding.

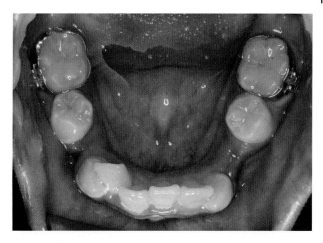

Figure 14.8 Occlusal view of the mandibular arch exhibiting a U-shaped form and severe crowding.

Maxillary Arch (Figure 14.7)

- Broad, U-shaped symmetric arch form with severe crowding and appliances in place
- No caries

Mandibular Arch (Figure 14.8)

- U-shaped, symmetric arch form with severe crowding and partial appliance in place
- No caries

Function

- Maximum opening = 40 mm
- Centric relation-centric occlusion: coincident
- Maximum excursive movements: right = 7 mm; left = 8 mm; protrusive = 6 mm
- Temporomandibular joint palpation: normal
- Late mixed dentition with maxillary appliance in place
- Supernumerary teeth present in maxillary right and left second molar sites and between the mandibular right first permanent molar and second premolar (Figure 14.9)
- Impeded eruption of maxillary right and left second molars due to supernumerary teeth
- Root length and periodontium appear normal
- Condyles appear normal

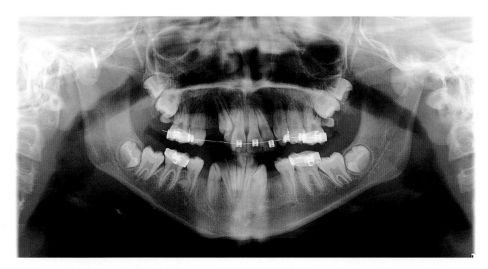

Figure 14.9 Panoramic radiograph exhibiting a late mixed dentition with supernumerary teeth present in the maxillary first molar area, extraction sites for the maxillary and mandibular first premolars, and normal periodontium and condyles.

Diagnosis and Treatment Plan

The patient presents with a mild Class III skeletal malocclusion, a Class I dental malocclusion, severe crowding, moderate overbite due to the extremely upright maxillary and mandibular incisors, and supernumerary teeth. The face is symmetric but hyperdivergent. The soft tissues are esthetic and balanced (Figures 14.10; Tables 14.1 and 14.2).

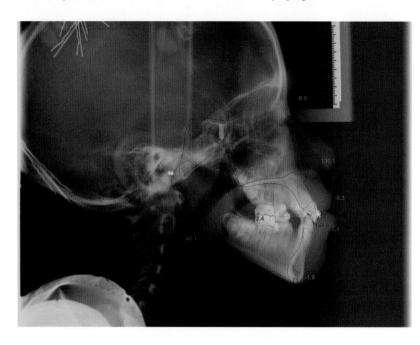

Figure 14.10 Digitized cephalogram exhibiting a Class III skeletal relationship, high mandibular plane angle, and upright maxillary and mandibular incisors with excessive mandibular soft tissue drape.

Table 14.1 Significant cephalometric values

	Norm	Patient pre-treatment
SNA	80°	83.5°
SNB	78°	78.3°
ANB	2°	+5.3°
WITS appraisal	−1 to +1 mm	−2.9 mm
FMA	21°	30.4°
SN-GoGn	32°	45.1°
Maxillary incisor to SN	105°	94.7°
Mandibular incisor to GoGn	95°	71.4°
Soft tissue		
Lower lip to E-plane	−2 mm	+5.0 mm
Upper lip to E-plane	−1.6 mm	−0.3 mm

SNA, sella-nasion-A point; SNB, sella-nasion-B point; ANB, A point-nasion-B point; WITS appraisal, Witwatersrand appraisal; FMA, Frankfort horizontal-mandibular plane; SN-GoGn, sella nasion-gonion gnathion.

Table 14.2 The patient's problem list in three dimensions

	Transverse	Sagittal	Vertical
Soft tissue	Normal	Convex profile; normal nasolabial angle	Hyperdivergent
Dental	Crossbite of right and left maxillary lateral incisors	Late mixed dentition; Class I molar; crossbite of lateral incisors	4 mm overbite; extremely upright maxillary and mandibular incisors
Skeletal	Normal	Mild Class III	Hyperdivergent

Treatment Objectives

The patient began treatment in another office where the four first premolars were extracted. The goal of treatment was to maintain the Class I occlusion with maximum anchorage conservation and to allow the child to grow normally. The incisor angulation was to be corrected; however, due to the hyperdivergent growth pattern, an open bite relationship needed to be avoided. The supernumerary teeth that were impeding the eruption of the maxillary second molars required removal, while the mandibular supernumerary tooth was to be observed for further root formation and development. Extraction would be postponed so as not to devitalize the existing second premolar.

Treatment Options

1) No treatment was not an alternative as the parent had already committed to treatment via the extraction of permanent teeth (Figures 14.11 and 14.12).
2) Alternate extraction patterns might have been indicated in an attempt to anecdotally close the mandibular plane angle, but the level of anterior crowding justified the removal of the first premolars.
3) Growth modification with the use of high pull headgear in concert with extraction therapy was advised – both anchorage and vertical control could be augmented, but the patient refused to wear this appliance.
4) Maximum anchorage would be attained with the placement of a Nance appliance on the maxilla and a lingual arch on the mandible.

Option 4 was chosen.

First Active Appointment

As option 4 was chosen, the existing appliances were removed. New bands were fitted and impressions were taken to construct a Nance appliance and a mandibular lingual arch to enhance anchorage. Elastic separators were placed for appliance cementation at the next appointment.

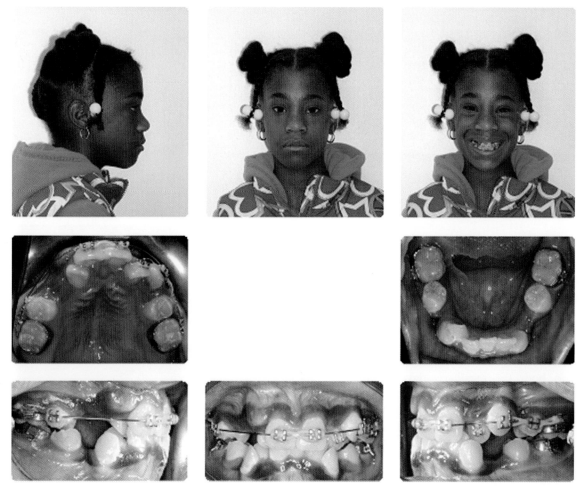

Figure 14.11 Pre-treatment extraoral and intraoral composite photograph.

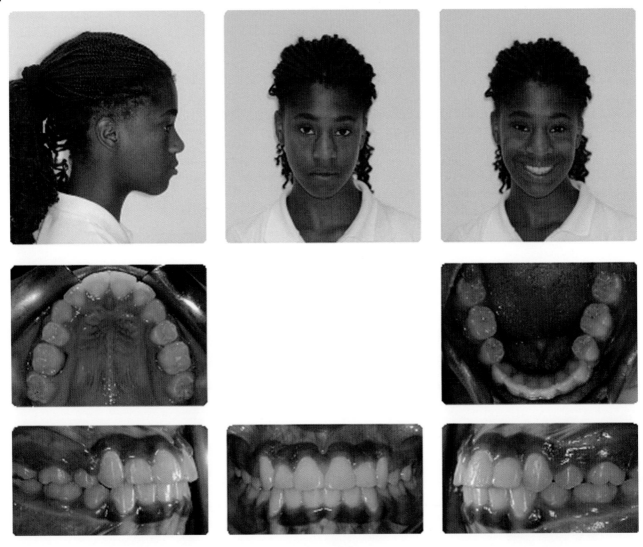

Figure 14.12 Post-treatment extraoral and intraoral composite photograph.

Second Active Appointment

The Nance appliance and lingual arch were cemented with glass ionomer. The remaining teeth, except for the maxillary right lateral incisor, were bonded with a bi-dimensional appliance. A .016 × .022 β-titanium sectional arch was placed from the maxillary right molar to the right canine and an elastomeric chain was attached for canine retraction. A .016 nickel-titanium arch wire was ligated to both the maxillary and mandibular teeth except for the mandibular right lateral incisor. Elastomeric chain was placed from the mandibular right molar to the second premolar for rotation and from the mandibular left molar and canine for retraction (Figures 14.13–14.17).

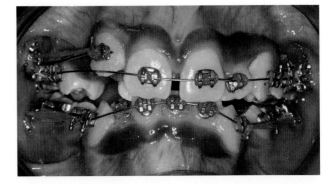

Figure 14.13 Anterior view of the dentition at the second active appointment. Maxillary and mandibular .016 nickel-titanium arch wires have been placed. A sectional .016 × .022 β-titanium wire was placed on the maxillary right molar to canine for retraction of the canine.

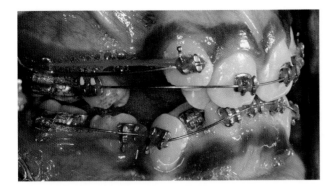

Figure 14.14 Right buccal view of the dentition exhibiting sectional retraction of the maxillary canine with elastomeric chain and rotation of the mandibular second premolar with elastomeric chain.

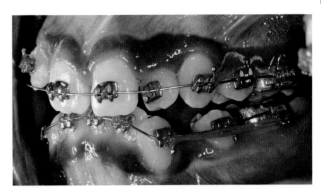

Figure 14.15 Left buccal view of the dentition exhibiting retraction of the mandibular canine with elastomeric chain.

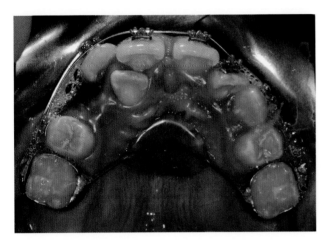

Figure 14.16 Occlusal view of the maxillary arch on the second active appointment displaying the Nance appliance used for anchorage.

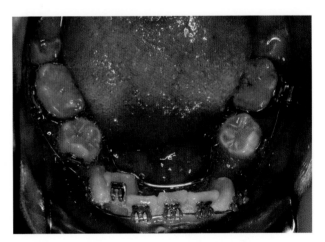

Figure 14.17 Occlusal view of the mandibular arch on the second active appointment displaying the lingual arch used for anchorage.

Third Active Appointment

Four weeks later both the maxillary and mandibular arch wires were changed to .016 × .022 nickel-titanium. An open coil spring was placed between the mandibular right central incisor and the right canine to create space for the blocked-out lateral incisor and to shift the midline to the left. Elastomeric chain was placed between the maxillary central incisors, the maxillary right canine to first molar, and from the mandibular left canine to the first molar (Figures 14.18–14.22).

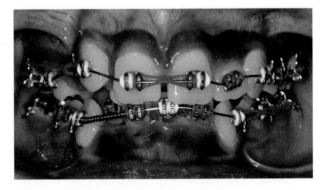

Figure 14.18 Anterior view of the dentition 4 weeks later. Both the maxillary and mandibular arch wires were changed to .016 × .022 nickel-titanium. An open coil spring was placed between the mandibular right canine and central incisor to make space and shift the midline to the left. Elastomeric chain was used to consolidate space between the maxillary central incisors.

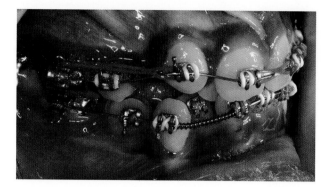

Figure 14.19 Right buccal view of the dentition 4 weeks later. The maxillary canine was being retracted and the open coil spring between the mandibular canine and central incisor was used to open space and to shift the midline.

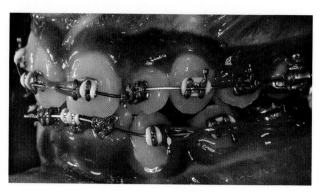

Figure 14.20 Left buccal view of the dentition 4 weeks later. Elastomeric chain was being used to retract the canine.

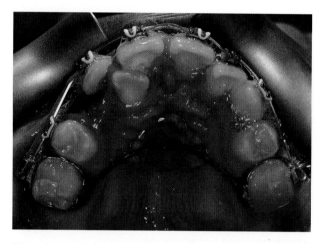

Figure 14.21 Occlusal view of the maxillary arch 4 weeks later.

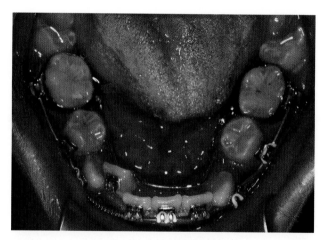

Figure 14.22 Occlusal view of the mandibular arch 4 weeks later.

Fourth Active Appointment

Eight weeks later (Figures 14.23–14.27) the maxillary and mandibular arch wires were changed to .017 × .025 nickel-titanium and the mandibular right lateral incisor was engaged with a .014 nickel-titanium overlay (arrow in Figure 14.27). A button was bonded to the lingual of the maxillary right lateral incisor and an elastomeric chain was stretched from the labial of the maxillary right central incisor and labial of the maxillary right canine to labialize the lateral incisor. An open coil spring was also placed between the maxillary canine to the central incisor to help open space for the lateral incisor. Elastomeric chain was also ligated from the maxillary right first molar to the right canine for retraction.

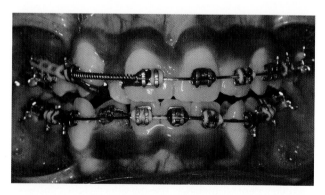

Figure 14.23 Eight weeks later, the maxillary and mandibular arch wires were changed to .017 × .025 nickel-titanium. An open coil spring was placed between the maxillary right central incisor and canine to create space. A button was bonded to the lingual of the maxillary right lateral incisor and an elastomeric chain stretched from the right canine to the lingual button of the lateral incisor and to the right central incisor to labialize the lateral incisor. A .014 nickel-titanium overlay wire was placed on the mandibular right lateral incisor to bring the tooth into the arch form.

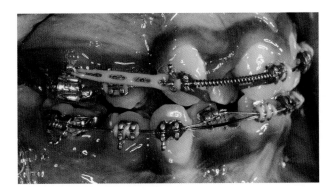

Figure 14.24 Right buccal view of the dentition 8 weeks later. The maxillary canine was being retracted with elastomeric chain with an open coil spring between the canine and the central incisor. The mandibular .014 nickel-titanium overlay was being used to bring the lateral incisor into the arch form.

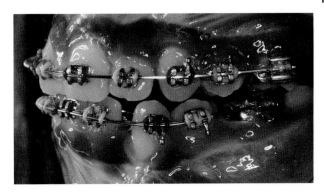

Figure 14.25 Left buccal view of the dentition 8 weeks later.

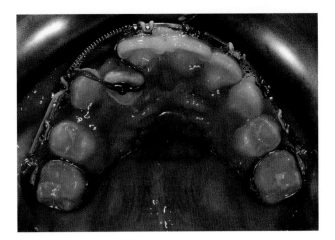

Figure 14.26 Occlusal view of the maxillary arch displaying the elastomeric chain in place to labialize the right lateral incisor.

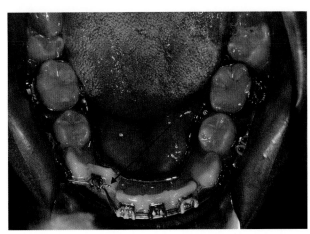

Figure 14.27 Occlusal view of the mandibular arch 8 weeks later exhibiting the .014 nickel-titanium overlay wire (arrow).

Fifth Active Appointment

Four weeks later, the patient returned and the oral hygiene was considered poor, such that a gingivectomy via laser would have been indicated at the following appointment if no improvement was noted. The Nance button was removed (Figures 14.28–14.32). Note the irritation on the maxilla due to the palatal button (arrow in Figure 14.31). The mandibular wire was changed to .016 × .022 nickel-titanium. The elastomeric chain and open coil spring were continued on the maxillary arch as per the previous appointment.

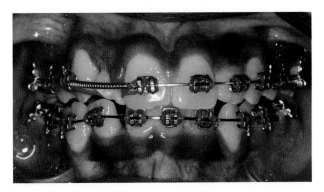

Figure 14.28 Anterior view of the dentition 4 weeks later at the fifth active appointment. The mandibular wire was changed to .016 × .022 nickel-titanium and the overlay was removed. Mechanics on the maxillary arch remained the same as per the previous visit for lateral incisor labialization. The canine retraction via elastomeric chain was removed.

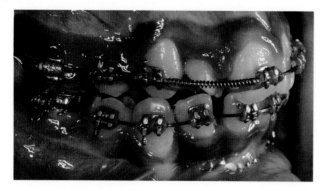

Figure 14.29 Right buccal view of the dentition 4 weeks later at the fifth active appointment.

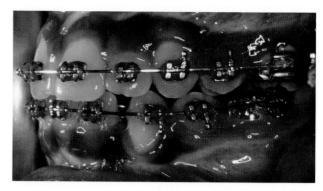

Figure 14.30 Left buccal view of the dentition 4 weeks later at the fifth active appointment.

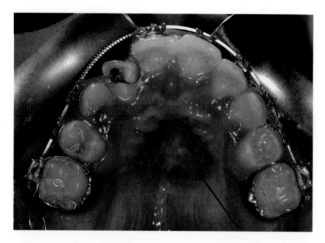

Figure 14.31 Occlusal view of the maxillary arch 4 weeks later at the fifth active appointment. The Nance appliance was removed. Note the palatal irritation from the acrylic button (arrow).

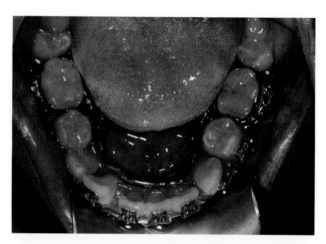

Figure 14.32 Occlusal view of the mandibular arch 4 weeks later at the fifth appointment. Note the improvement in arch form.

Sixth Active Appointment

Four weeks later the lingual button on the maxillary right lateral incisor was removed and a bracket was bonded to the labial surface. The mandibular lingual arch was removed (Figures 14.33–14.37). Note the healing of the palatal inflammation (arrow in Figure 14.36) when compared to Figure 14.31. A mandibular .017 × .025 stainless steel wire was ligated to the arch. The maxillary arch wire was changed to .017 × .025 stainless steel and a .014 nickel-titanium overlay was placed to engage the maxillary right lateral incisor.

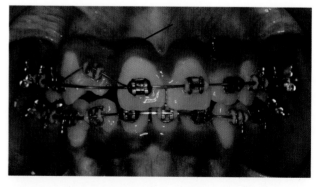

Figure 14.33 Anterior view of the dentition 4 weeks later. Both maxillary and mandibular arch wires have been changed to .017 × .025 stainless steel. The lingual button on the maxillary right incisor was removed. A .014 nickel-titanium overlay wire was "piggybacked" (arrow) to the maxillary wire to engage the right lateral incisor.

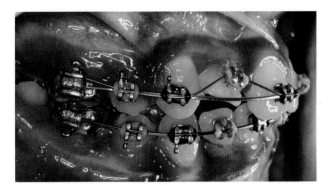

Figure 14.34 Right buccal view of the dentition 4 weeks later.

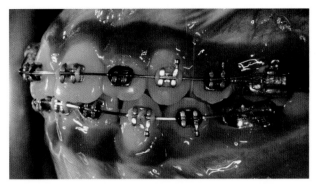

Figure 14.35 Left buccal view of the dentition 4 weeks later.

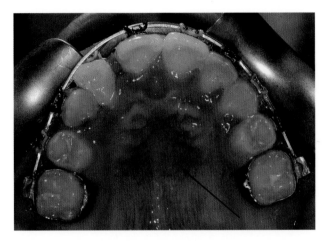

Figure 14.36 Occlusal view of the maxillary arch 4 weeks later. Note the healing of the palate once the acrylic button was removed (arrow).

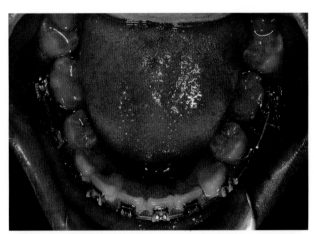

Figure 14.37 Occlusal view of the mandibular arch 4 weeks later. The lingual arch was removed.

Seventh Active Appointment

Four weeks later, the maxillary right lateral incisor bracket was removed and rebonded upside down to reverse the torque prescription in order to move the root more to the labial direction. The maxillary arch wire was changed to .016 × .022 nickel-titanium, while the mandibular arch wire remained the same as per the previous appointment. Elastomeric chain was placed on the mandibular arch from the left first molar to the left central incisor to help shift the mandibular midline to the left (Figures 14.38–14.42).

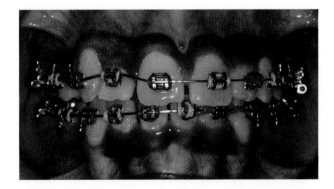

Figure 14.38 Anterior view of the dentition at the seventh active appointment 4 weeks later. The maxillary right lateral incisor bracket was replaced upside down to reverse the torque prescription. The maxillary arch wire was changed to .016 × .022 nickel-titanium. Elastomeric chain was placed from the left mandibular molar to the left central incisor to shift the midline to the left.

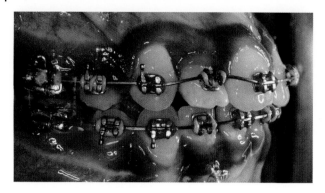

Figure 14.39 Right buccal view of the dentition 4 weeks later.

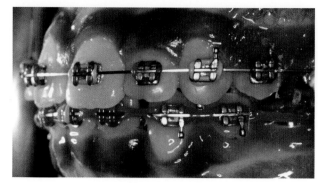

Figure 14.40 Left buccal view of the dentition 4 weeks later.

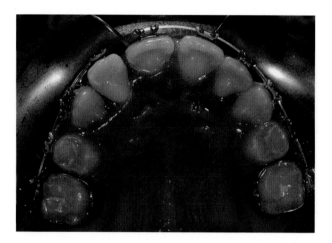

Figure 14.41 Occlusal view of the maxillary arch 4 weeks later.

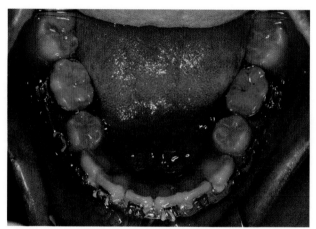

Figure 14.42 Occlusal view of the mandibular arch 4 weeks later with elastomeric chain attached to the left molar through the central incisor to shift the midline to the left.

Eighth Active Appointment

Four weeks later, the maxillary arch wire was changed to .017 × .025 nickel-titanium. Elastomeric chain was placed from the maxillary right first molar to the maxillary left first molar for space consolidation and from the mandibular left first molar to the right central incisor to move the midline to the left. A triangle elastic was placed from the maxillary left canine to the mandibular left canine and second premolar to settle the occlusion, and a Class II elastic was placed from the maxillary right canine to the mandibular right first molar (3/16", 4.5 oz.) to correct the Class II relationship. The patient was instructed to change the elastics daily (Figures 14.43–14.47).

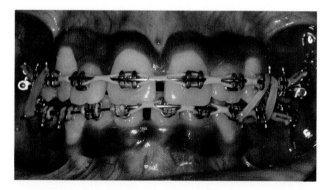

Figure 14.43 Anterior view of the dentition 4 weeks later at the eighth active appointment. The maxillary arch wire was changed to .017 × .025 nickel-titanium. Elastomeric chain was attached from maxillary right first molar to the maxillary left first molar for space consolidation, and from the mandibular left first molar to the right central incisor to shift the midline.

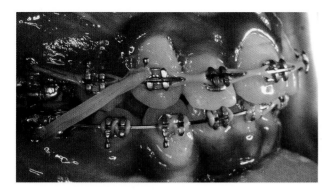

Figure 14.44 Right buccal view of the dentition 4 weeks later. The Class II elastic was used to establish a Class I canine and molar relationship and to shift the midline to the left.

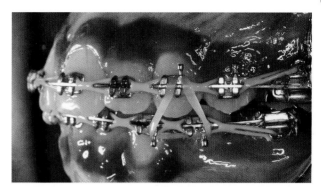

Figure 14.45 Left buccal view of the dentition 4 weeks later. A triangle elastic was used to settle the occlusion.

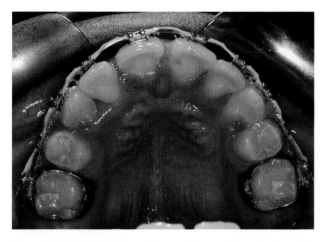

Figure 14.46 Occlusal view of the maxillary arch 4 weeks later with the elastomeric chain extending from first molar to first molar.

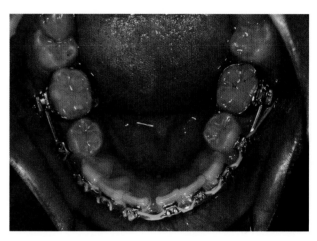

Figure 14.47 Occlusal view of the mandibular arch 4 weeks later.

Ninth Active Appointment

Five weeks later, the elastomeric chain on the mandibular arch was removed and each tooth was individually ligated. Elastomeric chain was replaced on the maxillary arch. A triangular Class II elastic was worn from the maxillary right canine to the mandibular first molar and second premolar (for Class II correction and settling of the occlusion) and a triangle elastic was worn from the maxillary left canine to the mandibular left canine and second premolar (3/16″, 4.5 oz.). These elastics were to be changed daily (Figures 14.48–14.52).

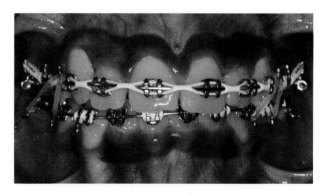

Figure 14.48 Anterior view of the dentition 5 weeks later. Elastomeric chain was replaced from the maxillary first molar to first molar. The mandibular teeth were individually ligated.

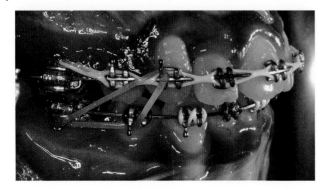

Figure 14.49 Anterior view of the dentition 5 weeks later. Elastomeric chain was replaced from the maxillary first molar to first molar. The mandibular teeth were individually ligated.

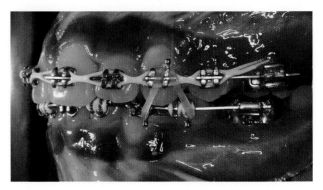

Figure 14.50 Left buccal view of the dentition 5 weeks later with a triangle elastic placed.

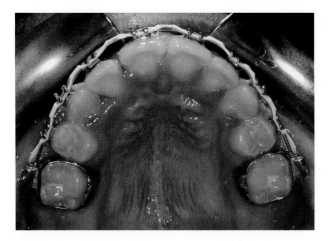

Figure 14.51 Occlusal view of the maxillary arch 5 weeks later with elastomeric chain in place.

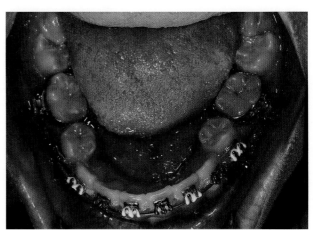

Figure 14.52 Occlusal view of the mandibular arch 5 weeks later.

Tenth Active Appointment

Six weeks later, elastomeric chain was placed from the maxillary right canine to the left canine. Elastic wear was continued as per the previous appointment. (Figures 14.53–14.55) An evaluation was made regarding the remaining supernumerary tooth The oral surgeon recommended that the tooth be left in place as it showed no significant signs of change and its removal could jeopardize the mandibular right first molar and second premolar (Figure 14.56). The supernumerary tooth was scheduled for periodic monitoring.

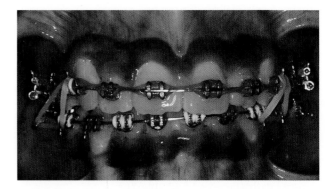

Figure 14.53 Anterior view of the dentition 6 weeks later at the 10th active appointment. Elastomeric chain was replaced from maxillary right canine to left canine.

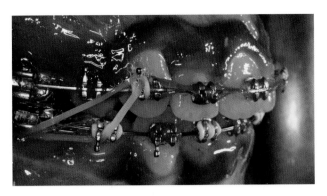

Figure 14.54 Right buccal view of the dentition 6 weeks later with the triangular Class II elastic in place.

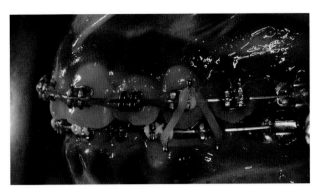

Figure 14.55 Left buccal view of the dentition 6 weeks later with a triangle elastic in place.

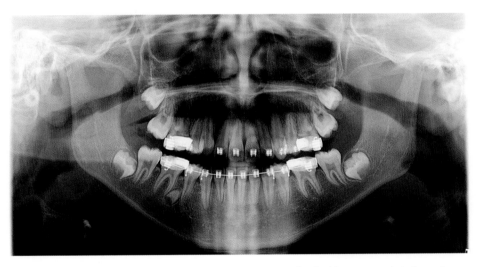

Figure 14.56 Panoramic view at the 10th active appointment. The decision was made to leave the supernumerary tooth in the mandibular right quadrant in place and to observe periodically for changes.

Eleventh to 12th Active Appointments

Four weeks later, the same procedure was performed and elastic wear was continued. At the following appointment in 5 weeks, tubes were placed on all four second molars. The mandibular incisor brackets were removed and bonded upside down to reverse the torque prescription and to allow for better labial positioning of the crowns of these teeth. The maxillary arch wire was changed to .018 nickel-titanium, while the mandibular arch wire was changed to .016 × .022 nickel-titanium. Triangle elastics (3/16", 4.5 oz.) were placed on the maxillary right canine to the mandibular right canine and second premolar, and on the maxillary left canine to the mandibular left canine and second premolar for settling (Figures 14.57–14.61).

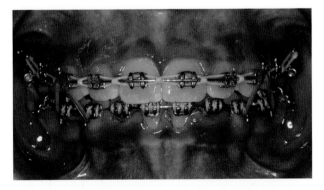

Figure 14.57 Anterior view of the dentition at the 12th active appointment. The maxillary arch wire was changed to .018 nickel-titanium and the mandibular wire was changed to .016 × .022 nickel-titanium. The mandibular incisor brackets were removed and placed upside down to reverse the torque prescription and to improve the overjet relationship.

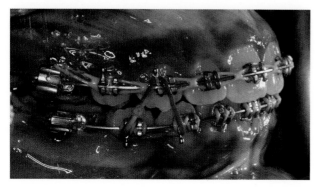

Figure 14.58 Right buccal view of the dentition at the 12th active appointment. The triangle elastic was used to settle the occlusion.

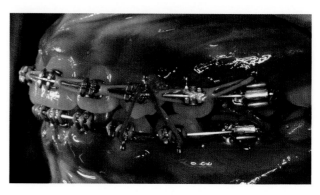

Figure 14.59 Left buccal view of the dentition at the 12th active appointment. The triangle elastic was used to settle the occlusion.

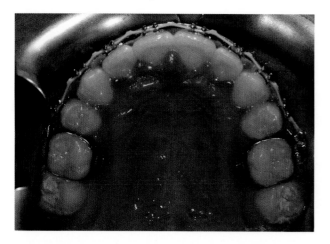

Figure 14.60 Occlusal view of the maxillary arch at the 12th active appointment. Elastomeric chain was placed from first molar to first molar.

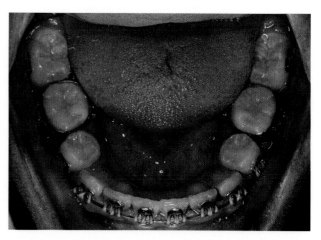

Figure 14.61 Occlusal view of the mandibular arch at the 12th active appointment.

Thirteenth Active Appointment

Four weeks later, both maxillary and mandibular arch wires were changed to .017 × .025 nickel-titanium. A triangle elastic (3/16", 4.5 oz.) was worn from the maxillary left canine to the mandibular left canine and second premolar, and a triangular Class II elastic was worn from the maxillary right canine to the mandibular first molar and second premolar (Figures 14.62–14.64). An elastomeric chain was ligated from the maxillary first molar to first molar.

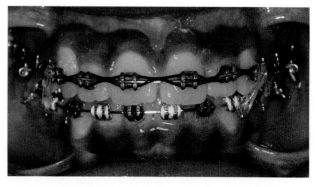

Figure 14.62 Anterior view of the dentition 4 weeks later. Both the maxillary and mandibular arch wires were changed to .017 × .025 nickel-titanium. Elastomeric chain was placed from maxillary first molar to first molar.

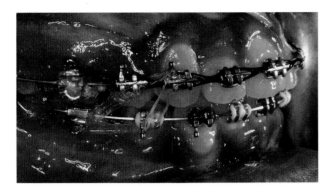

Figure 14.63 Right buccal view of the dentition 4 weeks later. A triangular Class II elastic was being worn.

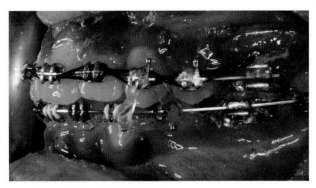

Figure 14.64 Left buccal view of the dentition 4 weeks later. A triangle elastic was being worn.

Fourteenth Active Appointment

Four weeks later, the maxillary arch wire was sectioned distal to the lateral incisors and the mandibular wire was sectioned distal to the canines. Settling elastics (1/4", 4 oz.) were placed and the patient was instructed to replace them daily. An elastomeric chain was placed between the maxillary incisors (Figures 14.65–14.67).

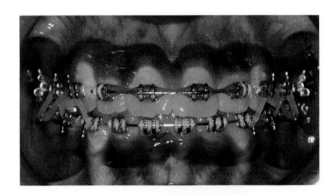

Figure 14.65 Anterior view of the dentition at the 14th active appointment 4 weeks later. The maxillary arch wire was sectioned distal to the maxillary lateral incisors and the mandibular arch wire was sectioned distal to the mandibular canines. Elastomeric chain was placed on the maxillary right lateral incisor to the left lateral incisor.

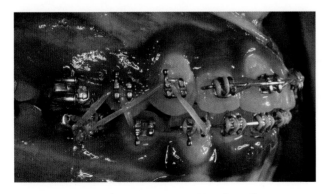

Figure 14.66 Right buccal view of the dentition at the 14th active appointment with settling elastics in place.

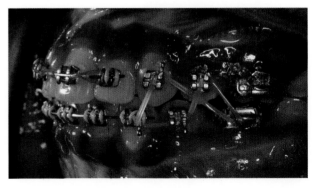

Figure 14.67 Left buccal view of the dentition at the 14th active appointment with settling elastics in place.

Fifteenth Appointment

Five weeks later the patient was debonded. The patient's occlusion was Class I with a normal overjet and overbite relationship. The arch forms were broad and U-shaped. The soft tissues were esthetic and balanced for the patient's ethnicity (Figures 14.68–14.75). Impressions were taken for immediate Essix retainers (DENTSPLY Raintree Essix, Sarasota, FL, USA). An iTero scan (Align Technology, Inc, San Jose, CA, USA), photographs, and a cephalogram were taken. The patient was instructed to wear the retainers at night and during sleep and would be observed every 3 months during the first year after the completion of treatment. Examination of the supernumerary tooth would be done on an annual basis. The total treatment time was 21 months.

Upon measurement, the skeletal relationship of the maxilla to the mandible improved slightly, while the incisor positioning and relationship appeared normal (Figure 14.76; Table 14.3).

The overall superimposition indicated that the majority of growth that occurred was in the horizontal vector. The Nance appliance and lingual arch appeared to maintain the molar anchorage. Regional superimposition indicated that bite opening had occurred through molar extrusion. The incisor relationships improved by tipping the crowns in the labial direction (Figure 14.77).

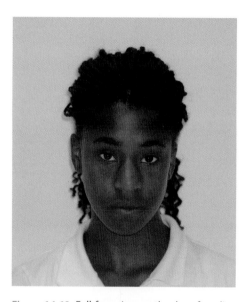

Figure 14.68 Full-face view on the day of appliance removal.

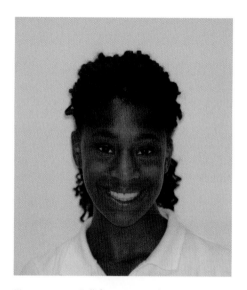

Figure 14.69 Full-face view with smile on the day of appliance removal.

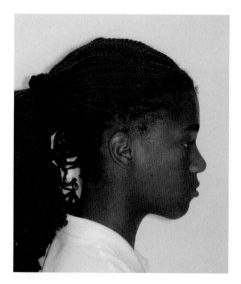

Figure 14.70 Right lateral view of profile on the day of appliance removal.

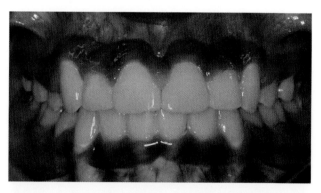

Figure 14.71 Anterior view of the dentition on the day of appliance removal with coincident midlines and normal overbite and overjet relationships.

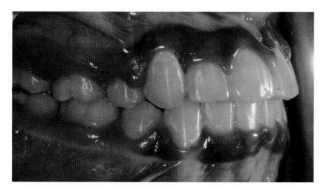

Figure 14.72 Right buccal view of the dentition on the day of appliance removal with molar and canine in Class I occlusion.

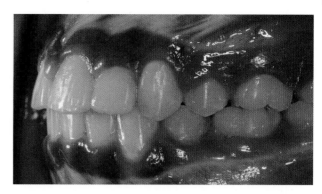

Figure 14.73 Left buccal view of the dentition on the day of appliance removal with molar and canine in Class I occlusion.

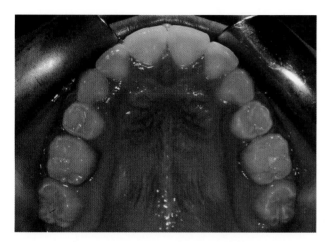

Figure 14.74 Occlusal view of the maxillary arch on the day of appliance removal.

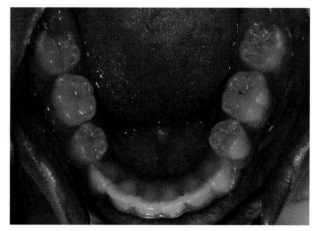

Figure 14.75 Occlusal view of the mandibular arch on the day of appliance removal.

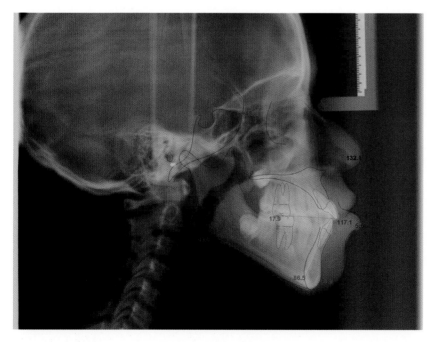

Figure 14.76 Digitized cephalogram on the day of appliance removal. The skeletal and incisal relationships have improved.

Table 14.3 Significant pre-treatment and post-treatment cephalometric values

	Norm	Pre-treatment	Post-treatment
SNA	82°	83.5°	83.1°
SNB	80°	78.3°	79.7°
ANB	2°	+5.3°	+3.4°
WITS appraisal	−1 to +1 mm	−2.9 mm	−0.9 mm
FMA	21°	30.4°	32.0°
SN-GoGn	32°	45.1°	43.0°
Maxillary incisor to SN	105°	94.7°	113.5°
Mandibular incisor to GoGn	95°	71.4°	86.5°
Soft tissue			
Lower lip to E-plane	−2.0 mm	+5.0 mm	+5.5 mm
Upper lip to E-plane	−1.6 mm	−0.3 mm	+1.0 mm

SNA, sella-nasion-A point; SNB, sella-nasion-B point; ANB, A point-nasion-B point; WITS appraisal, Witwatersrand appraisal; FMA, Frankfort horizontal-mandibular plane; SN-GoGn, sella nasion-gonion gnathion.

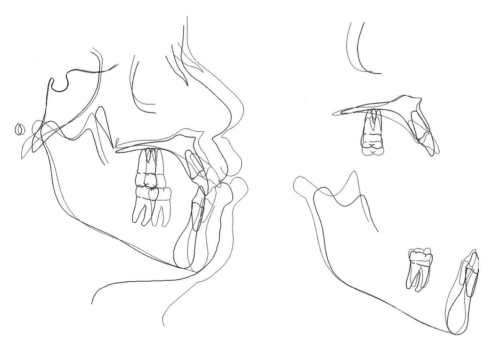

Figure 14.77 Overall superimposition indicating that the majority of growth was in the horizontal vector. Regional superimposition indicates that the incisor relationship improved by crown tipping and that the Nance appliance and lingual arch maintained molar anchorage. Bite opening occurred through molar extrusion.

Commentary

Transfer cases very often become eyebrow-raising when examined in the new treatment office and even more so when four premolars have been extracted with very little prior orthodontic corrections attained. With cooperation from the patient, a successful event can be achieved within the requisite time period for care.

Review Questions

1 How was maximum anchorage attained in this patient?

2 Open coil springs provided two functions in this patient. What were these functions?

3 Rather than closing space, elastomeric chain provided two other additional functions. What were they?

4 Where was patient compliance demonstrated in this case?

Suggested References

Andrews LF. The six keys to normal occlusion. Am J Orthod 62: 296–309, 1972.

Dean, JA, Jones, JE, Vinson LAW. Managing the developing dentition. In: McDonald and Avery's Dentistry for the Child and Adolescent, 10th edn. Elsevier, 2016; pp. 415–432.

Nance HN. The limitations of orthodontic treatment. Mixed dentition diagnosis and treatment. Am J Orthod 33: 177–223, 1947.

Ngan P, Alkire RG, Fields H Jr. Management of space problems in the primary and mixed dentitions. J Am Dent Assoc 130: 1330–1339, 1999.

Sonis A, Ackerman M. E-space preservation: Is there a relationship to mandibular second molar impaction? Angle Orthod 81(6): 1045–1049, 2011.

15

Class III Surgical

Interview Data

The patient was in orthodontic care prior to this initial appointment. The previous orthodontist retired because of health reasons. The patient's chief complaint was "to continue with care and get ready for surgery."

- Development: 19-year-old post-pubertal male
- Motivation: excellent
- Medical history: mild aortic stenosis with no need for medication
- Dental history: a history of temporomandibular joint discomfort

- Family history: twin sister does not require orthodontic care; father's occlusion is edge to edge
- Habits: none
- Facial form: long, ovoid leptoprosopic facial form with asymmetry for the chin deviating to the right
- Facial proportions: long, lower facial height

Clinical Examination

- Incisor-stomion (Figures 15.1 and 15.2):
  – At rest: 2 mm
  – Smiling: 10 mm

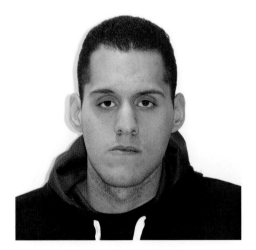

Figure 15.1 Full-face view displaying an asymmetric, leptoprosopic form with mandibular deviation to the right.

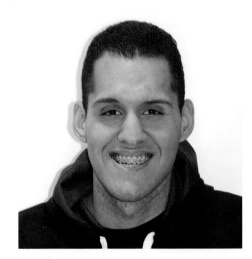

Figure 15.2 Full-face view with smile displaying 6 mm of gingiva.

Atlas of Orthodontic Case Reviews, First Edition. Marjan Askari and Stanley A. Alexander.
© 2017 John Wiley & Sons, Inc. Published 2017 by John Wiley & Sons, Inc.

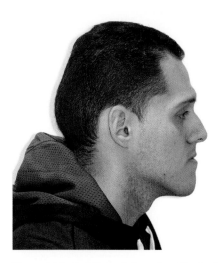

Figure 15.3 Right lateral view of profile displaying a concave pattern, obtuse nasolabial angle, and normal mandibular plane.

- Breathing: nasal
- Lips: together at rest
- Appliances are in place from the previous orthodontist
- Soft tissue profile: concave with prognathic mandible (Figure 15.3)
- Nasolabial angle: slightly obtuse
- High mandibular plane angle

Dentition (Figure 15.4)

- Teeth clinically present:

7654321	1234567
7654321	1234567

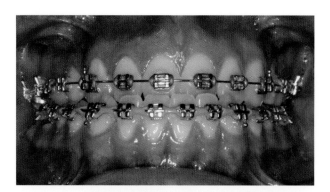

Figure 15.4 Anterior view of the dentition with prior appliances in place. The maxillary midline is shifted 1 mm to the left and the mandibular midline is shifted 3.5 mm to the right of the maxillary midline. An anterior crossbite is present.

- Overjet: −4 mm
- Overbite: 2 mm in anterior crossbite
- Midlines: maxillary midline is shifted 1 mm to left of facial midline; mandibular midline is 3.5 mm shifted to right of maxillary midline

Right Buccal View (Figure 15.5)

- Molar: Class III by 10 mm
- Canine: Class III
- Curve of Spee: flat
- Crossbite: posterior and anterior crossbite
- Caries: none

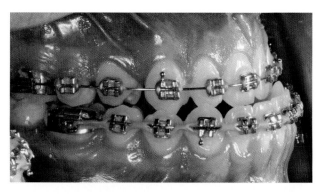

Figure 15.5 Right buccal view of the dentiton displaying a Class III molar and canine relationship, a flat curve of Spee, and anterior and posterior crossbites.

Left Buccal View (Figure 15.6)

- Molar: Class III by 12 mm
- Canine: Class III
- Curve of Spee: flat

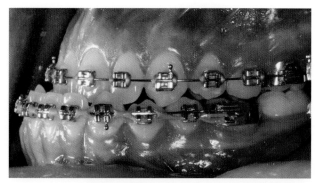

Figure 15.6 Left buccal view of the dentiton displaying a Class III molar and canine relationship, a flat curve of Spee, and anterior and posterior crossbites.

- Crossbite: anterior and posterior crossbite to first premolar
- Caries: none

Maxillary Arch (Figure 15.7)
- Symmetric, U-shaped arch form with appliances in place
- Slight rotation of right first premolar and left second premolar

Mandibular Arch (Figure 15.8)
- Tapered, U-shaped symmetric arch form

Function

- Centric relation-centric occlusion: coincident with appliance in place
- Maximum opening = 57 mm with clicking at 47 mm bilaterally; lateral excursions = 7 mm bilaterally; protrusive = 13 mm. There is a loud click on the right joint with no associated pain; there is no pain upon palpation
- Adult dentition with orthodontic appliances in place; third molars not present
- Root length and periodontium appear normal
- Condyles appear normal (Figure 15.9)

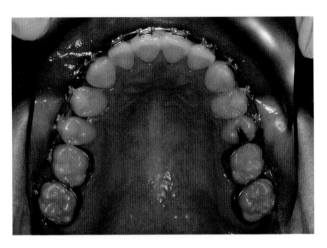

Figure 15.7 Occlusal view of the maxillary arch displaying a symmetric, U-shaped arch form.

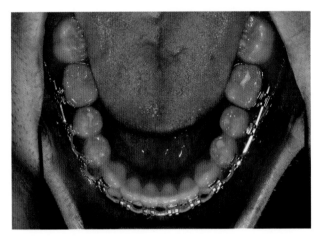

Figure 15.8 Occlusal view of the mandibular arch dispalying a tapered, U-shaped arch form.

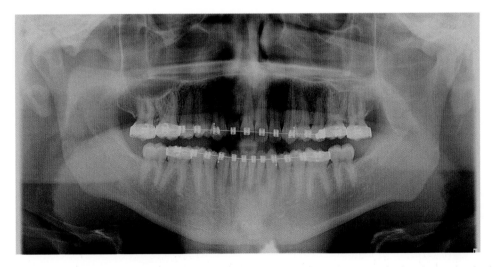

Figure 15.9 Panoramic radiograph exhibiting a full adult dentition with missing third molars and orthodontic appliances in place. The periodontium and condyles appear normal.

Diagnosis and Treatment Plan

The patient is currently wearing an orthodontic appliance for the treatment of a Class III skeletal and dental malocclusion, mid-face deficiency, mandibular prognathia, mandibular asymmetry, posterior crossbite, and anterior crossbite (Tables 15.1 and 15.2). The treatment plan consists of pre-surgical orthodontics followed by orthognathic surgery which will consist of a maxillary advancement and an asymmetric mandibular setback.

Table 15.1 Significant cephalometric values

	Norm	Patient pre-treatment
SNA	80°	76.9°
SNB	78°	83.6°
ANB	2°	−6.6°
WITS appraisal	−1 to +1 mm	−10.6 mm
FMA	21°	18.2°
SN-GoGn	32°	29.5°
Maxillary incisor to SN	105°	106.5°
Mandibular incisor to GoGn	95°	83.3°
Soft tissue		
Lower lip to E-plane	−2 mm	−2.4 mm
Upper lip to E-plane	−1.6 mm	−10.0 mm

SNA, sella-nasion-A point; SNB, sella-nasion-B point; ANB, A point-nasion-B point; WITS appraisal, Witwatersrand appraisal; FMA, Frankfort horizontal-mandibular plane; SN-GoGn, sella nasion-gonion gnathion.

Table 15.2 The patient's problem list in three dimensions

	Transverse	Sagittal	Vertical
Soft tissue	Asymmetric with mandibular shift to the right	Concave profile; slightly obtuse nasolabial angle; prognathic mandible	Appears hyperdivergent facially, but normal cephalometrically
Dental	Anterior and posterior crossbite	Adult dentition; Class III molar and canines and reverse overjet	2 mm overbite
Skeletal	Asymmetric with anterior and posterior crossbite	Class III	Normodivergent, yet appears vertically sensitive and hyperdivergent facially

Treatment Objectives

The patient's problem is predominantly skeletal in nature, and will require orthognathic surgery for correction of the mid-face deficiency and mandibular prognathia (Figures 15.10 and 15.11). The postero-anterior (PA) cephalogram in Figure 15.11 indicates the facial asymmetry due to the mandibular shift to the right. Pre-surgical orthodontics will be required and growth completed before the surgical correction is performed. Surgical movements of the maxilla and mandible were explained to the patient via Aquarium software (Dolphin Imaging and Management Solutions, Chatsworth, CA, USA).

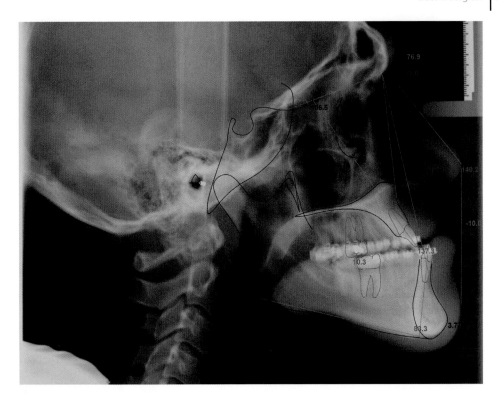

Figure 15.10 Digitized cephalogram exhibiting a severe Class III skeletal malocclusion. Normal mandibular plane angle, and normal incisal relationships with orthodontic appliances in place.

Treatment Options

1) No treatment.
2) Pre-surgical orthodontics followed by orthognathic surgery.
3) The option for camouflage was not discussed due to the severe skeletal deformity.

Option 2 was chosen as the patient was in prior orthodontic treatment with a surgical correction as part of the treatment plan (Figures 15.12 and 15.13). For proper band and bracket placement, it was decided to debond the existing appliance and place a bi-dimensional appliance for the pre-surgical phase of treatment.

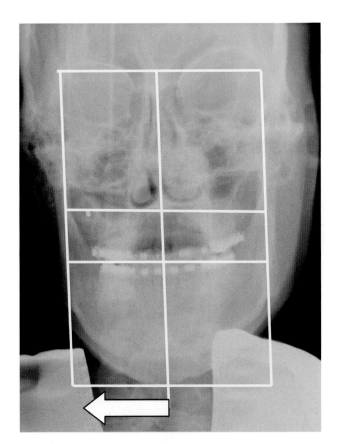

Figure 15.11 Postero-anterior (PA) cephalogram with gridlines demonstrating skeletal asymmetry.

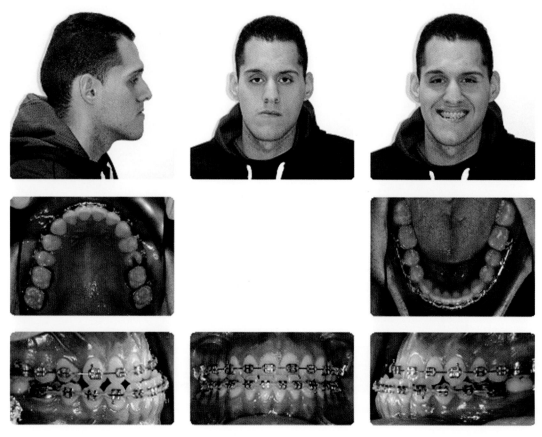

Figure 15.12 Pre-treatment extraoral and intraoral composite photograph with prior appliances in place.

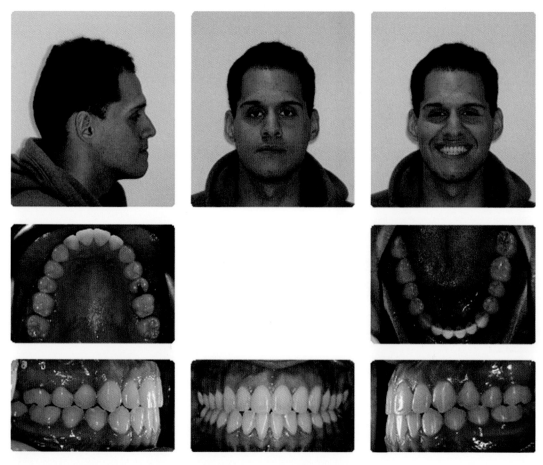

Figure 15.13 Post-treatment extraoral and intraoral composite photograph.

First Active Appointment

The patient's current appliance was completely debonded. Maxillary and mandibular first and second molars bands were fitted and cemented with glass ionomer. The remaining teeth were bonded with a bi-dimensional orthodontic appliance. Maxillary and mandibular .016 nickel-titanium wires were ligated (Figures 15.14–15.18).

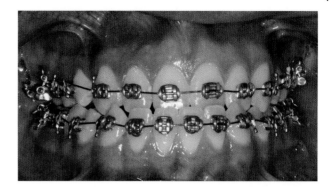

Figure 15.14 Anterior view of the dentition after new appliances were placed. Maxillary and mandibular .016 nickel-titanium arch wires were placed.

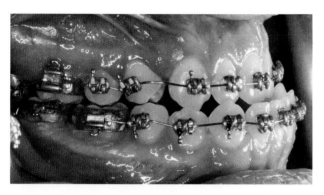

Figure 15.15 Right buccal view of the dentition after new bi-dimensional appliances were placed.

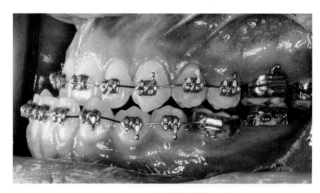

Figure 15.16 Left buccal view of the dentition after new bi-dimensional appliances were placed.

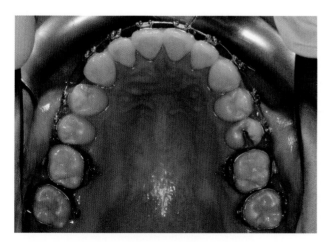

Figure 15.17 Occlusal view of the maxillary arch after new bi-dimensional appliances were placed.

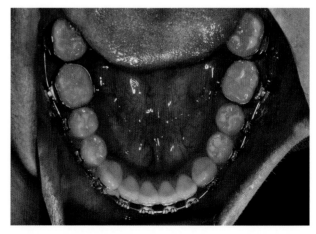

Figure 15.18 Occlusal view of the mandibular arch after new bi-dimensional appliances were placed.

Second and Third Active Appointments

Four weeks later, the maxillary and mandibular arch wires were changed to .016 × .022 nickel-titanium. During this month the patient consulted with the oral and maxillofacial surgeon, who indicated that the surgical procedure would require two-jaw surgery and a genioplasty. Five weeks later the arch wires were changed to .017 × .025 nickel-titanium.

Fourth Active Appointment

Four weeks after the third appointment, both arch wires were changed to .017 × .025 stainless steel and cinched. The remaining maxillary space was closed with elastomeric chain extending from first molar to first molar and from the right first premolar to the right canine for greater space closure in the maxillary right quadrant (Figures 15.19–15.21).

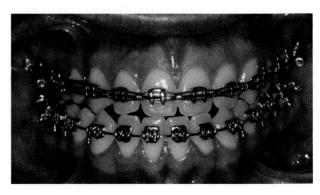

Figure 15.19 Anterior view of the dentition at the fourth active appointment 13 weeks later. Both maxillary and mandibular arch wires were changed to .017 × .025 stainless steel. Elastomeric chain was placed from the maxillary right first molar to the left first molar and from the maxillary right canine to the right first molar for space consolidation. Prior to this appointment, the arch wire sequence went from .016 × .022 nickel-titanium to .017 × .025 nickel-titanium.

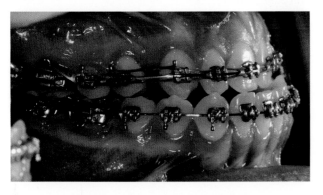

Figure 15.20 Right buccal view of the dentition at the fourth active appointment. In addition to the elastomeric chain extending from the maxillary right first molar to the left first molar, an addition chain was placed from the maxillary right canine to the right first molar.

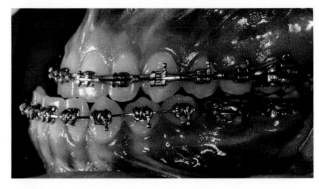

Figure 15.21 Left buccal view of the dentition at the fourth active appointment.

Fifth and Sixth Active Appointments

For the next 8 weeks, space closure was continued with elastomeric chain extending from the maxillary first molar to first molar and from maxillary right canine to maxillary first molar (Figures 15.22–15.26). Progress models, a progress lateral cephalogram to evaluate the removal of dental compensations, and a panoramic radiograph were taken to evaluate root morphology (Figures 15.27–15.29).

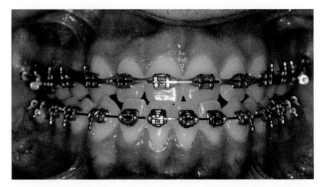

Figure 15.22 Anterior view of the dentition 8 weeks later. Space closure was continued in the maxillary arch as previously discussed.

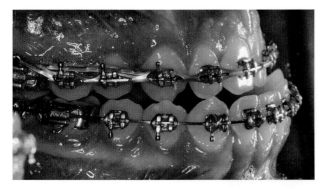

Figure 15.23 Right buccal view of the dentition 8 weeks later.

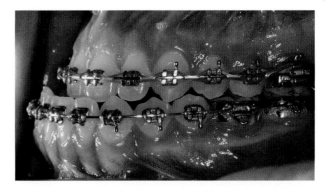

Figure 15.24 Left buccal view of the dentition 8 weeks later.

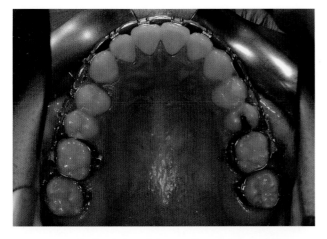

Figure 15.25 Occlusal view of the maxillary arch 8 weeks later.

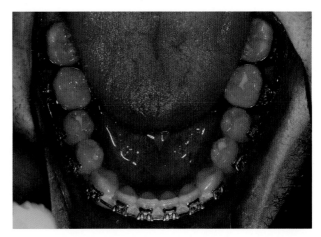

Figure 15.26 Occlusal view of the mandibular arch 8 weeks later.

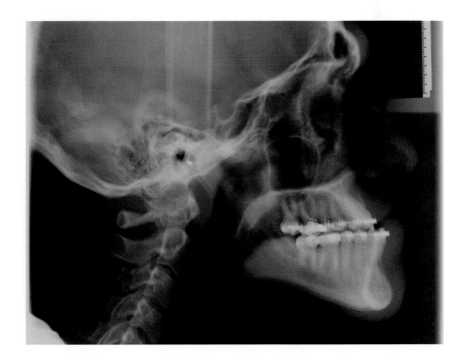

Figure 15.27 Progress cephalogram taken at the fourth active appointment to indicate the removal of dental compensations and root positions.

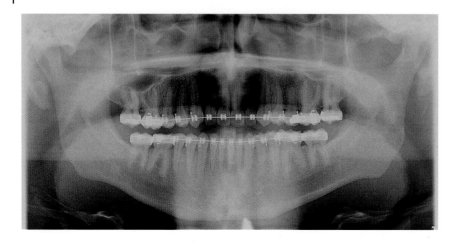

Figure 15.28 Panoramic radiograph taken at the fourth active appointment to evaluate root morphology and positions.

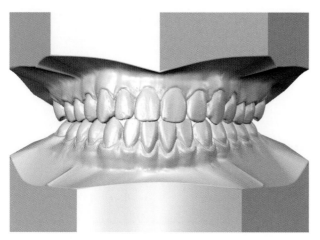

Figure 15.29 An iTero scan taken at the seventh active appointment, 12 weeks later, to evaluate arch coordination prior to surgery.

Seventh Active Appointment

Twelve weeks later an iTero scan (Align Technology, Inc, San Jose, CA, USA) was taken to evaluate arch coordination and to determine whether the patient was ready for surgery (Figure 15.29). The patient saw the oral and maxillofacial surgeon 1 month later, where the surgeon indicated that the patient was ready for the procedure.

Eighth Active Appointment

Two months later, surgical hooks were placed on the .017 × .025 stainless steel wires and all teeth were tied with stainless steel ligatures (Figures 15.30–15.34). The surgery was scheduled in two weeks.

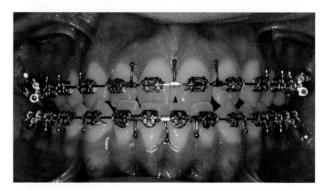

Figure 15.30 Anterior view of the dentition 2 months later at the eighth active appointment. Surgical hooks were placed on the maxillary and mandibular .017 × .025 stainless steel arch wires.

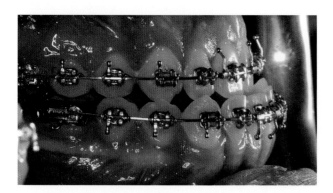

Figure 15.31 Right buccal view of the dentition 2 months later at the eighth active appointment.

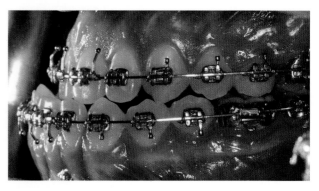

Figure 15.32 Left buccal view of the dentition 2 months later at the eighth active appointment.

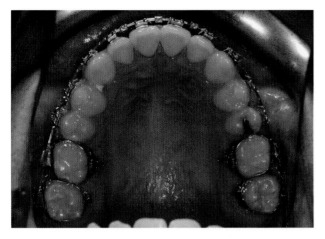

Figure 15.33 Occlusal view of the maxillary arch 2 months later at the eighth active appointment.

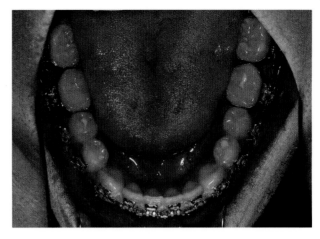

Figure 15.34 Occlusal view of the mandibular arch 2 months later at the eighth active appointment.

First Post-Surgical Appointment

Prior to this visit, the surgeon had seen the patient due to bleeding complications. Because of the distance from the hospital, the patient went to the emergency room of a local hospital where clots were removed from the maxillary sinus. The surgeon of record had seen the patient a short time thereafter when it was determined that a slight shifting of the mandible had taken place. As a result, the surgeon placed the patient on Class III elastics. Jaw exercises were continued, and the patient was now referred back to complete the post-surgical phase of treatment. The Class III elastics were discontinued. Both the parents and patient were happy with the surgical result.

The maxillary arch wire was changed to .017 × .025 nickel-titanium and the mandibular arch wire was changed to .016 × .022 nickel-titanium. Elastomeric chain was used for space consolidation between the maxillary canines and mandibular canines. A Class III triangular elastic (3/16", 4.5 oz.) from the maxillary left first molar to the mandibular left canine, and a short Class II elastic (3/16", 4.5 oz.) from the maxillary right canine to the mandibular right first and second premolars were to be placed until the next appointment (Figures 15.35–15.37). A post-surgical panoramic radiograph and cephalogram were taken (Figures 15.38 and 15.39). The patient was to return to the surgeon in 5 weeks for progress evaluation.

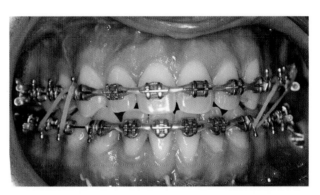

Figure 15.35 Anterior view of the dentition at the first post-surgical appointment. The maxillary arch wire was changed to .017 × .025 nickel-titanium and the mandibular arch wire was changed to .016 × .022 nickel-titanium. Elastomeric chain was used to consolidate space between the maxillary canines and mandibular canines. A Class III triangular elastic was placed from the maxillary left first molar to the mandibular left canine and a short Class II elastic was placed from the maxillary right canine to the mandibular first and second premolars. These elastics were used to correct the midline and to settle the occlusion.

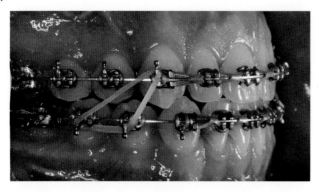

Figure 15.36 Right buccal view of the dentition at the first post-surgical appointment. A short Class II elastic was used to settle the occlusion and coordinate the midlines.

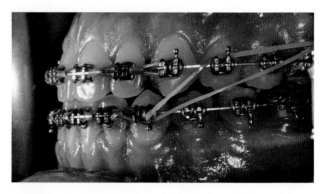

Figure 15.37 Left buccal view of the dentition at the first post-surgical appointment. A Class III triangular elastic was used to settle the occlusion and coordinate the midlines.

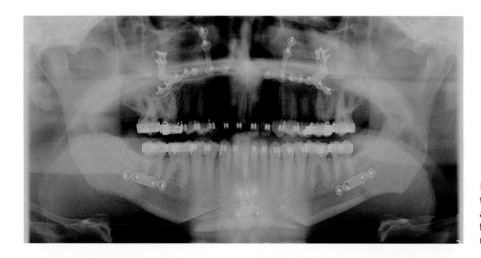

Figure 15.38 Panoramic radiograph taken at the first post-surgical appointment exhibiting the rigid fixation used to stabilize the maxillary, mandibular, and chin surgery.

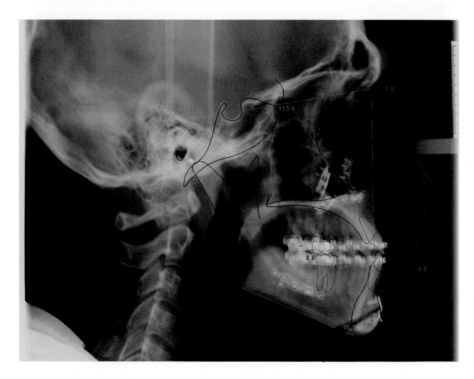

Figure 15.39 Digitized cephalogram taken at the first post-surgical appointment exhibiting the maxillary advancement, mandibular setback, and genioplasty.

Second Post-Surgical Appointment

Three weeks later, the patient returned and the mandibular arch wire was changed to .017 × .025 nickel-titanium. Elastomeric chain was used to consolidate space between the maxillary first molars. The patient was instructed to wear settling elastics (3/8", 4.5 oz.) and to return in 4 weeks for possible debonding of the appliances (Figures 15.40–15.42).

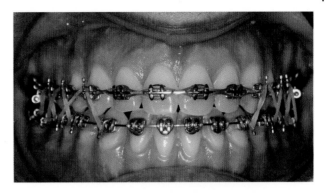

Figure 15.40 Anterior view of the dentition 3 weeks later at the second post-surgical appointment. The mandibular arch wire was changed to .017 × .025 nickel-titanium and settling elastics were used to improve intercuspation.

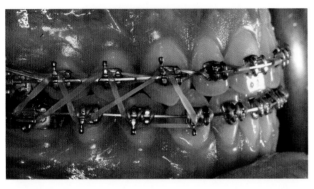

Figure 15.41 Right buccal view of the dentition at the second post-surgical appointment. Settling elastics were used to improve intercuspation.

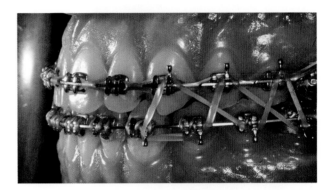

Figure 15.42 Left buccal view of the dentition at the second post-surgical appointment. Settling elastics were used to improve intercuspation.

Third Post-Surgical Appointment

The appliances were removed and photographs (Figures 15.43–15.50) and impressions were taken for immediate Essix retainers (DENTSPLY Raintree Essix, Sarasota, FL, USA). An iTero scan of the occlusion was done. The patient was instructed to wear the retainers at night and while sleeping. The patient's extraoral features improved. The smile is esthetic and the profile is straight with a strong chin button as a result of the genioplasty. The molar and canine occlusion is Class I and the arch forms are broad and U-shaped. There is a slight mandibular dental midline deviation to the right which does not affect the esthetics or function. The patient will be seen in 1 month and then every 3 months if retainer adjustments are required. During the course of treatment, no temporomandibular dysfunction was apparent; therefore no referral to a proper specialist became necessary. The total treatment time was 14 months.

Upon measurement, both the sella-nasion-A point (SNA) and sella-nasion-B point (SNB) improved due to surgical repositioning of the maxilla and mandible. The WITS appraisal also improved. Dental positions of the maxillary and mandibular incisors are acceptable for soft tissue support.

Overall superimposition of the pre-treatment (black), pre-surgical (green), and post-surgical (red) phases indicate that the dental compensations were removed prior to surgery, the maxilla was brought forward and the mandible was set back for a proper overjet appearance. The genioplasty maintained the strong chin position, but was masked by the mandibular surgery (Figure 15.51; Table 15.3).

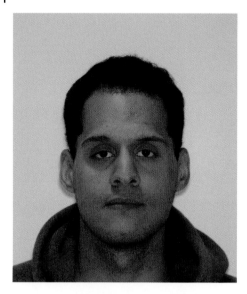

Figure 15.43 Full-face view at the third post-surgical appointment after appliance removal.

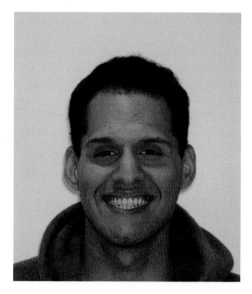

Figure 15.44 Full-face view with smile at the third post-surgical appointment after appliance removal.

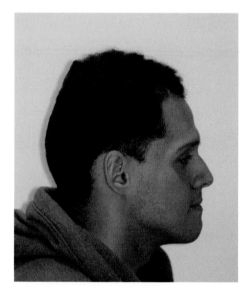

Figure 15.45 Right lateral view of the profile at the third post-surgical appointment after appliance removal.

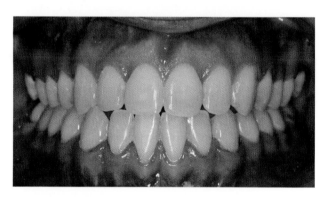

Figure 15.46 Anterior view of the dentition at the third post-surgical appointment after appliance removal.

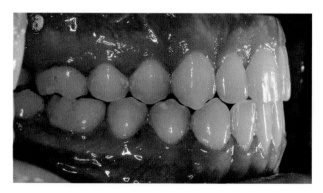

Figure 15.47 Right buccal view of the dentition at the third post-surgical appointment after appliance removal.

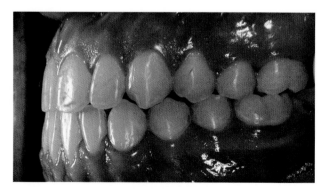

Figure 15.48 Left buccal view of the dentition at the third post-surgical appointment after appliance removal.

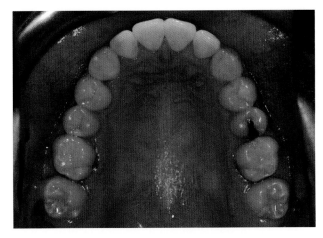

Figure 15.49 Occlusal view of the maxillary arch at the third post-surgical appointment after appliance removal.

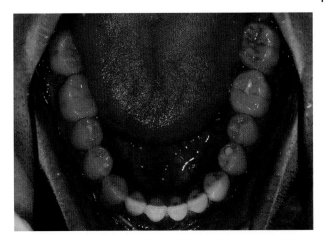

Figure 15.50 Occlusal view of the mandibular arch at the third post-surgical appointment after appliance removal.

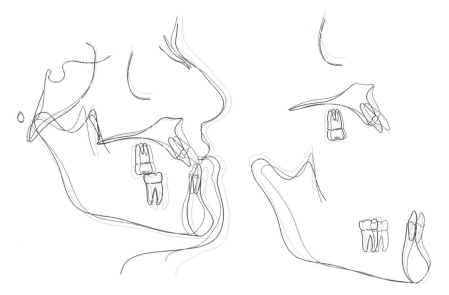

Figure 15.51 Overall and regional superimpositions of pre-treatment (black), pre-surgical (green), and post-surgical (red) phases. The skeletal relationships were improved due to the maxillary advancement and mandibular setback. Dental compensations were removed prior to surgery. The genioplasty was partially masked by the mandibular setback.

Table 15.3 Significant pre-treatment and post-treatment cephalometric values

	Norm	Pre-treatment	Post-treatment
SNA	82°	76.9°	81.3°
SNB	80°	83.6°	81.8°
ANB	2°	−6.6°	−0.5°
WITS appraisal	−1 to + 1 mm	−10.6 mm	−0.8 mm
FMA	21°	18.2°	17.1°
SN-GoGn	32°	29.1°	27.0°
Maxillary incisor To SN	105°	106.5°	113.9°
Mandibular incisor to GoGn	95°	83.3°	86.9°
Soft tissue			
Lower lip to E-plane	−2.0 mm	−2.4 mm	−5.6 mm
Upper lip to E-plane	−1.6 mm	−10.0 mm	−9.3 mm

SNA, sella-nasion-A point; SNB, sella-nasion-B point; ANB, A point-nasion-B point; WITS appraisal, Witwatersrand appraisal; FMA, Frankfort horizontal-mandibular plane; SN-GoGn, sella nasion-gonion gnathion.

Commentary

The orthodontic treatment of a true skeletal problem of the maxilla and mandible that affects daily function and the psyche of the patient due to the deformity requires the clinical skills of both the orthodontist and the oral and maxillofacial surgeon. Selective extraction and/or an attempt to camouflage the defect, and thus to avoid the necessary surgery, very often result in failure for both the patient and the clinician.

Review Questions

1 Are dental compensations removed or enhanced prior to orthognathic surgery?

2 What are the possible causes of a skeletal Class III malocclusion: maxillary deficiency or mandibular excess, or both anomalies?

3 Stainless steel arch wires are placed prior to surgery due to their stiffness as compared with nickel-titanium. True or false?

4 In most orthognathic surgical cases, growth should be completed prior to surgery. True or false?

Suggested References

Joondeph DR. Stability of orthognathic surgery. In: Huang GJ, Richmond S, Vig KWL, eds. Evidence Based Orthodontics. Ames, IA: Wiley Blackwell, 2011; 217–231.

McNamara JA Jr. Maxillary deficiency syndrome. In: Nanda R, Kapila S, eds. Current Therapy in Orthodontics. St Louis, MO: Mosby Elsevier, 2010; pp. 137–142.

Musich DR, Chemello PD. Orthodontic aspects of orthognathic surgery. In: Graber LW, Vanarsdall RL, Vig KWL, eds. Orthodontics Current Principles and Techniques, 5th edn. Philadelphia, PA: Elsevier Mosby, 2012; pp. 897–963.

Ngan P, He H. Effective maxillary protraction for Class III Patients. In: Nanda R, Kapila S, eds. Current Therapy in Orthodontics. St Louis, MO: Mosby Elsevier, 2010; pp. 143–158.

Stellzig-Eisenhauer A, Lux CJ, Schuster G. Treatment decision in adult patients with Class III malocclusion: orthodontic therapy or orthognathic surgery. Am J Orthod Dentofacial Orthop 122: 27–28, 2002.

Index

a

anterior crossbite   24, 186, 220,
    242–244
  correction   23–39, 174, 176
    dental compensation   189
    maxillary canine crossbite   208,
      210–211
    rapid palatal expander use
      25–36
  lateral incisor crossbite   24
anterior space closure *see* diastema;
    space closure; space
    consolidation
asymmetric mandibular
    setback   244–245
asymmetry   75–90, 93, 129, 244
  masking of   79–90
  see also midline discrepancies

b

bite opening   48, 59, 71, 121–122,
    142–143, 212, 236
blocked-out canines   57
  creation of space for   47–53,
    61–64
  mandibular   57
  maxillary   41–53, 93–94
buccal crossbite   35, 64, 102
  correction   36, 64–66, 102–104
button   114–115, 226
  palatal irritation   227–229

c

canines
  blocked-out   57
    creation of space for   47–53,
      61–64
    mandibular   57
    maxillary   41–53, 93–94
  eruption   68–69, 98–100, 135, 137
    forced eruption   100

indication for extraction of
    primary teeth   9
maxillary canine crossbite
    correction   208, 210–211
  retraction   132–134, 137–138,
    154–157, 224–227
cervical headgear   109, 113–114
  non-compliance   116
Class I dental pattern   3–4, 14, 44
  asymmetry   75–90
  blocked-out canines   41–53,
    57–58
  deep bite   55–74
  malocclusion   26, 57
  molar   24, 42, 56
  posterior and anterior
    crossbites   23–39
Class I skeletal pattern   3–4, 14–15
  asymmetry   75–90
  blocked out canine   41–53
  deep bite   55–74
Class II dental pattern   203–216
  malocclusion   206
  mixed dentition   2
  non-compliant patient   109–126
  premolar extractions   91–108,
    127–146
Class II elastics   84–85, 117–118,
    121, 138–139, 162, 211–213,
    230–235, 251–252
Class II skeletal pattern
  non-compliant patient   109–126
  premolar extractions   91–108,
    127–146
class III dental pattern   169–183,
    185–201, 241–256
  camouflage through dental
    compensation   188–201
Class III elastics   82–85, 173,
    176–179, 191–194,
    251–252

Class III skeletal pattern   152,
    169–183, 185–201, 203–216,
    219–238, 241–256
  malocclusion   78, 188, 206,
    244–245
  dental compensation
    189–201
  posterior and anterior
    crossbites   26–27, 39
coil spring
  closed   61, 114–115, 132–135,
    156–157
  open   46–47, 61–63, 97, 134–135,
    225–227
compliance issues   109–126
  cervical headgear   116
  elastics wear   139–140, 143
  protraction face mask   32–33, 36
  see also oral hygiene problems
condyles
  asymmetric   77, 86
  flattened   129
cross elastics   64–65
crossbite correction *see* anterior
    crossbite; buccal crossbite;
    posterior crossbite
crowding   43, 57, 78, 94–96, 108,
    171
  blocked-out canines   41–53, 57,
    93–94, 128–130
  creation of space for   47–53,
    61–64
  severe   128–131, 152–153,
    221–222
curve of Spee
  accentuated   142, 161
  deep   56, 110, 128, 170,
    186, 220
  flat   2, 12, 24, 42, 150, 242
  moderate   76, 92
  severe   204

Atlas of Orthodontic Case Reviews, First Edition. Marjan Askari and Stanley A. Alexander.
© 2017 John Wiley & Sons, Inc. Published 2017 by John Wiley & Sons, Inc.

d

deep bite   55–74, 112, 128, 130
  correction   59–74
dental hygiene problems *see* oral hygiene problems
diagonal elastic   105
diastema   2
  closure   29–30, 32
    see also space closure; space consolidation
  rapid palatal expander as cause   9–10, 32

e

elastics
  Class II elastics   84–85, 117–118, 121, 138–139, 162, 211–213, 230–235, 251–252
  Class III elastics   82–85, 173, 176–179, 191–194, 251–252
  cross elastics   64–65
  diagonal elastics   105
  settling elastics   70, 104–105, 122, 143, 179–180, 196–198, 235, 253
  triangle elastics
    Class I skeletal and Class I dental   47–48, 62–63, 66–69, 80–85
    Class II skeletal and Class II dental   100–104, 119–121, 142–143
    Class III skeletal and Class I dental   159–162, 230–235
    Class III skeletal and Class II dental   211–212
    Class III skeletal and Class III dental   176–179, 192–193, 195–196
    Class III surgical   251–252
elastomeric chain
  canine retraction   132–134, 137–138, 154–157, 224–227
  incisor labialization   226–227
  midline shift   229–230
  molar alignment   138–139
    rotation correction   114–116
  premolar rotation correction   114–116, 174–177, 224–225
  space closure   19, 29, 32–38, 69–70, 101–104, 160–163, 177–179, 248
  space consolidation   81–85, 116–122, 134–143, 156–158, 160, 176, 179–180, 190–197, 211–212, 225, 230, 251–253

eruption
  canines   68–69, 98–100, 135, 137
    forced   100
    indication for extraction of primary teeth   9
  premolar   117–118
Essix retainers   49, 71, 86, 105, 122, 143, 163, 180, 198, 213, 236, 253
extractions
  extraction sites   97, 155
    healed   156
  premolars   127–146, 219–223
    first premolars   91–108, 149–167
  primary teeth   9

f

flaring of the incisors   38, 45, 59, 71, 212
  avoidance of   154
forced canine eruption   100
Forsus spring   118–119, 140–141
Frankel III retainer   39

g

genioplasty   252–253, 255
glass ionomer build-up   68–69, 137–138, 190–194, 208–210

h

Hawley retainer   36
headgear, cervical   109, 113–114
  non-compliance   116
hygiene problems *see* oral hygiene problems
Hyrax appliance   153–155

i

incisors
  alignment   156–158
  angulation improvement   134, 223
  anterior crossbite   24
  diastema   2
    closure   29–30, 32
  flaring of   38, 45, 59, 71, 212
    avoidance   154
  intrusion   134–139
  labialization   226–227
  non-ligation   154–155
  rotation   13
  severely flared   206
  see also anterior crossbite; space closure; space consolidation

interceptive treatment
  anterior space closure   18–21
  posterior crossbite   5–10, 14–21
interproximal reduction (IPR)   173

l

lingual holding arch   2–3, 6–7, 33, 36–38, 109, 111–115, 151, 153–154
  maximum anchorage attainment   223–225

m

malocclusion
  Class I   26, 57
  class II   206
  class III   78, 188, 206, 244–245
mandibular arch
  ovoid   3
  U-shaped   13, 43, 77, 111, 129, 187, 221
    broad   25, 205
    tapered   57, 93, 151, 171, 243
mandibular prognathia   244
mandibular setback   252
mandibular shift *see* asymmetry; midline discrepancies
maxillary advancement   244, 252
maxillary arch
  asymmetric   77, 93, 129
  catenary   3, 129
  levelling   18
  ovoid   13, 171
  U-shaped   77, 93, 151, 243
    broad   20, 38, 43, 111, 187, 205, 221
    narrow   25
    tapered   57
maxillary constriction   1, 14
maxillary intrusion   135–139
maxillary shift *see* asymmetry; midline discrepancies
maximum anchorage attainment   223–224
mid-face deficiency   244
midline discrepancies
  left mandibular shift   2, 56, 61, 110, 186, 204
  left maxillary shift   42, 76, 110, 204, 242
  right mandibular shift   11, 12, 17, 24, 75–90, 135, 220, 225, 229–231, 241–244
  right maxillary shift   220
  see also asymmetry

mixed dentition 1–10, 150–152, 187, 221
  blocked-out canines 57, 93
  posterior crossbite correction 1–10, 11–21, 23–39
  supernumerary teeth 221–223, 232
molars
  alignment 138–139
  Class I pattern 24, 42, 56
  Class II pattern 2
  rotation 3, 7, 13–14
    elastomeric chain use 114–116
    quad-helix appliance use 5, 15, 17

n
Nance appliance 96–97, 132–136, 151
  maximum anchorage attainment 223–225
nasolabial angle
  acute 170, 186
  normal 76, 204
  obtuse 2, 12, 24, 92, 110, 150, 242
non-compliance *see* compliance issues

o
open coil spring 46–47, 61–63, 97, 134–135, 225–227
opening space *see* space creation
oral hygiene problems 53, 85, 98–103, 206, 227
orthognathic surgery 244, 251–252
over expansion correction 64–66
overbite
  improvement 56–74, 83, 87, 120, 136–138, 162–164
  palatal impingement 56–58, 128–130
overjet
  improvement 32, 83, 87, 102, 106, 138–141
  overcorrection 119, 142
  positive overjet creation 175–178
  severe 128, 130, 206
overlay wire 47–48, 66, 134, 226–228

p
PA radiograph 5
palatal expansion
  over-expansion correction 64–66
  radiograph 5

rapid palatal expander (RPE) 26–36
  diastema risk 9–10, 32
  slow-expansion device 9
    quad-helix appliance 3, 5–7, 14–18, 60–65
  space closure following 32–37, 69
  surgically assisted rapid palatal expansion (SARPE) 10
palatal impingement 56–58, 128–130
  quad-helix appliance 17
  rapid palatal expander 35
palatal irritation by button 227–229
piggyback wire 134, 137, 228
posterior crossbite 2, 12, 24, 242–244
  interceptive correction 5–10, 14–21
    over-correction 7–9, 17–18
    quad-helix appliance 3, 5–7, 14–18
    rapid palatal expander 26–36
  mixed dentition 1–10, 11–21, 23–39
premolars
  eruption 117–118
  extractions 127–146, 219–223
    extraction sites 97, 155–156
    first premolars 91–108, 149–167
  rotation 114–116, 159, 174–177, 224–225
protraction face mask 31–33, 36
  compliance issues 32–33, 36

q
quad-helix appliance
  crowding correction 60–64
  molar rotation 5, 15, 17
  palatal expansion 3, 5–7, 14–18, 60–65
  posterior crossbite correction 3, 5–7, 14–18

r
rapid palatal expander (RPE)
  crossbite correction 26–36
  diastema risk 9–10, 32
  surgically assisted rapid palatal expansion (SARPE) 10
retainers
  Essix 49, 71, 86, 105, 122, 143, 163, 180, 198, 213, 236, 253
  Frankell III 39
  Hawley 36

retraction, canines 132–134, 137–138, 154–157, 224–227
roller-coaster effect 205
rotation
  incisors 13
  molars 3, 7, 13–14
    elastomeric chain use 114–116
    quad-helix appliance use 15, 17
  premolars 114–116, 159, 174–177, 224–225

s
settling elastics 70, 104–105, 122, 143, 179–180, 196–198, 235, 253
  see also triangle elastics
shim 141
slow-expansion device 9
  see also quad-helix appliance
space closure 18–21, 29, 32–38, 69–70, 101–104, 160–163, 177–179, 248
  following palatal expansion 32–37, 69
space consolidation 81–85, 116–122, 134–143, 156–157, 160, 176, 179–180, 190–197, 211–212, 225, 230, 251–253
space creation 97, 225–226
  for blocked-out canines 47–53, 61–64
supernumerary teeth 221–223, 232–233
surgical hooks 250
surgically assisted rapid palatal expansion (SARPE) 10

t
tooth extractions *see* extractions
triangle elastics
  Class I skeletal and Class I dental 47–48, 62–63, 66–69, 80–85
  Class II skeletal and Class II dental 100–104, 119–121, 142–143
  Class III skeletal and Class I dental 159–162, 230–235
  Class III skeletal and Class II dental 211–212
  Class III skeletal and Class III dental 176–179, 192–193, 195–196
  Class III surgical 251–252